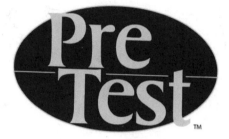

Obstetrics and Gynecology
PreTest™ Self-Assessment and Review

Notice

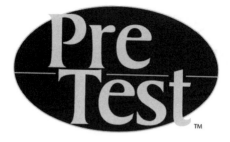

Obstetrics and Gynecology
PreTest™ Self-Assessment and Review
Eleventh Edition

Karen M. Schneider, M.D.
Assistant Professor
Department of Obstetrics, Gynecology and Reproductive Sciences
University of Texas Medical School—Houston
Houston, Texas

Stephen K. Patrick, M.D.
Assistant Professor
Department of Obstetrics, Gynecology and Reproductive Sciences
University of Texas Medical School—Houston
Houston, Texas

McGraw-Hill
Medical Publishing Division

New York   Chicago   San Francisco   Lisbon   London   Madrid   Mexico City
Milan   New Delhi   San Juan   Seoul   Singapore   Sydney   Toronto

The **McGraw-Hill** Companies

Obstetrics and Gynecology: PreTest™ Self-Assessment and Review, Eleventh Edition

PreTest is a trademark of The McGraw-Hill Companies, Inc.

2 3 4 5 6 7 8 9 0   DOC/DOC   0 9 8 7 6

ISBN 0-07-145810-7

This book was set in Berkeley by North Market Street Graphics.
The editor was Catherine A. Johnson.
The production supervisor was Sherri Souffrance.
Project management was provided by North Market Street Graphics.
The cover designer was Mary McKeon.
RR Donnelley was printer and binder.

This book is printed on acid-free paper.

Library of Congress Cataloging-in-Publication Data

Obstetrics and gynecology : PreTest self-assessment and review.—11th ed. / [edited by]
    Karen M. Schneider, Stephen K. Patrick.
        p. ; cm.
    Includes bibliographical references and index.
    ISBN 0-07-145810-7
        1. Obstetrics—Examinations, questions, etc. 2. Gynecology—Examinations, questions, etc. I. Schneider, Karen M. II. Patrick, Stephen K.
    [DNLM: 1. Gynecology—Examination Questions.
    2. Obstetrics—Examination Questions. WP 18.2 O14 2006]
    RG111.W88 2006
    616.076—dc22   2005056204

Student Reviewers

Spencer Behr
Tufts University School of Medicine
Class of 2005

Sarah Harper
University of Pittsburgh School of Medicine
Class of 2005

Sunitha J. Moonthungal
St. George's University School of Medicine
Class of 2006

Anand Shah
University of Pennsylvania School of Medicine
Class of 2007

Contents

Obstetrics

Preconception Counseling, Genetics, and Prenatal Diagnosis

Maternal-Fetal Physiology and Placentation

Antepartum Care and Fetal Surveillance

Obstetrical Complications of Pregnancy

Medical and Surgical Complications of Pregnancy

Normal and Abnormal Labor and Delivery

Gynecology

Ethical and Legal Issues in Obstetrics and Gynecology

Introduction

Obstetrics and Gynecology: PreTest™ Self-Assessment and Review, Eleventh Edition, is intended to provide medical students, as well as physicians, with a convenient tool for assessing and improving their knowledge of obstetrics and gynecology. The 500 questions in this book are similar in format and complexity to those included in Step 2 of the United States Medical Licensing Examination (USMLE). They may also be a useful study tool for Step 3.

Each question in this book has a corresponding answer, a reference to a text that provides background for the answer, and a short discussion of various issues raised by the question and its answer. A listing of references for the entire book follows the last chapter.

To simulate the time constraints imposed by the qualifying examinations for which this book is intended as a practice guide, the student or physician should allot about one minute for each question. After answering all questions in a chapter, as much time as necessary should be spent reviewing the explanations for each question at the end of the chapter. Attention should be given to all explanations, even if the examinee answered the question correctly. Those seeking more information on a subject should refer to the reference materials listed or to other standard texts in medicine.

Obstetrics

Preconception Counseling, Genetics, and Prenatal Diagnosis

Questions

DIRECTIONS: Each item below contains a question followed by suggested responses. Select the **one best** response to each question.

1. After an initial pregnancy resulted in a spontaneous loss in the first trimester, your patient is concerned about the possibility of this recurring. Which of the following is an appropriate answer regarding the chance of recurrence?

a. It depends on the genetic makeup of the prior abortus
b. It is no different than it was prior to the miscarriage ✓
c. It is increased to approximately 50%
d. It is increased most likely to greater than 50%
e. It depends on the sex of the prior abortus

2. A 24-year-old woman has had three first-trimester spontaneous abortions. Which of the following statements concerning chromosomal aberrations in abortions is true?

a. 45,X is more prevalent in chromosomally abnormal term babies than in abortus products
b. Approximately 20% of first-trimester spontaneous abortions have chromosomal abnormalities
c. Trisomy 21 is the most common trisomy in abortuses
d. Despite the relatively high frequency of Down syndrome at term, most Down fetuses abort spontaneously
e. Stillbirths have twice the incidence of chromosomal abnormalities as live births

3. A 29-year-old G3P0 presents to your office for preconception counseling. All of her pregnancies were lost in the first trimester. She has no significant past medical or past surgical history. She should be counseled that without evaluation and treatment her chance of having a live birth is which of the following?

a. <20%
b. 20 to 35%
c. 40 to 50% ✓
d. 70 to 85%
e. >85%

4. A 26-year-old G3P0030 has had three consecutive spontaneous abortions in the first trimester. As part of an evaluation for this problem, which of the following tests is most appropriate in the evaluation of this patient?

a. Hysterosalpinogram
b. Chromosomal analysis of the couple
c. Cervical biopsy in the luteal phase
d. Postcoital test
e. Cervical length by ultrasonography

5. A 30-year-old G1P0 at 8 weeks gestation presents for her first prenatal visit. She has no significant past medical or surgical history. A friend of hers just had a baby with Down syndrome. The patient denies any family history of genetic disorders or birth defects. You should tell her that she has an increased risk of having a baby with Down syndrome in which of the following circumstances?

a. The age of the father of the baby is 40 years or older
b. Her pregnancy has been achieved by induction of ovulation by menotropins (e.g., Follistin, Gonal-F)
c. She has an incompetent cervix
d. She has a luteal phase defect
e. She has had three first-trimester spontaneous abortions

6. A 20-year-old female presents to your office for routine well-woman examination. She has a history of acne, for which she takes minocycline and isotretinoin on a daily basis. She also has a history of epilepsy that is well controlled on valproic acid. She also takes a combined oral contraceptive birth control pill containing norethindrone acetate and ethinyl estradiol. She is a nonsmoker but drinks alcohol on a daily basis. She is concerned about the effectiveness of her birth control pill, given all the medications that she takes. She is particularly worried about the effects of her medications on a developing fetus in the event of an unintended pregnancy. Which of the following drugs has the lowest potential to cause birth defects?

a. Alcohol
b. Isotretinoin (Accutane)
c. Tetracyclines
d. Progesterones
e. Valproic acid (Depakote)

7. A 24-year-old woman is in a car accident and is taken to an emergency room, where she receives a chest x-ray and a film of her lower spine. It is later discovered that she is 10 weeks pregnant. Which of the following is the most appropriate statement to make to the patient?

a. The fetus has received 50 rads
b. Either chorionic villus sampling (CVS) or amniocentesis is advisable to check for fetal chromosomal abnormalities
c. At 10 weeks, the fetus is particularly susceptible to derangements of the central nervous system
d. The fetus has received less than the assumed threshold for radiation damage
e. The risk that this fetus will develop leukemia as a child is raised

8. One of your patients, a 25-year-old G0, comes to your office for pre-conception counseling. She is a long-distance runner and wants to continue to train during her pregnancy. This patient wants to know whether there are any potential adverse effects to her fetus if she pursues a program of regular exercise throughout gestation. You advise her of which of the following true statements regarding exercise and pregnancy?

a. During pregnancy, women should stop exercising because such activity is commonly associated with intrauterine growth retardation in the fetus
b. Exercise is best performed in the supine position to maximize venous return and cardiac output
c. It is acceptable to continue to exercise throughout pregnancy as long as the maternal pulse does not exceed 160
d. Non-weight-bearing exercises are optimal because they minimize the risks of maternal and fetal injuries
e. Immediately following delivery, patients can continue to exercise at prepregnancy levels

9. A 47-year-old woman has achieved a pregnancy via in vitro fertilization (IVF) using donor eggs from a 21-year-old donor and sperm from her 46-year-old husband. She has a sonogram performed at 7 to 12 weeks gestational age that shows a quintuplet pregnancy. A 5-mm nuchal translucency is discovered in one of the embryos. Implications of this include which of the following?

a. The embryo has a high risk of neural tube defect
b. The embryo has a high risk of cardiac malformation
c. The nuchal translucency will enlarge by 20 weeks
d. If the nuchal translucency resolves, the risk of a chromosome abnormality is comparable to that of other embryos
e. If the embryo is aneuploid, the most likely diagnosis is Turner syndrome

10. Your patient presents for preconception counseling. She is 27 years old and has never been pregnant. Her husband is an achondroplastic dwarf. Which of the following statements is true regarding achondroplasia?

a. The inheritance pattern is autosomal recessive
b. It is rarely caused by a new genetic mutation
c. Affected women have a low incidence of cesarean section
d. Affected women rarely live to reproductive age
e. Spinal cord compression is common

11. A 25-year-old G3P0 presents for preconception counseling. She has had three first-trimester pregnancy losses. As part of her evaluation for recurrent abortion, she had karyotyping done on herself and her husband. Her husband is 46,XY. She was found to carry a balanced 13;13 translocation. What is the likelihood that her next baby will have an abnormal karyotype?

a. <5%
b. 10%
c. 25%
d. 50%
e. 100%

12. A 31-year-old G1P0 presents to your office at 22 weeks gestation for a second opinion. She was told that her baby has a birth defect. She has copies of the ultrasound films and asks you to review them for her. The ultrasound image below shows the birth defect. Which of the following is the most likely defect?

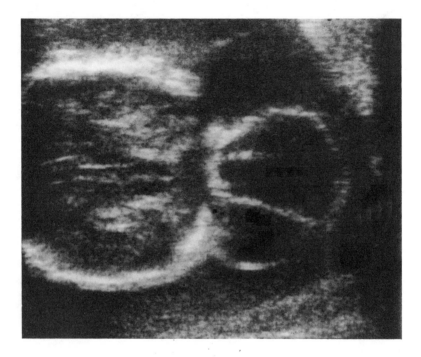

a. A cystic hygroma
b. An encephalocele
c. Hydrocephaly
d. Anencephaly
e. An oomphalocele

13. A 24-year-old white woman has a maternal serum α-fetoprotein (MSAFP) at 17 weeks gestation of 6.0 multiples of the median (MOM). Which of the following is the most appropriate next step in management?

a. A second MSAFP test
b. Ultrasound examination
c. Amniocentesis
d. Amniography
e. Recommendation of termination

14. A 40-year-old woman pregnant at 6 weeks gestation presents to your office for prenatal care. She is interested in prenatal testing for genetic abnormalities. She read on the Internet that an ultrasound measurement of the neck of the fetus can be used in prenatal diagnosis. Which of the following is correct information to tell your patient regarding ultrasound measurement of the fetal nuchal translucency for prenatal diagnosis?

a. It is a simple way to screen for Turner's syndrome
b. It can be performed by anyone trained in basic fetal ultrasonography
c. It should be offered only to pregnant women under the age of 35
d. It can be performed at any gestational age
e. It is a screening test for Down syndrome performed between 10 and 13 weeks of pregnancy

15. A 41-year-old had a baby with Down syndrome 10 years ago. She is anxious to know the chromosome status of her fetus in her current pregnancy. Which of the following tests has the fastest lab processing time for karyotype?

a. Amniocentesis
b. Maternal serum screen
c. Chorionic villus sampling (CVS)
d. Doppler flow ultrasound
e. Cystic hygroma aspiration

16. A 39-year-old wants first-trimester prenatal diagnosis. Which of the following is an advantage of amniocentesis over CVS?

a. Amniocentesis can be performed earlier in pregnancy
b. Amniocentesis is usually less painful
c. Second-trimester diagnosis allows for safer termination of pregnancy when termination is chosen by the patient
d. CVS has a higher complication rate than midtrimester amniocentesis
e. CVS has a higher complication rate than first-trimester amniocentesis

17. A patient presents for prenatal care in the second trimester. She was born outside the United States and has never had any routine vaccinations. Which of the following vaccines is contraindicated in pregnancy?

a. Hepatitis A
b. Tetanus
c. Typhoid
d. Hepatitis B
e. Measles

18. During preconception counseling, a woman has a question for you regarding immunizations. Correct advice for this patient includes which of the following?

a. Inactivated vaccines are hazardous to the mother
b. Congenital rubella syndrome is common in fetuses born to mothers who were immunized early in pregnancy for rubella
c. Inactivated vaccines are hazardous to the fetus
d. The polio virus has the ability to spread from a vaccinated individual to susceptible persons in the immediate environment
e. Hepatitis B vaccine crosses the placenta and causes neonatal jaundice

19. A patient presents to your office at term with no prenatal care. An ultrasound is ordered and shows the fetus to have multiple congenital anomalies, including microcephaly, cardiac anomalies, and growth retardation. You should question the patient if she has abused which of the following substances during her pregnancy?

a. Amphetamines
b. Barbiturates
c. Heroin
d. Methadone
e. Alcohol

20. Your 25-year-old patient is pregnant at 36 weeks gestation. She has an acute urinary tract infection. Which of the following medications is contraindicated in the treatment of the UTI in this patient?

a. Ampicillin
b. Nitrofurantoin
c. Bactrim
d. Keflex
e. Augmentin

21. You diagnose a 21-year-old woman at 12 weeks gestation with gonor-rhea cervicitis. Which of the following is the most appropriate treatment for her infection?

a. Doxycycline
b. Chloramphenicol
c. Tetracycline
d. Minocycline
e. Ceftriaxone

22. You see a healthy 40-year-old multiparous patient for preconception counseling. She is extremely worried about her risk of having a baby with spina bifida. Five years ago, this patient delivered a baby with anencephaly who died shortly after birth. How should you counsel this woman regarding future pregnancies?

a. She does not have a recurrence risk of a neural tube defect above that of the general population
b. She has an increased risk of having another baby with anencephaly because she is over 35 years old
c. When she becomes pregnant, she should undergo diagnostic testing for fetal neural tube defects with a first-trimester chorionic villus sampling
d. When she becomes pregnant, she should avoid hyperthermia in the first trimester because both maternal fevers and the use of hot tubs have been asso-ciated with an increased risk of neural tube defects
e. She has a recurrence risk of having another baby with a neural tube defect of less than 1%

23. A 36-year-old G1 undergoes a triple screen test at 16 weeks of preg-nancy to evaluate her risk of having a baby with Down syndrome because she is worried about being of "advanced maternal age." Her maternal serum AFP level comes back elevated. This patient is extremely concerned and comes into your office to get additional counseling and recommenda-tions. Which of the following is the best advice to give this patient?

a. An elevated serum AFP level indicates that she is at risk for having a baby with Down syndrome
b. An ultrasound should be performed to confirm the gestational age of the fetus and to rule out any fetal anomalies
c. She is probably going to have twins
d. Unexplained elevated MSAFP levels have no prognostic value for her pregnancy
e. Most women who have an elevated MSAFP have a fetus with a neural tube defect

24. An obese, 25-year-old G1P0 comes to your office at 8 weeks gestational age for her first prenatal visit. She is delighted to be pregnant and wants to do whatever is necessary to ensure a healthy pregnancy. She is currently 5 ft 2 in. tall and weighs 300 lb. She is concerned because she is overweight and wants you to help her with a strict exercise and diet regimen so that she can be more healthy during the pregnancy. Which of the following should you tell your patient regarding obesity and pregnancy?

a. Marked obesity in pregnancy decreases the risk of developing diabetes, hypertension, and fetal macrosomia
b. She should gain at least 25 lb during the pregnancy because nutritional deprivation can result in impaired fetal brain development and intrauterine fetal growth retardation
c. Obese women will still have adequate fetal growth in the absence of any weight gain during pregnancy
d. She should immediately initiate a vigorous exercise program to get in shape
e. Being obese places her at a decreased risk of needing a cesarean section for delivery

25. A 26-year-old G1P1 comes to see you in your office for preconception counseling because she wants to get pregnant again. She denies a history of any illegal drug use but admits to smoking a few cigarettes each day and occasionally drinking some beer. When you advise her not to smoke or drink at all during this pregnancy, she gets defensive because she smokes and drinks very little, and she did the same during her previous pregnancy 2 years ago and her baby was just fine. Which of the following statements is true regarding the effects of tobacco and alcohol on pregnancy?

a. Small amounts of alcohol, such as a glass of wine or beer a day at dinnertime, are safe; only binge drinking of large amounts of alcohol has been associated with fetal alcohol syndrome
b. Fetal alcohol syndrome can be diagnosed prenatally via identifying fetal anomalies on sonogram done antenatally
c. Cigarette smoking is associated with an increased risk of spontaneous abortion
d. In most studies, cigarette smoking has been associated with an increased risk of congenital anomalies
e. Tobacco use in pregnancy is a common cause of mental retardation and developmental delay in neonates

26. A 36-year-old G0 who has been epileptic for many years is contemplating pregnancy. She wants to go off her phenytoin because she is concerned about the adverse effects that this medication may have on her unborn fetus. She has not had a seizure in the past five years. Which of the following is the most appropriate statement to make to the patient?

a. Babies born to epileptic mothers have an increased risk of structural anomalies even in the absence of anticonvulsant medications
b. She should see her neurologist to change from phenytoin to valproic acid because valproic acid is not associated with fetal anomalies
c. She should discontinue her phenytoin because it is associated with a 1 to 2% risk of spina bifida
d. Vitamin C supplementation reduces the risk of congenital anomalies in fetuses of epileptic women taking anticonvulsants
e. The most frequently reported congenital anomalies in fetuses of epileptic women are limb defects

27. A patient who works as a nurse in the surgery intensive care unit at a local community hospital comes to see you for her annual gynecologic exam. She tells you that she plans to go off her oral contraceptives because she plans to attempt pregnancy in the next few months. This patient has many questions regarding updating her immunizations and whether or not she can do this when pregnant. Which of the following is the most appropriate recommendation?

a. The patient should be checked for immunity against the rubella (German measles) virus prior to conception because the rubella vaccine contains a live virus and should not be given during pregnancy
b. The patient should be given the tetanus toxoid vaccination prior to becoming pregnant because it is a live virus vaccine that has been associated with multiple fetal anomalies when administered during pregnancy
c. The Centers for Disease Control and Prevention recommends that all pregnant women should be vaccinated against the influenza virus during the first trimester
d. If she is exposed to chicken pox while she is pregnant she can be immunized at that time since the chicken pox vaccine is safe during pregnancy
e. Because of her occupation, the patient is at high risk for hepatitis B; she should complete the hepatitis B vaccination series before she conceives, since that vaccine has been associated with neonatal jaundice

28. A patient comes to see you in the office because she has just missed her period and a home urine pregnancy test reads positive. She is extremely worried because last week she had a barium enema test done as part of a workup for blood in her stools. She is also concerned because her job requires her to sit in front of a computer screen all day and she uses the microwave oven on a regular basis. The patient is concerned regarding the deleterious effects of radiation exposure on her fetus. Which of the following statements is true regarding the effects of exposure to radiation and electromagnetic fields during pregnancy?

a. There is ample evidence in humans and animals that exposure to electromagnetic fields such as from high-voltage power lines, electric blankets, microwave ovens, and cellular phones causes adverse fetal outcomes
b. There are documented adverse fetal effects with exposure to radiation doses of less than 5 rads
c. A single diagnostic procedure, such as a barium enema, results in a radiation dose that will adversely affect the embryo or fetus
d. There is no consistent data that exposure to radiation used for a single diagnostic study is associated with an increased risk of childhood leukemia in the fetus
e. There is an increased risk of mental retardation when radiation exposure occurs at less than 8 weeks, even with low doses of radiation

29. A Jewish couple comes in to see you for preconception counseling. They are concerned that they might be at an increased risk of certain genetic diseases because of their ethnic background. The woman is 38 years old and tells you that in neither side of the family is there a family history of any genetic disorders. Which one of the following statements is a correct recommendation for this couple?

a. They are at an increased risk of having a β thalassemia, and they should both undergo screening tests with a hemoglobin electrophoresis prior to conception
b. They are at an increased risk of having a baby born with a neural tube defect and should undergo amniocentesis in the second trimester of pregnancy for a definitive diagnosis
c. They do not need to undergo screening for Tay-Sachs disease if there is no history of affected children in their families
d. The American College of Obstetrics and Gynecology recommends that all Jewish couples be screened for cystic fibrosis
e. Canavan's disease has a carrier frequency of 1 in 40 in the Jewish population, and the couple therefore should be screened for this genetic disease prior to conception

30. You have a patient who is very health-conscious and regularly ingests a large number of vitamins in megadoses and herbal therapies on a daily basis. She is a strict vegetarian as well. She is going to attempt pregnancy and wants your advice regarding her diet and nutrition intake. Which of the following is true regarding diet recommendations in pregnancy?

a. Because herbal medications are natural, there is no reason to avoid these dietary supplements in pregnancy
b. It is recommended that in pregnancy the majority of the protein consumed be supplied from animal sources
c. Routine supplementation of vitamin A is necessary during pregnancy because dietary intake alone does not provide sufficient amounts needed during pregnancy
d. During pregnancy, vegetarians obtain sufficient amounts of vitamin B_{12} in their diet needed for the fetus
e. Vitamin C supplementation in pregnancy is to be avoided because excessive levels can result in fetal malformations

31. A patient of yours has a history of multiple substance abuse. She is now pregnant again and tells you that she has a 2-year-old little boy who is slow in school and has difficulty concentrating. Which of the following substances has been associated with behavioral and developmental abnormalities in children?

a. Tobacco
b. Cocaine
c. Caffeine
d. Marijuana
e. LSD

32. A 20-year-old G2P1 patient comes to see you at 17 weeks gestational age to review the results of her triple test done 1 week ago. You tell the patient that her MSAFP level is 2.0 MOM. The patient's obstetrical history consists of a term vaginal delivery 2 years ago without complications. Which of the following is correct advice for your patient regarding how to proceed next?

  a. Explain to the patient that the blood test is diagnostic of a neural tube defect and she should consult with a pediatric neurosurgeon as soon as possible
  b. Tell the patient that the blood test result is most likely a false-positive result and she should repeat the test at 20 weeks
  c. Refer the patient for an ultrasound to confirm dates
  d. Offer the patient immediate chorionic villus sampling to obtain a fetal karyotype
  e. Recommend to the patient that she undergo a cordocentesis to measure fetal serum AFP levels

33. You see a 42-year-old patient in your office who is now 5 weeks pregnant with her fifth baby. She is very concerned regarding the risk of Down syndrome because of her advanced maternal age. After extensive genetic counseling, she has decided to undergo a second-trimester amniocentesis to determine the karyotype of her fetus. You must obtain informed consent prior to the procedure. During your discussion you should tell the patient which of the following?

  a. Transient leakage of amniotic fluid is common after amniocentesis so she should not be concerned if she notices a watery vaginal discharge for a few days
  b. Chorioamnionitis, although an uncommon complication of amniocentesis, can be treated with broad spectrum oral antibiotics
  c. Fetal loss rate after amniocentesis is around 5%
  d. Amniocentesis has not been associated with fetal limb reduction defects
  e. Karyotyping may not be possible as cell culture failure of the amniocytes occurs frequently

DIRECTIONS: Each group of questions below consists of lettered options followed by a set of numbered items. For each numbered item, select the **one** lettered option with which it is **most** closely associated. Each lettered option may be used once, more than once, or not at all.

Questions 34–37

Match each clinical situation described, with the appropriate inheritance pattern.

a. Autosomal dominant
b. Autosomal recessive
c. X-linked recessive
d. Codominant
e. Multifactorial

34. A pregnant patient presents to you for prenatal care. Her parents are from Greece. She has a 2-year-old son who was diagnosed with hemolytic anemia after he was treated for otitis media with a sulfonamide antibiotic. Her pediatrician gave her a list of antibiotics and foods that trigger her son's anemia.

35. A patient presents to you for a well-woman examination. On physical examination she has a café au lait lesion on her back, along with multiple smooth, flesh-colored, dome-shaped papules scattered over her entire body.

36. A patient has a 2-year-old son with chronic pulmonary disease. His recent sweat test showed an elevated chloride level.

37. Your patient's father was just diagnosed with dementia associated with emotional disturbances and choreic body movements. She was told his disease is hereditary.

Questions 38–46

For each ultrasonogram, select one diagnosis or diagnostic indicator.

a. Obstructed urethra and bladder
b. Nonspinal marker for spina bifida
c. Indication of highest likelihood of a chromosomal abnormality
d. Marker for Down syndrome (trisomy 21)
e. Common marker for trisomies 18 and 21
f. Osteogenesis imperfecta
g. Mesomelic dwarfism
h. Anencephaly
i. Prune belly syndrome
j. Hydrocephalus
k. Spina bifida with meningocele

38.

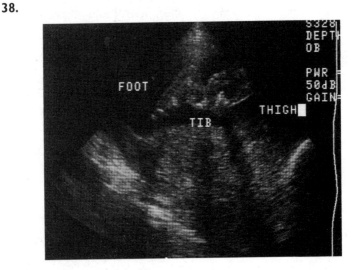

39.

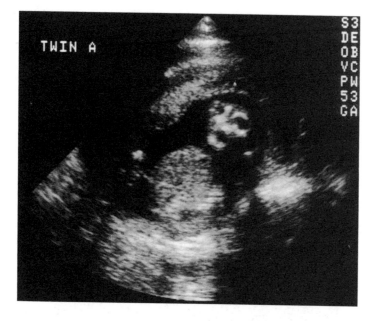

40.

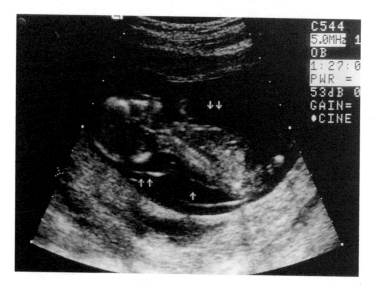

41.

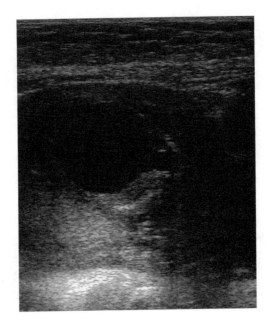

42.

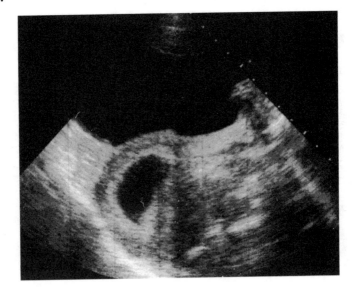

43.

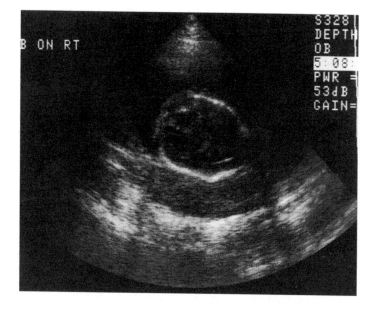

44.

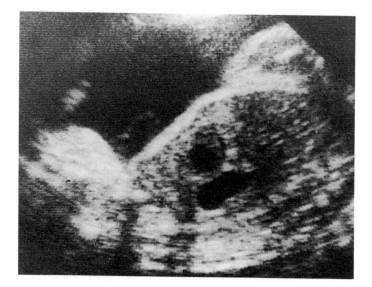

45.

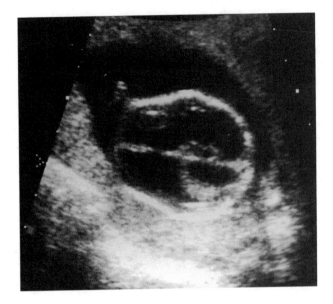

46.

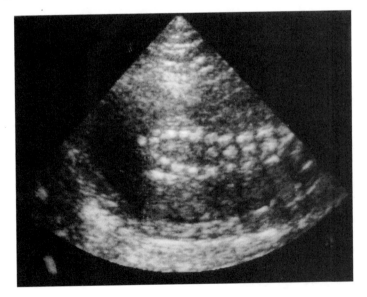

Questions 47–50

Match the appropriate scenario with the antibiotic most likely responsible for the clinical findings presented.

a. Tetracycline
b. Streptomycin
c. Nitrofurantoin
d. Chloramphenicol
e. Sulfonamides

47. At 1 year of age, a child has six deciduous teeth, which are discolored and have hypoplasia of the enamel.

48. A 2-week-old baby boy is brought in to the emergency department by his mother. For the past few days he has been lethargic. Yesterday he did not eat well and this morning he started vomiting. On the way to the hospital the baby had a seizure. On examination, the baby is jaundiced.

49. During routine auditory testing of a 2-day-old baby, the baby failed to respond to high-pitched tones.

50. A 2-week-old neonate who delivered at 28 weeks gestation developed pallid cyanosis, abdominal distension, and vascular collapse after exposure to an antibiotic. A few days later the baby died.

Questions 51–55

For each disease, select the recommendation regarding vaccination during pregnancy with which it is most likely to be associated.

a. Recommended if the underlying disease is serious
b. Recommended after exposure or before travel to endemic areas
c. Not routinely recommended, but mandatory during an epidemic
d. Contraindicated unless exposure to the disease is unavoidable
e. Contraindicated

51. Poliomyelitis

52. Mumps

53. Influenza

54. Rubella

55. Hepatitis A

Preconception Counseling, Genetics, and Prenatal Diagnosis

Answers

1. The answer is b. (*Adashi, pp 2245–2255.*) An initial spontaneous abortion, irrespective of the karyotype or sex of the child, does not change the risk of recurrence in a future pregnancy. The rate is commonly quoted as 15% of all known pregnancies.

2. The answer is d. (*Keye, pp 230–245. Speroff, p 1045.*) Chromosomal abnormalities are found in approximately 50% of spontaneous abortions, 5% of stillbirths, and 0.5% of live-born babies. In spontaneous losses, trisomy 16 is the most common trisomy, with 45,X the most common single abnormality found. At term, trisomy 16 is never seen, and 45,X is seen in approximately 1 in 2000 births. It is estimated that 99% of 45,X and 75% of trisomy 21 conceptuses are lost before term.

3. The answer is c. (*Speroff, pp 1069–1101.*) Miscarriage risk rises with the number of prior spontaneous abortions. Without treatment the live birth rate approaches 50%. With treatment successful pregnancy rates of 70 to 85% are possible in a patient with a diagnosis of habitual abortion. When cervical incompetence is present and a cerclage is placed, success rates range as high as 90%.

4. The answer is b. (*Speroff, pp 1069–1101.*) A major cause of spontaneous abortions in the first trimester is chromosomal abnormalities. The causes of losses in the second trimester are more likely to be uterine or environmental in origin. Patients should also be screened for thyroid function, diabetes mellitus, and collagen vascular disorders. There is also a correlation between patients with a positive lupus anticoagulant and recurrent miscarriages. For recurrent second-trimester losses, a hysterosalpingogram should be ordered to rule out uterine structural abnormalities, such as bicornuate uterus, septate uterus, or unicornuate uterus. Endometrial biopsy is performed to rule out an insufficiency of the luteal phase or evidence of chronic endometritis. A cervical biopsy would be of no value in the workup of recurrent pregnancy losses. A postcoital test is useful for couples who cannot conceive, but does not address postconception losses. Measuring the cervical length by ultrasonography is helpful in the management of patients with recurrent second-trimester losses due to cervical incompetence.

5. The answer is e. (*Gleicher, pp 173–178. Speroff, pp 1069–1101.*) The risk of aneuploidy is increased with multiple miscarriages not attributable to other causes such as endocrine abnormalities or cervical incompetence. Paternal age does not contribute significantly to aneuploidy until probably age 55, and most risks of paternal age are for point mutations. A 45,X karyotype results from loss of chromosome material and does not involve increased risks for nondisjunctional errors. Similarly, induced ovulation does not result in increased nondisjunction, and hypermodel conceptions (triploidy) do not increase risk for future pregnancies.

6. The answer is d. (*Cunningham, pp 346–355. Gleicher, pp 263–267.*) Alcohol is an enormous contributor to otherwise preventable birth defects. Sequelae include retardation of intrauterine growth, craniofacial abnormalities, and mental retardation. The occasional drink in pregnancy has not been proved to be deleterious. Isotretinoin (Accutane) is a powerful drug for acne that has enormous potential for producing congenital anomalies when ingested in early pregnancy; it should never be used in pregnancy. Tetracyclines interfere with development of bone and can lead to stained teeth in children. Progesterones have been implicated in multiple birth defects, but controlled studies have failed to demonstrate a significant association with increased risk. Patients who have inadvertently become pregnant while on birth control pills should be reassured that the incidence of birth defects is no higher for them than for the general population. Phenytoin (Dilantin) is used for epilepsy and can be associated with a spectrum of abnormalities, including digital hypoplasia and facial abnormalities.

7. The answer is d. (*Gleicher, p 163.*) While a 50-rad exposure in the first trimester of pregnancy would be expected to entail a high likelihood of serious fetal damage and wastage, the anticipated fetal exposure for chest x-ray and one film of the lower spine would be less than 1 rad. This is well below the threshold for increased fetal risk, which is generally thought to be 10 rads. High doses of radiation in the first trimester primarily affect developing organ systems such as the heart and limbs; in later pregnancy, the brain is more sensitive. The chromosomes are determined at the moment of conception. Radiation does not alter the karyotype, and determination of the karyotype is not normally indicated for a 24-year-old patient. The incidence of leukemia is raised in children receiving radiation therapy or those exposed to the atomic bomb, but not from such a minimal exposure as here.

8. The answer is d. (*Cunningham, pp 219–220.*) Women with uncomplicated pregnancies can continue to exercise during pregnancy if they had previously been accustomed to exercising prior to becoming pregnant. Studies indicate that well-conditioned women who maintain an antepartum exercise program consisting of aerobics or running have improved pregnancy outcomes in terms of shorter active labors, fewer cesarean section deliveries, less meconium-stained amniotic fluid, and less fetal distress in labor. On average, women who run regularly during pregnancy have babies that weigh 310 g less than women who do not exercise during pregnancy. Even though birth weight is reduced in exercising pregnant women, there is not an increased incidence of intrauterine growth retardation. The American College of Obstetricians and Gynecologists recommends that women avoid exercising while in the supine position to avoid a decrease in venous return to the heart, which results in decreased cardiac output. In addition, women should modify their exercise based on symptoms. There is not set pulse above which exercise is to be avoided; rather, women should decrease exercise intensity when experiencing symptoms of fatigue. Non-weight-bearing exercises will minimize the risk of injury. Since the physiologic changes associated with pregnancy will persist from 4 to 6 weeks following delivery, women should not resume the intensity of prepregnancy exercise regimens immediately following delivery.

9. The answer is b. (*Gleicher, pp 203–204.*) It has been shown in numerous studies that nuchal translucency measured between 10 and 13 weeks is a useful marker for increased risk of chromosome abnormalities such as, but not limited to, Down syndrome. The larger the nuchal translucency, the greater the risk of other adverse pregnancy outcomes, including fetal demise, cardiac abnormalities, and other genetic syndromes, even if the karyotype is normal. The nuchal translucency will almost always disappear by 15 weeks; this does not reduce the risk of there being an aneuploid condition, although cystic hygromas in the second trimester are primarily associated with Turner syndrome. In the first trimester, nuchal translucencies most likely indicate Down syndrome, followed by trisomy 18 and then Turner syndrome.

10. The answer is e. (*Jones, pp 346–351.*) Achondroplasia, a congenital disorder of cartilage formation characterized by dwarfism, is associated with an autosomal dominant pattern of inheritance. However, mutations account for 90% of all cases of the disorder. Affected women almost always require cesarean section because of the distorted shape of the pelvis. Achondroplastic fetuses, when prenatally diagnosed, should also be delivered by cesarean section to minimize trauma to the fetal neck. Women who have achondroplasia and receive adequate treatment for its associated complications, including the neurologic signs of cord compression due to spinal deformity, generally have a normal life expectancy.

11. The answer is e. (*Korf, pp 143–144, 187–189.*) Carriers of balanced translocations of the same chromosome are phenotypically normal. However, in the process of gamete formation (either sperm or ova), the translocated chromosome cannot divide, and therefore the meiosis products end up with either two copies or no copies of the particular chromosome. In the former case, fertilization leads to trisomy of that chromosome. Many trisomies are lethal in utero. Trisomies of chromosomes 13, 18, and 21 lead to classic syndromes. In the latter case, a monosomy is produced, and all except for monosomy X (Turner syndrome) are lethal in utero.

12. The answer is b. (*Fleisher, pp 216–223. Timor-Tritsch, p 325.*) An encephalocele is an outpouching of neural tissue through a defect in the skull. A cystic hygroma, with which encephalocele can often be confused on ultrasound, emerges from the base of the neck with an intact skull present. Hydrocephalus is related to the size of the lateral ventricles. Anencephaly would require absence of a much larger proportion of the skull with diminished neural tissues. An omphalocele is a defect in the abdominal wall at the insertion of the umbilical cord, which may lead to herniation of the abdominal contents. Omphaloceles are associated with various other birth defects and chromosomal abnormalities.

13. The answer is b. (*Gleicher, pp 199–205.*) The maternal serum α-fetoprotein (MSAFP) may be performed between 15 and 21 weeks gestation to screen for neural tube defects. The recommended sequence for an MSAFP screening program for 1000 hypothetical patients would normally produce about 30 with an elevated level (2.5 MOM) on the first MSAFP. If the patient does not have an extremely elevated value (i.e., the value is <4.0 MOM) and is relatively early in pregnancy (<19 weeks gestation), a second MSAFP value is usually drawn. About two-thirds of these patients will have an elevated test. Those who are normal a second time drop back into the normal population. However, if the value is extremely high ($\geq$4.0 MOM) or if the gestational age is approaching the limit of options for termination of pregnancy (19+ weeks), most programs then skip a second test and go directly on to ultrasound and possibly amniocentesis. A thorough ultrasound on patients with two elevations or one very high elevation will reveal an obvious reason for the elevation in about 10 of 30 patients. These reasons may include anencephaly, twins, wrong gestational age of the fetus, or fetal demise. The approximately 20 patients with no obvious cause for their elevations should then be offered counseling and amniocentesis. Of patients without a benign explanation, about 5% have an elevated amniotic fluid α-fetoprotein (AFP) and positive acetylcholinesterase. Such patients will have a greater than 99% chance of having a baby with an open neural tube defect or other serious malformations, such as a ventral wall defect. Amniography is an outmoded procedure in which radiopaque dye is injected into the amniotic cavity for the purpose of taking x-rays. Under no circumstances whatsoever should termination of pregnancy be recommended on the basis of MSAFP testing alone. MSAFP is only a screening test used to define who is at risk and requires further testing; it is never diagnostic per se.

14. The answer is e. (*Gleicher, pp 203–205. Cunningham, pp 321–328.*) The ultrasound nuchal translucency (NT) is now appreciated as a sensitive marker for Down syndrome and other aneuploidies between 10 and 13 weeks. Outside that range, the NT disappears. Although some centers have had superb results, others have not done well. Blood-free β-hCG and PAPP-A in the first trimester and double (AFP and hCG) or triple (AFP, hCG, and estriol at 15 to 20 weeks) evaluations are statistically comparable. The combination of NT and first-trimester biochemistry will likely be the optimal approach. Biochemistry does not work well for multiple gestations. Ultrasound can also detect structural anomalies, but often high-quality ultrasound services require patients to travel long distances, whereas blood can be shipped from essentially anywhere to a competent lab. Measurement of the nuchal translucency should be performed only by persons certified for the procedure. NT screening may be used in women of all ages.

15. The answer is c. (*Gleicher, pp 178–190.*) Amniocentesis, cordocentesis, cystic hygroma aspiration, and chorionic villus sampling are techniques of obtaining fetal tissues that are amenable to cytogenetic analysis. Amniotic fluid cells require tissue culture to obtain adequate cell numbers for analysis. Chorionic villi can be harvested directly for extremely rapid diagnosis or can be cultured for higher banding (increased detail). Fetal blood obtained by percutaneous umbilical blood sampling (PUBS) requires 2 to 3 days of culturing before a karyotype is obtained. Doppler flow ultrasound is used to assess blood flow through fetal vessels, but is not a substitute for direct analysis of tissue.

16. The answer is d. (*Gleicher, pp 178–190.*) Chorionic villus sampling (CVS) has many theoretical and practical advantages over amniocentesis, including its earlier performance and quicker results. CVS is performed as a transcervical catheter procedure the majority of the time; therefore, there are no needles and the procedure is painless. Suction terminations during the first trimester are safer than prostaglandin and other second-trimester techniques. However, CVS does have a somewhat higher complication rate. In the most experienced hands, midtrimester genetic amniocentesis probably carries about a 1/300 risk and CVS probably has a 1/150 to 1/200 risk. Early or first-trimester amniocentesis has a complication rate higher than that for CVS, and has been shown to have an increased risk of talipes.

17. The answer is e. (*Gleicher, pp 595–597.*) Immunization in pregnancy often brings about much concern for both patient and physician. Teratogenic concerns regarding the vaccine must be weighed against the potential for harm from the infectious agent. In the case of hepatitis A and B, rabies, tetanus, and varicella, patients may be treated with hyperimmunoglobulin or pooled immune serum globulin. Inactivated bacterial vaccines can be used for cholera, plague, and typhoid, as appropriate. Vaccines for measles and mumps are generally considered to be contraindicated, as these are live viruses, although the rubella vaccine, which is known to have been administered inadvertently to more than 1000 pregnant women, has never caused a problem and in fact can be used in selected circumstances of exposure.

18. The answer is d. *(Gleicher, pp 594–597.)* Inactivated or formalin-killed vaccines such as those for influenza, typhoid fever, tetanus, pertussis, diphtheria toxoid, rabies, poliomyelitis, cholera, plague, and Rocky Mountain spotted fever are probably not hazardous for either the mother or the fetus. Among the live viral vaccines, such as those for measles, mumps, and poliomyelitis, only the rubella vaccine theoretically may retain its teratogenic properties. There is a 5 to 10% risk of fetal infection when the vaccine is administered during the first trimester. However, no cases of congenital rubella syndrome have been reported in this group of patients. Of the commonly administered attenuated live viral vaccines, only the polio virus has the ability to spread from a vaccine to susceptible persons in the immediate environment. Therefore, the risk of infection for the pregnant mother who has been exposed to children who have recently been vaccinated for measles, mumps, and rubella is probably minimal.

19. The answer is e. *(Gleicher, pp 263–267.)* Chronic alcohol abuse, which can cause liver disease, folate deficiency, and many other disorders in a pregnant woman, also can lead to the development of congenital abnormalities in the child. The chief abnormalities associated with the fetal alcohol syndrome are microcephaly, growth retardation, and cardiac anomalies. Chronic abuse of alcohol may also be associated with an increased incidence of mental retardation in the children of affected women.

20–21. The answers are 20-c, 21-e. *(Reece, pp 398–401.)* Tetracycline may cause fetal dental anomalies and inhibition of bone growth if administered during the second and third trimesters, and it is a potential teratogen to first-trimester fetuses. Administration of tetracyclines can also cause severe hepatic decompensation in the mother, especially during the third trimester. Chloramphenicol may cause the gray baby syndrome (symptoms of which include vomiting, impaired respiration, hypothermia, and, finally, cardiovascular collapse) in neonates who have received large doses of the drug. No notable adverse effects have been associated with the use of penicillins or cephalosporins. Trimethoprim-sulfamethoxazole (Bactrim) should not be used in the third trimester because sulfa drugs can cause kernicterus.

22. The answer is d. *(Cunningham, pp 302–304, 326–331.)* The incidence of neural tube defects in the general population is approximately 1.4 to 2.0/1000. It is a multifactorial defect and is not influenced by maternal age. Women who have a previously affected child have a neural tube defect recurrence risk of about 3 to 4%. This patient is at increased risk of having another child with a neural tube defect and therefore should be offered prenatal diagnosis with an amniocentesis and targeted ultrasound. A chorionic villus sampling will determine a fetus's chromosomal makeup but will give no information regarding AFP levels or risk for a neural tube defect. Hyperthermia at the time of neural tube formation in the embryo, as can occur with maternal fever or sauna baths, can increase the relative risk of a neural tube defect up to sixfold.

23. The answer is b. *(Cunningham, pp 318–324.)* Down syndrome is associated with decreased levels of maternal serum AFP levels. An elevated maternal serum AFP screening test requires further workup to rule out a fetal abnormality such as a neural tube or abdominal wall defect, which would allow leakage of this fetal protein into the maternal circulation. Elevated maternal AFP levels can also be found in multifetal gestations or can be due to incorrect dating of the pregnancy. Amniotic fluid AFP levels are obtained via an amniocentesis if a targeted ultrasound does not indicate a fetal anomaly that would explain the elevated AFP levels obtained on triple test. Maternal serum AFP screening will pick up 90% of neural tube defects, but its positive predictive value is only 2 to 6%. Therefore most pregnant women with elevated serum AFP levels will not have fetuses with neural tube defects. Studies indicate that unexplained high serum AFP levels (i.e., no obvious fetal malformations detected on sonogram) are associated with adverse pregnancy outcomes such as low birth weight, placental abruption, oligohydramnios, and fetal death in utero.

24. The answer is c. *(Cunningham, pp 1007–1016.)* Women who are markedly obese are at increased risk of developing complications during pregnancy. Obese women are more likely to develop diabetes and hypertension during pregnancy. In addition, these women are more likely to develop fetal macrosomia and undergo cesarean section for delivery. Morbidly obese women who do not gain weight during pregnancy are not at risk for having a fetus with growth abnormalities, and therefore they do not need to gain the 25 to 35 lb recommended for women of normal weight.

Although it is not recommended that obese women gain weight during pregnancy, diet restriction and weight loss are to be avoided. In addition, as with all women, it is not recommended that obese women initiate a rigorous exercise program during pregnancy.

25. The answer is c. *(Cunningham, pp 346–355.)* Alcohol is a potent teratogen. Fetal alcohol syndrome is the most common cause of mental retardation in the United States and consists of a constellation of fetal defects including craniofacial anomalies, growth restriction, behavioral disturbances, brain defects, cardiac defects, and spinal defects. Alcohol use in pregnancy has a prevalence of 1 to 2%, and the incidence of fetal alcohol syndrome is approximately 6 in 10,000 births. No safe threshold for alcohol use during pregnancy has been established. Fetal injury can occur with as little as one drink per day, but women who engage in binge drinking are at the greatest risk. There is no way to diagnose fetal alcohol syndrome prenatally. There are many potential teratogens in cigarette smoke, including nicotine, carbon monoxide, cadmium, lead, and hydrocarbons. Smoking has been shown to cause fetal growth restriction and to be related to increased incidences of subfertility, spontaneous abortions, placenta previa, abruption, and preterm delivery. The mechanisms for these adverse effects include increased fetal carboxyhemoglobin levels, reduced uteroplacental blood flow, and fetal hypoxia. Most studies do not indicate that tobacco use is related to an increased risk of congenital malformations. Alcohol consumption in pregnancy, not tobacco use, is a common cause of mental retardation and developmental day. However, tobacco use has been associated with attention deficit hyperactivity disorder and behavioral and learning problems.

26. The answer is a. *(Cunningham, pp 347–349, 1231–1233.)* Offspring of women with epilepsy have 2 to 3 times the risk of congenital anomalies even in the absence of anticonvulsant medications, because seizures cause a transient reduction in uterine blood flow and fetal oxygenation. When anticonvulsant medications are used, pregnant women have an even greater risk of congenital malformations. It is recommended that women undergo a trial of being weaned off their medications prior to becoming pregnant. If antiseizure medications must be used, monotherapy is preferred to minimize the risk to the fetus, since the incidence of fetal anomalies increases as additional anticonvulsants are consumed. Many anticonvulsants have been found to impair folate metabolism, and folate supplementation in pregnancy has been associated with a decreased incidence of congenital anomalies in epileptic women taking antiseizure medications. Fetal exposure to valproic acid has been associated with a 1 to 2% risk of spina bifida.

27. The answer is a. (*Cunningham, pp 221–223.*) Immunizations in pregnancy with toxoids (tetanus) or killed bacteria or viruses (influenza, hepatitis B) have not been associated with fetal anomalies or adverse outcomes. The varicella, rubella, measles, mumps, and polio vaccines consist of attenuated live viruses and should not be administered during pregnancy because of a theoretic risk to the fetus. The Centers for Disease Control recommends that women wait 3 months to conceive after receiving immunization with a live attenuated virus, and that all women receive the influenza vaccine after the first trimester of pregnancy.

28. The answer is d. (*Cunningham, pp 235, 977–986, 1258.*) Most of the data regarding the harmful fetal effects of ionizing radiation has been obtained from animal studies and from human studies involving Japanese atomic bomb survivors and women receiving radiation as treatment for malignancies and uterine myomas. Current evidence suggests that there are no adverse fetal effects when pregnant women are exposed to radiation doses less than 5 rads. The American College of Radiology states that not enough radiation is caused by any single diagnostic procedure to result in adverse embryo or fetal effects. Such diagnostic procedures include fluoroscopic procedures (barium swallow, barium enema, cerebral/cardiac angiography, IVP), plain films (chest/abdominal/pelvic x-rays), computed tomography studies, and nuclear medicine studies (ventilation-perfusion lung scans). Diagnostic ultrasound, used commonly in obstetrics, involves sound wave transmission at low intensity range; this modality has not been associated with any fetal risks in over 35 years of use. Magnetic resonance imaging (MRI) involves the use of strong magnetic fields. There are currently no teratogenic effects associated with the use of MRI, but its safety in pregnant women cannot be assured until additional studies are available for outcome analysis. Electromagnetic waves generated in conjunction with power lines, electric blankets, microwave ovens, and cell phones readily traverse tissue but have no teratogenic potential. Human data indicates that exposure to large amounts of radiation between 8 and 15 weeks results in an increased risk of microcephaly and mental retardation. Fetuses less than 8 weeks or greater than 25 weeks gestational age are not at increased risk of mental retardation even when radiation doses exceed 50 rads.

29. The answer is e. (*Cunningham, pp 192–193, 318, 325–326, 1155–1156.*) Individuals of Jewish ancestry are at increased risk for Tay-Sachs disease (carrier frequency 1/30), Canavan's disease (carrier frequency 1/40), and Gaucher's disease (carrier frequency 1/12 to 1/25). The American College of Obstetricians and Gynecologists recommends screening all Jewish couples for Tay-Sachs and Canavan's disease. Whites of Northern European descent are at an increased risk of cystic fibrosis, which has a carrier frequency of 1/25 in white Americans. ACOG does not recommend widespread screening for cystic fibrosis. Individuals who have a first- or second-degree affected relative should be counseled and offered screening. β thalassemias are hemoglobinopathies especially prevalent in individuals of Mediterranean or Asian heritage. Neonates who are homozygous for thalassemia major (Cooley's anemia) suffer from intense hemolysis and anemia. The couple described is not at an increased risk of β thalassemias and therefore does not need to undergo screening with hemoglobin electrophoresis. Based on maternal age or ethnic background, this couple is not at increased risk of having a baby born with a neural tube defect. Neural tube defects follow a multifactorial inheritance pattern.

30. The answer is b. (*Cunningham, pp 215–218, 361–362.*) The use of herbal remedies is not recommended during pregnancy because such products are classified as dietary supplements and therefore are not FDA-regulated for purity, safety, and efficacy. In fact, the actual ingredients of many herbal substances are not even known. There is almost no data regarding the teratogenic potential of herbal medications in humans. It is not recommended that women assume a vegetarian diet during pregnancy, because animal sources of protein such as meat, poultry, fish, and eggs contain amino acids in the most desirable combinations. In addition, strict vegetarians can give birth to infants who are low in vitamin B_{12} stores, because vitamin B_{12} occurs naturally only in foods of animal origin. Pregnant women do not need to take vitamin A supplements because adequate amounts can be obtained in the diet; in addition, a very high intake of vitamin A has been associated with the type of congenital malformations seen with oral Accutane use. Adequate vitamin C levels needed for pregnancy can be provided in a reasonable diet. No known fetal anomalies have been reported with vitamin C supplementation in pregnancy.

31. The answer is a. *(Cunningham, pp 195, 209, 211–224, 342, 354–355, 363–364, 813–814, 899.)* Moderate consumption of coffee has not been associated with any fetal risks. Consumption of more than five cups of coffee a day has been shown to be associated with a slightly increased risk of spontaneous abortion in some studies. Cocaine use has been associated with an increased incidence of placental abruption and a constellation of congenital anomalies (skull defects, disruptions in urinary tract development, limb defects, and cardiac anomalies). Marijuana has not been associated with any adverse fetal effects. Lysergic acid diethylamide (LSD) has not been found to be a human teratogen. Tobacco use has been associated with a number of adverse pregnancy outcomes, including spontaneous abortion, preterm labor, growth restriction, placental abruption, placenta previa, and attention deficit disorder and behavior and learning problems.

32. The answer is c. *(Cunningham, pp 319–324, 329–331.)* The multiple marker screening test, also referred to as the expanded AFP test or triple screen, consists of maternal serum measurements of estriol, human chorionic gonadotropin, and α-fetoprotein. The multiple marker screening test is used to determine a pregnant patient's risk of having a baby with aneuploidy and a neural tube defect. The AFP test has the greatest sensitivity when done between 16 and 18 weeks. A maternal serum AFP level that is greater than or equal to 2.0 to 2.5 MOM indicates an elevated risk for a neural tube defect and indicates that further workup and evaluation are needed. The first step when an elevated serum AFP result is obtained is to have the patient undergo an ultrasound to verify that the gestational age of the pregnancy is correct. The sonogram can also identify a fetal death in utero, multiple gestation, or a neural tube or abdominal defect, which could all explain the elevated AFP level. A repeat serum AFP test can be done, because at a level of 2.0 MOM there is some overlap between normal and affected pregnancies. The repeat test should be done as soon as possible; waiting until 20 weeks decreases the sensitivity of the test and wastes valuable time in the workup. An amniocentesis is recommended if a neural tube defect is suspected in order to measure amniotic fluid levels of AFP and therefore confirm the findings of the maternal serum AFP. The physician would not immediately refer the patient for a chorionic villus sampling because this procedure obtains placental tissue for fetal karyotyping and does not add to information regarding the presence of a neural tube defect. A cordocentesis, or percutaneous umbilical cord blood sampling (PUBS), is a procedure whereby the umbilical vein is punctured under ultrasonic guidance and a fetal blood sample is obtained. Usually a PUBS is performed when rapid fetal karyotyping must be done, such as in a situation where severe growth restriction exists. PUBS is most commonly used in situations where fetal hydrops exists to obtain information regarding fetal platelet counts and fetal hematocrits.

33. The answer is d. (*Cunningham, pp 319–324, 329–331.*) Amniocentesis performed in the second trimester has been associated with a 1 to 2% risk of amniotic fluid leakage, a fetal loss rate of less than 0.5%, transient transvaginal spotting, a less than 0.1% risk of chorioamnionitis, and a rare risk of cell culture failure. There has not been an association of amniocentesis in the second trimester with fetal limb reduction defects. Chorionic villus sampling performed at a gestational age of less than 9 weeks has been associated with fetal limb reduction defects.

34–37. The answers are 34-c, 35-a, 36-b, 37-a. (*Korf, pp 5, 132–161.*) Glucose-6-phosphate dehydrogenase (G6PD) deficiency is X-linked recessive and is found predominantly in males of African and Mediterranean origin. Although the causes of clinical manifestations in G6PD deficiency are multifactorial (e.g., sulfa drugs), the inheritance is not. Neurofibromatosis, whose occurrence is often sporadic (i.e., a spontaneous mutation in 50%), is inherited as an autosomal dominant trait once the gene is in a family. The severity of the condition can be quite variable even within the same family. The human leukocyte antigens (HLAs) (four from each parent) are all expressed and therefore do not show any dominance in their expression. Certain combinations of haplotypes are associated with some disease conditions (such as 21-hydroxylase deficiency congenital adrenal hyperplasia, which is autosomal recessive) in that they occur much more commonly than would be expected by chance; however, such associations do not, alone, define inheritance. Cystic fibrosis is the most common autosomal recessive disorder in the white European population, and Huntington's disease is autosomal dominant.

38–46. The answers are 38-f, 39-h, 40-e, 41-a, 42-c, 43-b, 44-d, 45-j, 46-k. *(Benacerraf, pp 229–235. Fleisher, pp 471–472.)* The diagnosis of osteogenesis imperfecta can be made by visualizing fractures in utero by ultrasound. The ultrasound in question 38 shows a crumpling of the tibia and fibula and curvature of the thigh such that proper extension of the foot does not occur.

The ultrasonogram in question 39 was done at approximately 15 weeks gestation and shows two orbits, a mouth, and a central nose, but there is clearly no forehead and no cranial contents. Even a relatively inexperienced sonographer using average equipment available in the early 1990s would be able to pick up anencephaly. Anencephaly is, of course, incompatible with life and is the only condition for which a termination of pregnancy is generally permissible at any gestational age.

The ultrasonogram in question 40 shows a 13-week-old fetus with a large nuchal translucency (double arrows) and beginning hydrops, sometimes called a cystic hygroma. Increasing experience with early ultrasonograms has demonstrated that cystic hygromas occur in 1 to 2% of patients. In the second and third trimesters, cystic hygromas are commonly associated with Turner syndrome (45,X). The earlier in pregnancy they are seen, however, the more likely it is that the diagnosis is related to trisomy 21, trisomy 18, or trisomy 13, which are collectively found on karyotype in approximately 50% of cases. Of those cases that are chromosomally normal, most of these nuchal translucencies disappear and the fetus goes on to have perfectly normal development.

In question 41, the transverse cut through the bladder shows megacystis (i.e., the bladder is markedly enlarged) and the distal portion of the urethra can be visualized up to the point of urinary blockage. The blocked urethra acts as a dam that causes the bladder to fill up, then the ureters, and finally the kidneys (hydronephrosis). There is oligohydramnios noted in this picture because by 16 weeks—the gestational age at which this picture was taken—the vast majority of amniotic fluid comes from fetal urine. Left untreated, these babies will often develop prune belly syndrome and show kidney and abdominal wall damage. The cause of death, however, is pulmonary, because the oligohydramnios does not allow for proper lung development. When these babies are born, they die from pulmonary causes; they do not live long enough to die from renal causes.

The ultrasonogram in question 42 was performed at approximately 8 weeks after the last menstrual period and shows a placenta but no fetal pole—the classic blighted ovum. Traditionally, 50% of first-trimester spontaneous abortions are said to be chromosomally abnormal. However, more recent evidence suggests that, particularly with advancing age of the mother (i.e., in women who are likely to have early ultrasonography for potential CVS), the risk of fetal chromosomal abnormalities is in fact much higher, in many cases approaching even 90% of first-trimester spontaneous abortions.

The cross-section through the fetal head in question 43 shows a classic lemon sign; that is, there is a frontal bosselation of the forehead such that the sides of the forehead are actually pulled in. This is because of the pull on the cisterna magna from spina bifida that is distorting the intracranial contents. This so-called lemon sign has a very high degree of sensitivity, although it is not perfect. The lemon sign disappears in the third trimester and is therefore not useful late in pregnancy.

The longitudinal ultrasonogram in question 44 shows the double bubble related to duodenal atresia. The two bubbles are the stomach and the jejunum. This finding is classic for trisomy 21. Approximately one-third of fetuses who have this finding will in fact be found to have trisomy 21. This risk, of course, is very high and is an automatic indication for offering prenatal diagnosis by amniocentesis, CVS, or cordocentesis to document the chromosomes regardless of any other indication the patient may have.

The ultrasound in 45 demonstrates dilation of the lateral ventricles consistent with hydrocephalous. In 46 the ultrasound shows splaying of the lumbar spine consistent with spina bifada.

47–50.   The answers are 47-a, 48-e, 49-b, 50-d. (*Zatuchni, pp 81–88.*) Fetal exposure to an antibiotic depends on many factors, such as gestational age, protein binding, lipid solubility, pH, molecular weight, degree of ionization, and concentration gradient. Some antibiotics are even concentrated in the fetal compartment. Tetracycline is contraindicated in all three trimesters. It has been associated with skeletal abnormalities, staining and hypoplasia of budding fetal teeth, bone hypoplasia, and fatal maternal liver decompensation. Sulfonamides are associated with kernicterus in the newborn. They compete with bilirubin for binding sites on albumin, thereby leaving more bilirubin free for diffusion into tissues. Sulfonamides should be withheld during the last 2 to 6 weeks of pregnancy. With prolonged treatment of tuberculosis (TB) in pregnancy, streptomycin has been associated with fetal hearing loss. Its use is restricted to complicated cases of TB. Nitrofurantoins can cause maternal and fetal hemolytic anemia if glucose-

6-phosphate dehydrogenase deficiency is present. Chloramphenicol is noted for causing the gray baby syndrome. Infants are unable to properly metabolize the drug, which reaches toxic levels in about 4 days and can lead to neonatal death within 1 to 2 days.

51–55. The answers are 51-c, 52-e, 53-a, 54-e, 55-b. *(Scott, p 81.)* The recommendations concerning immunizations during pregnancy offered by the American College of Obstetricians and Gynecologists are as follows:

- Administration of influenza vaccine is recommended if the underlying disease is serious.

- Typhoid immunization is recommended on travel to an endemic region.

- Hepatitis A immunization is recommended after exposure or before travel to developing countries.

- Cholera immunization should be given only to meet travel requirements.

- Tetanus-diphtheria immunization should be given if a primary series has never been administered or if 10 years has elapsed without the patient receiving a booster.

- Immunization for poliomyelitis is mandatory during an epidemic but otherwise not recommended.

- Smallpox immunization is unnecessary since the disease has been eradicated.

- Immunization for yellow fever is recommended before travel to a high-risk area.

- Mumps and rubella immunizations are contraindicated.

- Administration of rabies vaccine is unaffected by pregnancy.

Maternal-Fetal Physiology and Placentation

Questions

DIRECTIONS: Each item below contains a question followed by suggested responses. Select the **one best** response to each question.

56. A 29-year-old caucasian primigravid patient is 20 weeks pregnant with twins. She found out today on her routine ultrasound for fetal anatomy that she is carrying two boys. In this patient's case, which of the following statements about twinning is true?

a. The twins must be monozygotic since they are both males
b. If division of these twins occurred after formation of the embryonic disk the twins will be conjoined
c. She has a higher incidence of having monzygotic twins since she is caucasian
d. If the ultrasound showed two separate placentas, the twins must be dizygotic
e. Twinning causes no appreciable increase in maternal morbidity and mortality over singleton pregnancies

57. A 24-year-old primigravida with twins presents for routine ultrasonography at 20 weeks gestation. Based on the ultrasound findings, the patient is diagnosed with dizygotic twins. Which of the following is true regarding the membranes and placentas of dizygotic twins?

a. They are dichorionic and monoamniotic only if the fetuses are of the same sex
b. They are dichorionic and monoamniotic regardless of the sex of the fetuses
c. They are monochorionic and monoamniotic if they are conjoined twins
d. They are dichorionic and diamniotic regardless of the sex of the twins
e. They are monochorionic and diamniotic if they are of the same sex

58. After delivery of a term infant with Apgar scores of 2 at one minute and 7 at five minutes, you ask that umbilical cord blood be collected for pH. The umbilical arteries carry which of the following?

a. Oxygenated blood to the placenta
b. Oxygenated blood from the placenta
c. Deoxygenated blood to the placenta
d. Deoxygenated blood from the placenta

59. During the routine examination of the umbilical cord and placenta after a spontaneous vaginal delivery you notice that the baby had only one umbilical artery. Which of the following is true regarding the finding of a single umbilical artery?

a. It is a very common finding and is insignificant
b. It is a rare finding in singleton pregnancies and is therefore not significant
c. It is an indicator of an increased incidence of congenital anomalies of the fetus
d. It is equally common in newborns of diabetic and nondiabetic mothers
e. It is present in 5% of all births

60. A 22-year-old G1P0 at 28 weeks gestation by LMP presents to labor and delivery complaining of decreased fetal movement. She has had no prenatal care. On the fetal monitor there are no contractions. The fetal heart rate is 150 beats per minute and reactive. There are no decelerations in the fetal heart tracing. An ultrasound is performed in the radiology department and shows a 28-week fetus with normal-appearing anatomy and size consistent with dates. The placenta is implanted on the posterior uterine wall and its margin is well away from the cervix. A succenturiate lobe of the placenta is seen implanted low on the anterior wall of the uterus. Doppler flow studies indicate a blood vessel is traversing the cervix connecting the two lobes. This patient is at risk for which of the following?

a. Premature rupture of the membranes
b. Fetal exsanguination after rupture of the membranes
c. Torsion of the umbilical cord due to velamentous insertion of the umbilical cord
d. Amniotic fluid embolism
e. Placenta accreta

61. A healthy 25-year-old G1P0 at 40 weeks gestational age comes to your office to see you for a routine OB visit. The patient complains to you that on several occasions she has experienced dizziness, light-headedness, and feeling as if she is going to pass out when she lies down on her back to take a nap. What is the appropriate plan of management for this patient?

a. Do an ECG
b. Monitor her for 24 h with a Holter monitor to rule out an arrhythmia
c. Do an arterial blood gas analysis
d. Refer her immediately to a neurologist
e. Reassure her that nothing is wrong with her and encourage her not to lie flat on her back

62. A 42-year-old primigravida presents to your office for a routine OB visit at 34 weeks gestational age. She voices concern because she has noticed an increasing number of spidery veins appearing on her abdomen. She is upset with the unsightly appearance of these veins and wants to know what you recommend to get rid of them. Which of the following is the best advice to give this patient?

a. Tell her that this is not a serious condition and give her a referral to a vascular surgeon to have the veins removed
b. Tell her that you are concerned that she may have serious liver disease and order liver function tests
c. Refer her to a dermatologist for further workup and evaluation
d. Tell her that the appearance of these blood vessels is a normal occurrence with pregnancy and will resolve spontaneously after delivery
e. Recommend that she wear an abdominal support to relieve pressure from her abdomen and cause resolution of the blood vessels

63. A 32-year-old G2P1001 at 20 weeks gestational age presents to the emergency room complaining of constipation and abdominal pain for the past 24 h. The patient also admits to bouts of nausea and emesis since eating a very spicy meal at a new Thai restaurant the evening before. She denies a history of any medical problems. During her last pregnancy, the patient underwent an elective cesarean section at term to deliver a fetus in the breech presentation. The emergency room doctor who examines her pages you and reports that the patient has a low-grade fever of 100°F, with a normal pulse and blood pressure. She is minimally tender to deep palpation with hypoactive bowel sounds. She has no rebound tenderness. The patient has a WBC of 13,000, and electrolytes are normal. Which of the following is the most appropriate next step in the management of this patient?

a. The history and physical exam are consistent with constipation, which is commonly associated with pregnancy; the patient should be discharged with reassurance and instructions to give herself a soapsuds enema and follow a high-fiber diet with laxative use as needed
b. The patient should be prepped for the operating room immediately to have an emergent appendectomy
c. The patient should be reassured that her symptoms are due to the spicy meal consumed the evening before and should be given Pepto-Bismol to alleviate the symptoms
d. The patient should be sent to radiology for an upright abdominal x-ray
e. Intravenous antiemetics should be ordered to treat the patient's hyperemesis gravidarum

64. A healthy 34-year-old G1P0 patient comes to see you in your office for a routine OB visit at 12 weeks gestational age. She tells you that she has stopped taking her prenatal vitamins with iron supplements because they make her sick and she has trouble remembering to take a pill every day. A review of her prenatal labs reveals that her hematocrit is 39%. Which of the following statements is the correct way to counsel this patient?

a. Tell the patient that she does not need to take her iron supplements because her prenatal labs indicate that she is not anemic and therefore she will not absorb the iron supplied in prenatal vitamins
b. Tell the patient that if she consumes a diet rich in iron, she does not need to take any iron supplements
c. Tell the patient that if she fails to take her iron supplements, her fetus will be anemic
d. Tell the patient that she needs to take the iron supplements even though she is not anemic in order to meet the demands of pregnancy
e. Tell the patient that she needs to start retaking her iron supplements when her hemoglobin falls below 11 g/dL

65. A pregnant patient of yours goes to the emergency room at 20 weeks gestational age with complaints of hematuria and back pain. The emergency room physician orders an intravenous pyelogram (IVP) as part of a workup for a possible kidney stone. The radiologist indicates the absence of nephrolithiasis but reports the presence of bilateral hydronephrosis and hydroureter, which is greater on the right side than on the left. Which of the following statements is true regarding this IVP finding?

a. The bilateral hydronephrosis is of concern, and renal function tests, including BUN and creatinine, should be run and closely monitored
b. These findings are consistent with normal pregnancy and are not of concern
c. The bilateral hydronephrosis is of concern, and a renal sonogram should be ordered emergently
d. The findings indicate that a urology consult is needed to obtain recommendations for further workup and evaluation
e. The findings are consistent with ureteral obstruction, and the patient should be referred for stent placement

66. During a routine return OB visit, an 18-year-old G1P0 patient at 23 weeks gestational age undergoes a urinalysis. The dipstick done by the nurse indicates the presence of trace glucosuria. All other parameters of the urine test are normal. Which of the following is the most likely etiology of the increased sugar detected in the urine?

a. The patient has diabetes
b. The patient has a urine infection
c. The patient's urinalysis is consistent with normal pregnancy
d. The patient's urine sample is contaminated
e. The patient has kidney disease

67. A 29-year-old G1P0 patient at 15 weeks gestational age presents to your office complaining of some shortness of breath that is more intense with exertion. She has no significant past medical history and is not on any medication. The patient denies any chest pain but sometimes feels as though her heart is pounding. She is concerned because she has always been very athletic and cannot maintain the same degree of exercise that she was accustomed to prior to becoming pregnant. On physical exam, her pulse is 90/min. Her blood pressure is 90/50. On cardiac exam, a systolic ejection murmur is identified. The lungs are clear to auscultation and percussion. Which of the following is the most appropriate next step to pursue in the workup of this patient?

a. Refer the patient for a ventilation-perfusion scan to rule out a pulmonary embolism
b. Perform an arterial blood gas
c. Refer the patient to a cardiologist
d. Reassure the patient
e. Order an ECG

DIRECTIONS: Each group of questions below consists of lettered options followed by a set of numbered items. For each numbered item, select the **one** lettered option with which it is **most** closely associated. Each lettered option may be used once, more than once, or not at all.

Questions 68–70

Match the descriptions with the appropriate placenta type.

a. Fenestrated placenta
b. Succenturiate placenta
c. Vasa previa
d. Placenta previa
e. Membranaceous placenta
f. Placenta accreta

68. A 33-year-old G2P1 is undergoing an elective repeat cesarean section at term. The infant is delivered without any difficulties, but the placenta cannot be removed easily because a clear plane between the placenta and uterine wall cannot be identified. The placenta is removed in pieces. This is followed by uterine atony and hemorrhage.

69. A 22-year-old G3P2 undergoes a normal spontaneous vaginal delivery without complications. The placenta is spontaneously delivered and appears intact. The patient is brought to the postpartum floor, where she starts to bleed profusely. Physical exam reveals a boggy uterus, and a bedside sonogram indicates the presence of placental tissue.

70. A 34-year-old G2P1 presents to labor and delivery by ambulance at 28 weeks gestational age complaining of the sudden onset of profuse vaginal bleeding. The patient denies any abdominal pain or uterine contractions. Her OB history is significant for a previous cesarean section at term for fetal breech presentation. She admits to smoking several cigarettes a day, but denies any drug or alcohol use. Fetal heartrate tracing is normal.

Maternal-Fetal Physiology and Placentation

Answers

56. The answer is b. (*Cunningham, pp 912–920.*) The incidence of monozygotic twinning is constant at a rate of one set per 250 births around the world. It is unaffected by race, heredity, age, parity, or infertility agents. Examination of the amnion and chorion can be used to determine monozygosity only if one chorion is identified. Two identifiable chorions can occur in monozygotic or dizygotic twinning. The time of the division of a fertilized zygote to form monozygotic twins determines the placental and membranous anatomy. Late division after formation of the embryonic disk will result in conjoined twins.

57. The answer is d. (*Cunningham, pp 912–914.*) Dizygotic twins always have a dichorionic and diamniotic placenta regardless of the sex of the fetuses. The placentas of dizygotic twins may be totally separated or intimately fused. Monozygotic twins are always of the same sex but may be monochorionic or dichorionic depending upon when the separation of the twins occured. Of monozygotic twins, 20 to 30% have dichorionic placentation, the result of separation of the blastocyst in the first 2 days after fertilization. The majority of monozygotic twins have a diamniotic and monochorionic placenta. The least common type of placentation in monozygotic twins is the monochorionic and monoamniotic placenta; its incidence is only about 1%. Conjoined twins are always monozygotic.

58. The answer is c. (*Cunningham, pp 65, 68–69.*) Deoxygenated fetal blood is returned directly to the placenta through the umbilical branches of the two hypogastric arteries. The umbilical arteries exit through the abdominal wall at the umbilicus and continue by way of the umbilical cord to the placenta. Deoxygenated blood circulates through the placenta then returns, oxygenated, to the fetus via the umbilical vein. The umbilical arteries atrophy and obliterate within 3 to 4 days after birth; remnants are called *umbilical ligaments*.

59. The answer is c. (*Cunningham, pp 626.*) The absence of one umbilical artery occurs in 0.7 to 0.8% of all umbilical cords of singletons, in 2.5% of all abortuses, and in approximately 5% of at least one twin. The incidence of a single artery is significantly increased in newborns of diabetic mothers, and it occurs in white infants twice as often as in newborns of black women. The incidence of major fetal malformations when only one artery is identified has been reported to be as high as 18%, and there is an increased incidence of overall fetal mortality. The finding is an indication to offer amniocentesis, cordocentesis, or chorionic villus sampling to study fetal chromosomes, although there is debate about whether this should be done when there is only a truly isolated finding of single umbilical artery.

60. The answer is b. (*Cunningham, pp 627–628.*) With velamentous insertion of the cord, the umbilical vessels separate in the membranes at a distance from the placental margin, which they reach surrounded only by amnion. It occurs in about 1% of singleton gestations but is quite common in multiple pregnancies. Fetal malformations are more common with velamentous insertion of the umbilical cord. When fetal vessels cross the internal os (vasa previa), rupture of membranes may be accompanied by rupture of a fetal vessel, leading to fetal exsanguination. Vasa previa does not increase the risk for placenta accreta or amniotic fluid embolism. An increased risk of premature rupture of membranes and of torsion of the umbilical cord has not been described in association with velamentous insertion of the cord.

61. The answer is e. (*Cunningham, p 135. Beckmann, pp 57–58.*) Late in pregnancy, when the mother assumes the supine position, the gravid uterus compresses the inferior vena cava and decreases venous return to the heart. This results in decreased cardiac output and symptoms of dizziness, light-headedness, and syncope. This significant arterial hypotension resulting from inferior vena cava compression is known as supine hypotensive syndrome or inferior vena cava syndrome. Therefore, it is not recommended that women remain in the supine position for any prolonged period of time in the latter part of pregnancy. When patients describe symptoms of the supine hypotensive syndrome, there is no need to proceed with additional cardiac or pulmonary workup.

62. The answer is d. (*Cunningham, p 126.*) Vascular spiders, or angiomas, are common findings during pregnancy. They form as a result of the hyperestrogenemia associated with normal pregnancies and are of no clinical significance. The presence of these angiomas does not require any additional workup or treatment, and they will resolve spontaneously after delivery. Reassurance to the patient is all that is required.

63. The answer is d. (*Cunningham, pp 1118–1119, 1275–1281. Thompson, pp 1018–1019.*) This patient's history and physical exam are consistent with an intestinal obstruction. An intestinal obstruction must be ruled out because, if it goes undiagnosed and untreated, it can result in a bowel perforation. This patient has a history of a previous abdominal surgery, which places her at risk for adhesions. Beginning in the second trimester, the gravid uterus can push on these adhesions and result in a bowel strangulation. Common symptoms of intestinal obstruction include colicky abdominal pain, nausea, and emesis. Signs of a bowel obstruction include abdominal tenderness and decreased bowel sounds. Fever and an elevated white blood cell count are present with bowel strangulation and necrosis. This patient has a mild leukocytosis, which is also characteristic of normal pregnancy. In order to rule out an intestinal obstruction, an upright or lateral decubitus abdominal x-ray should be done to identify the presence of distended loops of bowel and air-fluid levels, which confirm the diagnosis. Treatment consists of bowel rest, intravenous hydration, and nasogastric suction; patients who do not respond to conservative therapy may require surgery. Bowel stimulants such as laxatives or enemas should not be administered. Pregnant women are predisposed to constipation secondary to decreased bowel motility induced by elevated levels of progesterone. The symptoms of nausea and emesis in this patient and the presence of a low-grade fever prompt further workup because her presentation is not consistent with uncomplicated constipation. In pregnancy, constipation can be treated with hydration, increased fiber in the diet, and the use of stool softeners. The patient's sudden onset of emesis and abdominal pain is not consistent with the normal presentation of hyperemesis gravidarum. Hyperemesis typically has an onset in the early part of the first trimester and usually resolves by 16 weeks. It is characterized by intractable vomiting causing severe weight loss, dehydration, and electrolyte imbalance. The ingestion of spicy foods during pregnancy can cause or exacerbate gastric reflux, or "heartburn," but would not cause the severity of the symptoms described in this patient's presentation. Dyspepsia during pregnancy can be treated with antacids. The patient with gastric reflux in pregnancy should also be counseled to eat smaller, more frequent meals and bland food.

64. The answer is d. (*Cunningham, p 1145.*) The amount of iron that can be mobilized from maternal stores and gleaned from the diet is insufficient to meet the demands of pregnancy. A pregnant woman with a normal hematocrit at the beginning of pregnancy who is not given iron supplementation will suffer from iron deficiency during the latter part of gestation. It is important to remember that the fetus will not have impaired hemoglobin production, even in the presence of maternal anemia, because the placenta will transport the needed iron at the expense of maternal iron store depletion.

65. The answer is b. (*Cunningham, pp 129–130.*) Bilateral hydronephrosis and hydroureter is a normal finding during pregnancy and does not require any additional workup or concern. When the gravid uterus rises out of the pelvis, it presses on the ureters, causing ureteral dilatation and hydronephrosis. It has also been proposed that the hydroureter and hydronephrosis of pregnancy may be due to a hormonal effect from progesterone. In the vast majority of pregnant women, ureteral dilatation tends to be greater on the right side due to dextrorotation of the uterus and/or cushioning of the left ureter provided by the sigmoid colon.

66. The answer is c. (*Cunningham, pp 137–138, 1171.*) The finding of glucosuria is common during pregnancy and usually is not indicative of any pathology. During pregnancy, there is an increase in the glomerular filtration rate and a decrease in tubular reabsorption of filtered glucose. In fact, one of six women will spill glucose in the urine during pregnancy. If the patient has risk factors for diabetes, such as obesity, previous macrosomic baby, advanced maternal age, or family history of diabetes, the physician may want to screen for diabetes with a glucose tolerance test. If the patient has a urinary tract infection, the dipstick will also show an increase in WBCs and blood. A contaminated urine sample would not be a cause of isolated glucosuria.

67. The answer is d. (*Cunningham, pp 137, 1018–1019, 1084–1088.*) The patient's symptoms and physical exam are most consistent with the physiologic dyspnea, which is common in pregnancy. The increased awareness of breathing that pregnant women experience, which can occur as early as the end of the first trimester, is due to an increase in lung tidal volume. The increase in minute ventilation that occurs during pregnancy may make patients feel as if they are hyperventilating and may also contribute to the feeling of dyspnea. The patient in this case needs to be reassured and counseled regarding these normal changes of pregnancy. She needs to understand that she may have to modify her exercise regimen accordingly. There is no need to refer this patient to a cardiologist or to order an ECG. Systolic ejection murmurs are common findings in pregnant women and are due to a normal increased blood flow across the aortic and pulmonic valves. The incidence of pulmonary embolism in pregnancy is about 1 in 6400. In many of these cases there is clinical evidence of a DVT. The most common symptoms of a PE are dyspnea, chest pain, apprehension, cough, hemoptysis, and tachycardia. On physical exam, there may be an accentuated pulmonic closure sound, rales, or a friction rub. A strong suspicion for a PE should be followed up with a ventilation-perfusion scan. Large perfusion defects and ventilation mismatches would suggest the presence of a PE.

68–70. The answers are 68-f, 69-b, 70-d. (Cunningham, pp 620–621, 810, 830–833.) A placenta accreta occurs when the trophoblastic tissue invades the superficial lining of the uterus. Therefore the placenta is abnormally adherent to the uterine wall and cannot be easily separated from it. A portion of the placenta may be removed, while other parts remain attached, resulting in hemorrhage. In placenta previa, the placenta is located very near or over the internal os. Painless hemorrhage can occur without warning in the antepartum period. The bleeding is due to tearing of the placental attachments at the time of formation of the lower uterine segment and cervical dilation. A history of previous cesarean section and maternal smoking have been associated with an increased risk of placenta previa. Succenturiate placenta is characterized by one or more smaller accessory lobes that develop in the membranes at a distance from the main placenta. A retained succenturiate lobe may cause uterine atony and be a cause of postpartum hemorrhage. Vasa previa occurs when there is a velamentous insertion of the cord and the fetal vessels in the membranes are located ahead of the presenting part. Fenestrated placenta is a rare anomaly where the central portion of the placenta is missing. In the membranaceous placenta, all fetal membranes are covered by villi, and the placenta develops as a thin membranous structure. This type of placenta is also known as placenta diffusa.

Antepartum Care and Fetal Surveillance

Questions

DIRECTIONS: Each item below contains a question followed by suggested responses. Select the **one best** response to each question.

71. The shortest distance between the sacral promontory and the symphysis pubis is called which of the following?

a. Interspinous diameter
b. True conjugate
c. Diagonal conjugate
d. Obstetric conjugate
e. Biparietal diameter

72. A patient presents in labor at term. Clinical pelvimetry is performed. She has an oval-shaped pelvis with the anteroposterior diameter at the pelvic inlet greater than the transverse diameter. The baby is occiput posterior. The patient most likely has what kind of pelvis?

a. A gynecoid pelvis
b. An android pelvis
c. An anthropoid pelvis
d. A platypelloid pelvis
e. An androgenous pelvis

73. On pelvic examination of a patient in labor at 34 weeks, the patient is noted to be 6 cm dilated, completely effaced with the fetal nose and mouth palpable. The chin is pointing toward the maternal left hip. This is an example of which of the following?

a. Transverse lie
b. Mentum transverse position
c. Occiput transverse position
d. Brow presentation
e. Vertex presentation

74. The labor nurse calls you in your office regarding your patient who is 30 weeks pregnant and complaining of decreased fetal movement. The fetus is known to have a ventricular septal defect of the heart. The nurse has performed a nonstress test on the fetus. No contractions are seen. She thinks the tracing shows either a sinusoidal or saltatory fetal heart rate (FHR) pattern. Without actually reviewing the FHR tracing what can you tell the nurse?

a. The FHR tracing is probably not a sinusoidal FHR pattern because this pattern can be diagnosed only if the patient is in labor
b. The FHR tracing is probably not a saltatory FHR pattern because this pattern is almost always seen during rather than before labor
c. The FHR tracing of the premature fetus should be analyzed by different criteria than tracings obtained at term
d. Fetuses with congenital anomalies of the heart will invariably exhibit abnormal FHR patterns
e. Neither sinusoidal nor saltatory fetal heart rate patterns are seen in premature fetuses because of the immaturity of their autonomic nervous systems

75. You are counseling a 24-year-old woman who is a G2P1 at 36 weeks gestation. She delivered her first baby at 41 weeks gestation by cesarean section due to fetal distress that occurred during an induction of labor for mild preeclampsia. She would like to know if she can have a trial of labor with this pregnancy. Which of the following is the best response to this patient?

a. No, since she has never had a vaginal delivery
b. Yes, but only if she had a low transverse cesarean section
c. No, because once she has had a cesarean section she must deliver all of her subsequent children by cesarean section
d. Yes, but only if her uterine incision was made in the uterine fundus
e. Yes, but only if she had a classical cesarean section

76. A 32-year-old poorly controlled diabetic G2P1 is undergoing amniocentesis at 38 weeks for fetal lung maturity prior to having a repeat cesarean section. Which of the following laboratory tests performed on the amniotic fluid best indicates that the fetal lungs are mature?

a. Phosphatidylglycerol is absent
b. Lecithin/sphingomyelin ratio of 1:1
c. Lecithin/sphingomyelin ratio of 1.5:1
d. Lecithin/sphingomyelin ratio of 2.0:1
e. Shake test is positive

77. A 26-year-old G1P0 patient at 34 weeks gestation is being evaluated with Doppler ultrasound studies of the fetal umbilical arteries. The patient is a healthy smoker. Her fetus has shown evidence of intrauterine growth restriction (IUGR) on previous ultrasound examinations. The Doppler studies currently show that the systolic to diastolic ratio (S/D) in the umbilical arteries is much higher than it was on her last ultrasound three weeks ago and there is now reverse diastolic flow. Which of the following is correct information to inform the patient?

a. The Doppler studies indicate that the fetus is doing well
b. With advancing gestational age the S/D ratio is supposed to rise
c. These Doppler findings are normal in someone who smokes
d. Reverse diastolic flow is normal as a patient approaches full term
e. The Doppler studies are worrisome and indicate that the fetal status is deteriorating

78. A 17-year-old primipara at 41 weeks wants an immediate cesarean section. She is being followed with biophysical profile testing. You correctly tell her which of the following?

a. Biophysical profile testing includes amniotic fluid volume, fetal breathing, fetal body movements, fetal body tone, and contraction stress testing
b. The false-negative rate of the biophysical profile is 10%
c. False-positive results on biophysical profile are rare
d. Spontaneous decelerations during biophysical profile testing are associated with significant fetal morbidity
e. A normal biophysical profile should be repeated in 1 week to 10 days in a post-term pregnancy

79. A patient comes to your office with LMP 4 weeks ago. She denies any symptoms such as nausea, fatigue, urinary frequency, or breast tenderness. She thinks that she may be pregnant because she has not gotten her period yet and is very anxious to find out because she has a history of a previous ectopic pregnancy and wants to be sure to get early prenatal care. Which of the following evaluation methods is most sensitive in diagnosing pregnancy?

a. No evaluation to determine pregnancy is needed because the patient is asymptomatic and therefore cannot be pregnant
b. Serum pregnancy test
c. Detection of fetal heart tones by Doppler equipment
d. Abdominal ultrasound
e. Bimanual exam to assess uterine size

80. A patient presents for her first initial OB visit after performing a home pregnancy test and gives a last menstrual period of about 8 weeks ago. She says she is not entirely sure of her dates, however, because she has a long history of irregular menses. Which of the following is the most accurate way of dating the pregnancy?

a. Determination of uterine size on pelvic examination
b. Quantitative serum HCG level
c. Crown-rump length on abdominal or vaginal ultrasound
d. Determination of progesterone level along with serum HCG level

81. A healthy 20-year-old G1P0 presents for her first OB visit at 10 weeks gestational age. She denies any significant medical history both personally and in her family. Which of the following tests is not part of the recommended first trimester blood testing for this patient?

a. Complete blood count (CBC)
b. Screening for human immunodeficiency virus (HIV)
c. Hepatitis B surface antigen
d. Blood type and screen
e. One-hour glucose challenge testing

82. Your patient is a healthy 28-year-old G2P1001 at 20 weeks gestational age. Two years ago, she vaginally delivered at term a healthy baby boy weighing 6 lb 8 oz. This pregnancy, she had a prepregnancy weight of 130 lb. She is 5 ft 4 in. tall. She now weighs 140 lb and is extremely nervous that she is gaining too much weight. She is worried that the baby will be too big and require her to have a cesarean section. How do you counsel this patient?

a. Her weight gain is excessive, and she needs to be referred for nutritional counseling to slow down her rate of weight gain
b. Her weight gain is excessive, and you recommend that she undergo early glucola screening to rule out gestational diabetes
c. She is gaining weight at a less than normal rate, and, with her history of a small-for-gestational-age baby, she should supplement her diet with extra calories
d. During the pregnancy she should consume an additional 300 kcal/day versus prepregnancy, and her weight gain so far is appropriate for her gestational age
e. During the pregnancy she should consume an additional 600 kcal/day versus prepregnancy, and her weight gain is appropriate for her gestational age

83. A healthy 31-year-old G3P2002 patient presents to the obstetrician's office at 34 weeks gestational age for a routine return visit. She has had an uneventful pregnancy to date. Her baseline blood pressures were 100–110/60–70, and she has gained a total of 20 lb so far. During the visit, the patient complains of bilateral pedal edema that sometimes causes her feet to ache at the end of the day. Her urine dip indicates trace protein, and her blood pressure in the office is currently 115/75. She denies any other symptoms or complaints. On physical exam, there is pitting edema of both legs without any calf tenderness. Which of the following is the most appropriate response to the patient's concern?

a. Prescribe Lasix to relieve the painful swelling
b. Immediately send the patient to the radiology department to have venous Doppler studies done to rule out deep vein thromboses
c. Admit the patient to L and D to rule out preeclampsia
d. Reassure the patient that this is a normal finding of pregnancy and no treatment is needed
e. Tell the patient that her leg swelling is due to too much salt intake and instruct her to go on a low-sodium diet

84. A 28-year-old G1P0 presents to your office at 18 weeks gestational age for an unscheduled visit secondary to right-sided groin pain. She describes the pain as sharp and occuring with movement and exercise. She denies any change in urinary or bowel habits. She also denies any fever or chills. The application of a heating pad helps alleviate the discomfort. As her obstetrician, what should you tell this patient is the most likely etiology of this pain?

a. Round ligament pain
b. Appendicitis
c. Preterm labor
d. Kidney stone
e. Urinary tract infection

85. A 19-year-old G1P0 presents to the obstetrician's office for a routine OB visit at 34 weeks gestation. Her pregnancy has been complicated by gestational diabetes requiring insulin for control. She has been noncompliant with diet and insulin therapy. She has had two prior normal ultrasounds at 20 and 28 weeks gestation. She has no other significant past medical or surgical history. During the visit, the fundal height measures 38 cm. Which of the following is the most likely explanation for the discrepancy between the fundal height and the gestational age?

a. Fetal hydrocephaly
b. Uterine fibroids
c. Polyhydramnios
d. Breech presentation
e. Undiagnosed twin gestation

86. A 43-year-old G1P0 who conceived via in vitro fertilization comes into the office for her routine OB visit at 38 weeks. She denies any problems since she was seen the week before. She reports good fetal movement and denies any leakage of fluid per vagina, vaginal bleeding, or regular uterine contractions. She reports that sometimes she feels crampy at the end of the day when she gets home from work, but this discomfort is alleviated with getting off her feet. The fundal height measurement is 36 cm; it measured 37 cm the week before. Her cervical exam is 2 cm dilated. Which of the following is the most appropriate next step in the management of this patient?

a. Instruct the patient to return to the office in 1 week for her next routine visit
b. Admit the patient for induction due to a diagnosis of fetal growth lag
c. Send the patient for a sonogram to determine the amniotic fluid index
d. Order the patient to undergo a nonstress test
e. Do a fern test in the office

87. A pregnant women who is 7 weeks from her LMP comes in to the office for her first prenatal visit. Her previous pregnancy ended in a missed abortion in the first trimester. The patient therefore is very anxious about the well-being of this pregnancy. Which of the following modalities will allow you to best document fetal heart action?

a. Regular stethoscope
b. Fetoscope
c. Special fetal Doppler equipment
d. Transvaginal sonogram

88. A 30-year-old G2P1001 patient comes to see you in the office at 37 weeks gestational age for her routine OB visit. Her first pregnancy resulted in a vaginal delivery of a 9-lb 8-oz baby boy after 30 min of pushing. On doing Leopold maneuvers during this office visit, you determine that the fetus is breech. Vaginal exam demonstrates that the cervix is 50% effaced and 1 to 2 cm dilated. The presenting breech is high out of the pelvis. The estimated fetal weight is about 7 lb. The patient denies having any contractions. You send the patient for a sonogram, which confirms a fetus with a double footling breech presentation. There is a normal amount of amniotic fluid present and the head is hyperextended in the "stargazer" position. Which of the following is the best next step in the management of this patient?

a. Allow the patient to undergo a vaginal breech delivery whenever she goes into labor
b. Send the patient to labor and delivery immediately for an emergent cesarean section
c. Schedule a cesarean section at or after 41 weeks gestational age
d. Schedule an external cephalic version in the next few days
e. Allow the patient to go into labor and do an external cephalic version at that time if the fetus is still in the double footling breech presentation

89. A healthy 23-year-old G1P0 has had an uncomplicated pregnancy to date. She is disappointed because she is 40 weeks gestational age by good dates and a first-trimester ultrasound and wants to have her baby. She feels like she has been pregnant forever, and wants to have her baby now. The patient reports good fetal movement; she has been doing kick counts for the past several days and reports that the baby moves about eight times an hour on average. On physical exam, her cervix is firm, posterior, 50% effaced, and 1 cm dilated, and the vertex is at a −1 station. As her obstetrician, which of the following should you recommend to the patient?

a. She should be admitted for an immediate cesarean section
b. She should be admitted for Pitocin induction
c. You will schedule a cesarean section in 1 week if she has not undergone spontaneous labor in the meantime
d. She should continue to monitor kick counts and to return to your office in 1 week to reassess the situation

90. A 29-year-old G1P0 presents to the obstetrician's office at 41 weeks gestation. On physical exam, her cervix is 1 centimeter dilated, 0% effaced, firm and posterior in position. The vertex is presenting at −3 station. Which of the following is the best next step in the management of this patient.

a. Send the patient to the hospital for induction of labor since she has a favorable Bishop score
b. Teach the patient to measure fetal kick counts and deliver her if at any time there are less than 20 perceived fetal movements in 3 hours
c. Order biophysical profile testing for the same or next day
d. Schedule the patient for induction of labor at 43 weeks gestation
e. Schedule cesarean delivery for the following day since it is unlikely that the patient will go into labor

91. Your patient had an ultrasound examination today at 39 weeks gestation for size less than dates. The ultrasound showed oligohydramnios with an amniotic fluid index of 1.5 centimeters. The patient's cervix is unfavorable. Which of the following is the best next step in the management of this patient?

a. Admit her to the hospital for cesarean delivery
b. Admit her to the hospital for cervical ripening then induction of labor
c. Write her a prescription for misoprostol to take at home orally every 4 hours until she goes into labor
d. Perform stripping of the fetal membranes and perform a biophysical profile in 2 days
e. Administer a cervical ripening agent in your office and have the patient present to the hospital in the morning for induction with oxytocin

92. A healthy 30-year-old G1P0 at 41 weeks gestational age presents to labor and delivery at 11:00 P.M. because she is concerned that her baby has not been moving as much as normal for the past 24 h. She denies any complications during the pregnancy. She denies any rupture of membranes, regular uterine contractions, or vaginal bleeding. On arrival to labor and delivery, her blood pressure is initially 140/90 but decreases with rest to 120/75. Her prenatal chart indicates that her baseline blood pressures are 100–120/60–70. The patient is placed on an external fetal monitor. The fetal heart rate baseline is 180 bpm with absent variability. There are uterine contractions every 3 min accompanied by late fetal heart rate decelerations. Physical exam indicates that the cervix is long/closed/–2. Which of the following is the appropriate plan of management for this patient?

a. Proceed with emergent cesarean section
b. Administer intravenous $MgSO_4$ and induce labor with Pitocin
c. Ripen cervix overnight with prostaglandin E_2 (Cervidil) and proceed with Pitocin induction in the morning
d. Admit the patient and schedule a cesarean section in the morning, after the patient has been NPO for 12 h
e. Induce labor with misoprostil (Cytotec)

93. A 27-year-old G3P2002 who is 34 weeks gestational age calls the on-call obstetrician on a Saturday night at 10:00 P.M. complaining of decreased fetal movement. She says that yesterday her baby has moved only once per hour. For the past 6 hours she has felt no movement. She is healthy, has had regular prenatal care, and denies any complications so far during the pregnancy. Which of the following is the best advice for the on-call physician to give the patient?

a. Instruct the patient to go to labor and delivery for a contraction stress test
b. Reassure the patient that one fetal movement per hour is within normal limits and she does not need to worry
c. Recommend the patient be admitted to the hospital for delivery
d. Counsel the patient that the baby is probably sleeping and that she should continue to monitor fetal kicks. If she continues to experience less than five kicks per hour by morning, she should call you back for further instructions
e. Instruct the patient to go to labor and delivery for a nonstress test

94. Your patient complains of decreased fetal movement at term. You recommend a modified biophysical profile test. Nonstress testing in your office was reactive. The next part of the modified biophysical profile is which of the following?

a. Contraction stress testing
b. Amniotic fluid index evaluation
c. Ultrasound assessment of fetal movement
d. Ultrasound assessment of fetal breathing movements
e. Ultrasound assessment of fetal tone

95. You are seeing a patient in the hospital for decreased fetal movement at 36 weeks gestation. She is healthy and has had no prenatal complications. You order a biophysical profile. The patient receives a score of 8 on the test. Two points were deducted for lack of fetal breathing movements. How should you counsel the patient regarding the results of the biophysical profile?

a. The results are equivocal, and she should have a repeat BPP within 24 hours
b. The results are abnormal, and she should be induced
c. The results are normal, and she can go home
d. The results are abnormal, and she should undergo emergent cesarean section
e. The results are abnormal, and she should undergo umbilical artery Doppler velocimetry

96. An 18-year-old G2P1001 with the first day of her last menstrual period of May 7 presents for her first OB visit at 10 weeks. What is this patient's estimated date of delivery?

a. February 10 of the next year
b. February 14 of the next year
c. December 10 of the same year
d. December 14 of the same year

97. A new patient presents to your office for her first prenatal visit. By her last menstrual period she is 11 weeks pregnant. This is the first pregnancy for this 36-year-old woman. She has no medical problems. At this visit you observe that her uterus is palpable midway between the pubic symphasis and the umbilicus. No fetal heart tones are audible with the Doppler stethoscope. Which of the following is the best next step in the management of this patient?

a. Reassure her that fetal heart tones are not yet audible with the Doppler stethoscope at this gestational age
b. Tell her the uterine size is appropriate for her gestational age and schedule her for routine ultrasonography at 20 weeks
c. Schedule genetic amniocentesis right away because of her advanced maternal age
d. Schedule her for a dilation and curettage because she has a molar pregnancy since her uterus is too large and the fetal heart tones are not audible
e. Schedule an ultrasound as soon as possible to determine the gestational age and viability of the fetus

98. A healthy 30-year-old G2P1001 presents to the obstetrician's office at 34 weeks for a routine prenatal visit. She has a history of a cesarean section (low transverse) performed secondary to fetal malpresentation (footling breech). This pregnancy, the patient has had an uncomplicated prenatal course. She tells her physician that she would like to undergo a trial of labor during this pregnancy. However, the patient is interested in permanent sterilization and wonders if it would be better to undergo another scheduled cesarean section so she can have a bilateral tubal ligation performed at the same time. Which of the following statements is true and should be relayed to the patient?

a. A history of a previous low transverse cesarean section is a contraindication to vaginal birth after cesarean section (VBAC)
b. Her risk of uterine rupture with attempted VBAC after one prior low transverse cesarean section is 4 to 9%
c. Her chance of having a successful VBAC is less than 60%
d. The patient should schedule an elective induction if not delivered by 40 weeks
e. If the patient desires a bilateral tubal ligation, it is safer for her to undergo a vaginal delivery followed by a postpartum tubal ligation rather than an elective repeat cesarean section with intrapartum bilateral tubal ligation

99. A 16-year-old primigravida presents to your office at 35 weeks gestation. Her blood pressure is 170/110 and she has 4+ proteinuria on a clean catch specimen of urine. She has significant swelling of her face and extremities. She denies having contractions. Her cervix is closed and uneffaced. The baby is breech by bedside ultrasonography. She says the baby's movements have decreased in the past 24 hours. Which of the following is the best next step in the management of this patient?

a. Send her to labor and delivery for a biophysical profile
b. Send her home with instructions to stay on strict bed rest until her swelling and blood pressure improve
c. Admit her to the hospital for enforced bed rest and diuretic therapy to improve her swelling and blood pressure
d. Admit her to the hospital for induction of labor
e. Admit her to the hospital for cesarean delivery

100. While you are on call at the hospital covering labor and delivery, a 32-year-old G3P2002 who is 35 weeks calls you complaining of lower back pain. The patient informs you that she had been lifting some heavy boxes while fixing up the baby's nursery. The patient's pregnancy has been complicated by diet-controlled gestational diabetes. The patient denies any regular uterine contractions, rupture of membranes, vaginal bleeding, or dysuria. She denies any fever, chills, nausea, or emesis. She reports that the baby has been moving normally. On physical exam, you note that the patient is obese; her cervix is long and closed. Her abdomen is soft and nontender with no palpable uterine contractions. No flank pain can be elicited. She is afebrile. The external fetal monitor indicates a reactive fetal heart rate strip; there are rare irregular uterine contractions demonstrated on toco. The patient's urinalysis comes back with trace glucose and protein, and is otherwise negative. The patient's most likely diagnosis is which of the following?

a. Labor
b. Musculoskeletal pain
c. Urinary tract infection
d. Chorioamnionitis
e. Round ligament pain

DIRECTIONS: Each group of questions below consists of lettered options followed by a set of numbered clinical scenarios. For each numbered scenario, select the **one** lettered option with which it is **most** closely associated. Each lettered option may be used once, more than once, or not at all.

Questions 101–105

Match each description with the appropriate fetal heart rate tracing. If none of the tracings apply, answer e (none).

a.

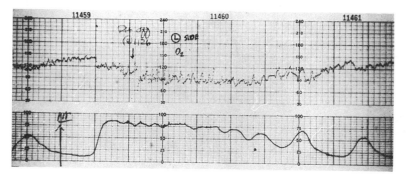

b.

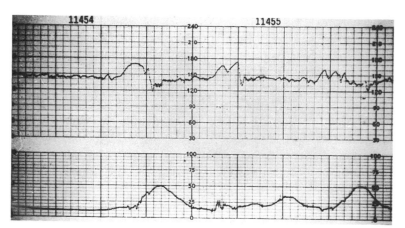

c.

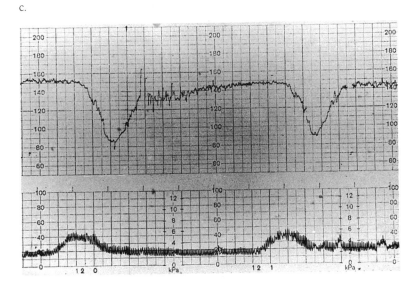

d.

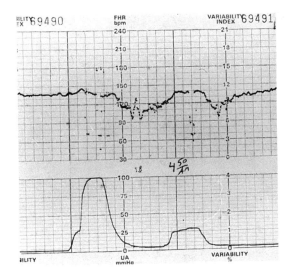

e. None

101. A 23-year-old G1P0 at 42 weeks is undergoing induction of labor. She is receiving intravenous oxytocin. She complains that her contractions are very painful and seem to be continuous.

102. A laboring patient has an internal fetal scalp electrode in place. Pelvic examination shows the patient to be 7 cm dilated with the fetal vertex at +1 station. The fetal heart rate tracing is consistent with fetal head compression.

103. A patient at 41 weeks is undergoing nonstress testing (NST). Her NST is reactive and reassuring.

104. A laboring patient at 40 weeks gestation presents with spontaneous rupture of membranes. Bedside ultrasonography shows no measurable pockets of amniotic fluid. With each contraction the fetal heart rate tracing shows evidence of umbilical cord compression.

105. A preeclamptic patient at 33 weeks gestation with intrauterine growth restriction is undergoing induction of labor. The fetal heart rate tracing shows evidence of uteroplacental insufficiency and is nonreassuring.

Antepartum Care and Fetal Surveillance

Answers

71. The answer is d. (*Cunningham, pp 33–37.*) The obstetric conjugate is the shortest distance between the promontory of the sacrum and the symphysis pubis. It generally measures 10.5 cm. Because the obstetric conjugate cannot be clinically measured, it is estimated by subtracting 1.5 to 2 cm from the diagonal conjugate, which is the distance from the lower margin of the symphysis to the sacral promontory. The true conjugate is measured from the top of the symphysis to the sacral promontory. The interspinous diameter is the transverse measurement of the midplane and generally is the smallest diameter of the pelvis.

72. The answer is c. (*Cunningham, pp 33–37.*) By tradition, pelves are classified as belonging to one of four major groups. The gynecoid pelvis is the classic female pelvis with a posterior sagittal diameter of the inlet only slightly shorter than the anterior sagittal diameter. In the android pelvis, the posterior sagittal diameter at the inlet is much shorter than the anterior sagittal diameter, limiting the use of the posterior space by the fetal head. In the anthropoid pelvis, the anteroposterior (AP) diameter of the inlet is greater than the transverse diameter, resulting in an oval with large sacrosciatic notches and convergent side walls. Ischial spines are likely to be prominent. The platypelloid pelvis is flattened with a short AP and wide transverse diameter. Wide sacrosciatic notches are common. The pelves of most women do not fall into a pure type and are blends of one or more of the above types.

73. The answer is b. (*Cunningham, pp 410–411.*) The lie of the fetus refers to the relation of the long axis of the fetus to that of the mother and is classified as longitudinal, transverse, or oblique. The presentation, or presenting part, refers to the portion of the baby that is foremost in the birth canal. The presentation may be cephalic, breech, or shoulder. Cephalic presentations are subclassified as vertex, brow, or face. The position is the relative relationship of the presenting part of the fetus to the mother. In this instance, the fetus is cephalic with the face presenting. The chin is the point of reference of the fetus when describing the position of the face. Since the chin (mentum) is pointing toward the mother's hip, the fetal position is described as mentum transverse.

74. The answer is b. (*Queenan, pp 177–179. Cunningham, pp 455–456.*) The sinusoidal pattern was first described in a group of severely affected Rh-isoimmunized fetuses. It has also been described, however, in normal fetuses and in association with maternal medication (e.g., alphaprodine). A saltatory pattern, which in the past was thought to be associated with depressed fetuses with low Apgar scores, is now thought to represent episodes of brief and acute hypoxia in the previously normally oxygenated fetus. This pattern is almost invariably seen during rather than before labor. The same relationship between the FHR pattern and the acid-base status has been documented in preterm and term fetuses. Thus, both the antepartum and the intrapartum FHR patterns of the premature fetus should be analyzed by the same criteria used at term. The vast majority of fetuses with congenital anomalies, including cardiac anomalies, have normal FHR patterns and a response to asphyxia similar to that of the normal fetus. Although no pathognomonic abnormal FHR patterns have been described for such fetuses, the rate of cesarean sections for fetal distress is reported to be significantly increased in this group. This may be explained by the oligohydramnios and fetal growth retardation that commonly occur in pregnancies affected by fetal congenital anomalies.

75. The answer is b. (*Hankins, pp 305–307. Cunningham, 610–613.*) Guidelines from the American College of Obstetricians and Gynecologists for vaginal birth after cesarean section (VBAC) state that a patient with a prior low transverse cesarean section may attempt a vaginal delivery following informed consent to the risks involved. A low transverse incision is cut transversely through the lower uterine segment, which does not actively contract during labor. A classical incision is made vertically on the uterus above the lower uterine segment through the myometrium, which actively contracts during labor. A prior classical incision on the uterus is a contraindication to a trial of labor because of a higher risk of uterine rupture. The risk of uterine rupture with a prior classical incision is 4 to 9% versus 0.2 to 1.5% with a prior low-transverse incision. Although a prior vaginal delivery increases the success rate for a successful VBAC, a prior vaginal birth is not a prerequisite for a VBAC attempt.

76. The answer is d. (*Reece, pp 109–111. Cunningham, 651–652.*) The lecithin-to-sphingomyelin (L/S) ratio in amniotic fluid is close to 1 until about 34 weeks of gestation, when the concentration of lecithin begins to rise. For pregnancies of unknown duration but otherwise uncomplicated, the risk of respiratory distress syndrome (RDS) is relatively minor when the L/S is at least 2:1. Maternal hypertensive disorders and fetal growth retardation may accelerate the rate of fetal pulmonary maturation, possibly as a result of chronic fetal stress. A delay in fetal pulmonary maturation is observed in pregnancies complicated by maternal diabetes or erythroblastosis fetalis. A risk of RDS of 40% exists with an L/S ratio of 1.5 to 2; when the L/S ratio is <1.5, the risk of RDS is 73%. When the L/S ratio is >2, the risk of RDS is slight. However, when the fetus is likely to have a serious metabolic compromise at birth (e.g., diabetes or sepsis), RDS may develop even with a mature L/S ratio (>2.0). This may be explained by lack of PG, a phospholipid that enhances surfactant properties. The identification of PG in amniotic fluid provides considerable reassurance (but not an absolute guarantee) that RDS will not develop. Moreover, contamination of amniotic fluid by blood, meconium, or vaginal secretions will not alter PG measurements.

77. The answer is e. (*Jaffe, pp 14–15, 252–254.*) Simple continuous-wave Doppler ultrasound can be used to display flow velocity waveforms as a function of time. With increased gestational age, in normal pregnancy there is an increase in end-diastolic flow velocity relative to peak systolic velocity, which causes the S/D ratio to decrease with advancing gestation. An increase in S/D ratio is associated with increased resistance in the placental vascular bed as can be noted in preeclampsia or fetal growth retardation. Nicotine and maternal smoking have also been reported to increase the S/D ratio. Many studies document the value of umbilical Doppler flow studies in recognition of fetal compromise. It seems that the S/D ratio increases as the fetal condition deteriorates; this is most severe in cases of absent or reversed diastolic flow. In normal twins, the S/D ratio falls within the normal range for singletons. Doppler studies have been used for intensive surveillance in cases of twin-to-twin transfusion.

78. The answer is d. (*Cunningham, pp 381–385.*) The biophysical profile is based on FHR monitoring (generally nonstress testing) in addition to four parameters observed on real-time ultrasonography: amniotic fluid volume, fetal breathing, fetal body movements, and fetal body tones. Each parameter gets a score of 0 to 2. A score of 8 to 10 is considered normal, a score of 6 is equivocal, and a score of 4 or less is abnormal and prompts delivery. The false-negative rate for the biophysical profile is less than 0.1%, but false-positive results are relatively frequent, with poor specificity. Oligohydramnios is an ominous sign, as are spontaneous decelerations. In patients with profile scores of 8 but with spontaneous decelerations, the rate of cesarean delivery indicated for fetal distress has been 25%. Testing more frequently than every 7 days is recommended in patients with post-term pregnancies, connective tissue disease, chronic hypertension, and suspected fetal growth retardation, as well as in patients with previous fetal death.

79. The answer is b. (*Cunningham, pp 204–207.*) Nausea, fatigue, breast tenderness, and urinary frequency are all common symptoms of pregnancy, but their presence cannot definitively make the diagnosis of pregnancy because they are nonspecific symptoms that are not consistently found in early pregnancy. On physical exam, the pregnant uterus enlarges and becomes more boggy and soft, but these changes are not usually apparent until after 6 weeks gestational age. In addition, other conditions such as ade-nomyosis, fibroids, or previous pregnancies can result in an enlarged uterus being palpated on physical exam. Abdominal ultrasound will not demon-strate a gestational sac until a gestational age of 5 to 6 weeks is reached. A Doppler instrument will detect fetal cardiac action usually no sooner than 10 weeks. A sensitive serum pregnancy test can detect placental HCG levels by 8 to 9 days postovulation, and it is therefore the most sensitive modality for detecting and diagnosing pregnancy.

80. The answer is c. (*Cunningham, pp 92, 96, 208, 212, 390–392, 882.*) Measurement of the fetal crown-rump length is the most accurate means of estimating gestational age. In the first trimester, this ultrasound measure-ment is accurate to within 3 to 5 days. Estimating the uterine size on phys-ical exam can result in an error of 1 to 2 weeks in the first trimester. Quantification of serum HCG cannot be used to determine gestational age, because at any gestational age the HCG number can vary widely in normal pregnancies. A single serum progesterone level cannot be used to date a pregnancy; however, it can be used to establish that an early pregnancy is developing normally. Serum progesterone levels less than 5 ng/mL usually indicate a nonviable pregnancy, while levels greater than 25 ng/mL indicate a normal intrauterine pregnancy. Progesterone levels in conjunction with quantitative HCG levels are often used to determine the presence of an ectopic pregnancy.

81. The answer is e. (*Cunningham, pp 208–212, 1171–1172.*) A 1-h glucose tolerance test should be performed between 24 and 28 weeks for women at risk for gestational diabetes. It is recommended that all women undergo tests for hepatitis B, HIV, type and screen, and CBC at the first prenatal visit.

82. The answer is d. (*Cunningham, pp 126–127, 213–219.*) The American College of Obstetrics and Gynecology supports the recommendation made by the Institute of Medicine in 1990 that women gain between 25 and 35 lb during pregnancy if they have a normal prepregnancy body mass index. Obese women with a BMI of >29 should not gain more than 15 lb, and women with a BMI of <19.8 can gain up to 40 lb. A daily increase in calories of 300 kcal is recommended. In the second and third trimesters, normal weight gain is about 1 lb/week. Low weight gain during pregnancy has been associated with infants that are small for gestational age; excessive weight gain has been associated with large-for-gestational-age infants and an increased risk for cesarean section. Sally had a previous delivery of an appropriate-size baby. Her weight gain this pregnancy has been appropriate, and she needs to continue to consume an additional 300 kcal daily to continue to gain appropriate weight.

83. The answer is d. (*Cunningham, pp 127, 135, 762–764, 1079–1084.*) Increased fluid retention manifested by pitting edema of the ankles and legs is a normal finding in pregnancy. During pregnancy, there is a decrease in colloid osmotic pressure and a fall in plasma osmolality. Moreover, there is an increase in venous pressure created by partial occlusion of the vena cava by the gravid uterus, which also contributes to pedal edema. Diuretics are sometimes given to pregnant women who have chronic hypertension, but this is not the case in this patient. More commonly, Lasix is used in the acute setting to treat pulmonary edema. This patient is not hypertensive and does not have any other signs or symptoms of preeclampsia and therefore does not need to be admitted for a further workup. Trace protein in the urine is common in normal pregnancies and is not of concern. Doppler studies of the lower extremities are not indicated in this patient since the history and exam (specifically, the lack of calf tenderness) are consistent with physiologic edema. The normal swelling detected in pregnancy is not prevented by a low-sodium diet or improved with a lower intake of salt.

84. The answer is a. (*Gabbe, pp 227. Cunningham, pp 22, 24, 867, 1119–1120.*) The patient is giving a classic description of round ligament pain. Each round ligament extends from the lateral portion of the uterus below the oviduct and travels in a fold of peritoneum downward to the inguinal canal and inserts in the upper portion of the labium majus. During pregnancy, these ligaments stretch as the gravid uterus grows farther out of the pelvis and can thereby cause sharp pains, particularly with sudden movements. Round ligament pain is usually more frequently experienced on the right side due to the dextrorotation of the uterus that commonly occurs in pregnancy. Usually this pain is greatly improved by avoiding sudden movements and by rising and sitting down gradually. Local heat and analgesics may also help with pain control. The diagnosis of appendicitis is not likely because the patient is not experiencing any fever or anorexia. In addition, because the gravid uterus pushes the appendix out of the pelvis, pregnant women with appendicitis often have pain located much higher than the groin area. The diagnosis of preterm labor is unlikely because the pain is localized to the groin area on one side and is alleviated with a heating pad, which would not be the case with labor contractions. In addition, when labor occurs, the pain would persist at rest, not just with movement. A urinary tract infection is unlikely because the patient has no urinary symptoms. A kidney stone is unlikely because usually the patient would complain of pain in the back, not low in the groin. In addition, with a kidney stone the pain would occur not only with movement, but would persist at rest as well.

85. The answer is c. (*Gabbe, p 230.*) The fundal height in centimeters has been found to correlate with gestational age in weeks with an error of 3 cm from 16 to 36 weeks. Uterine fibroids, polyhydramnios (excessive amniotic fluid), fetal macrosomia, and twin gestation are all plausible explanations of why the uterine size would measure larger than expected for the patient's dates. Breech presentation does not cause the uterus to be larger than expected for the gestational age. Since this patient has had two prior ultrasound examinations, hydrocephaly, fibroids, and twins would have previously been diagnosed. In this uncontrolled diabetic, the most likely cause for the excessive fundal height is polyhydramnios. Polyhydramnios is an excessive amount of amniotic fluid and is a sign of poor glucose control.

86. The answer is a. (*Cunningham, pp 208, 212, 377–380, 392–393, 425–426, 900–901.*) The decrease in fundal height between visits can be explained by engagement of the fetal head, which is verified on vaginal exam with determination of the presenting part at 0 station. Engagement of the fetal head commonly occurs before labor in nulliparous patients. Therefore it is appropriate for the patient to return for another scheduled visit in a week. Intrauterine growth lag is unlikely because there will usually be a greater discrepancy (>3 cm) between fundal height and gestational age. Therefore, the patient does not need to be induced. Since the patient has been reporting good fetal movement and is not postterm, there is no indication to do antepartum testing such as an NST. A fern test is not indicated since the patient has not reported leakage of fluid. An assessment of amniotic fluid to detect oligohydramnios is not indicated since the fundal height is appropriate for the patient's gestational age.

87. The answer is d. (*Cunningham, p 205.*) Vaginal ultrasound can detect fetal heart action as early as 5 weeks of amenorrhea. With a traditional, nonelectric fetal stethoscope, heart tones can be heard after 19 to 20 weeks gestational age. With appropriate Doppler equipment, fetal heart tones can be usually be detected by 10 weeks gestational age.

88. The answer is d. (*Cunningham, pp 570–572. Gabbe, pp 560–562.*) The patient who has a fetus with a breech presentation has the option of scheduling an external cephalic version, an elective cesarean section at or after 39 weeks, or can elect to have a vaginal breech delivery if certain conditions are met. It is inappropriate to electively deliver any patient prior to 39 weeks without a documentation of fetal lung maturity because of the risk of neonatal respiratory distress syndrome. Therefore, if a patient declines to undergo a vaginal breech delivery, an elective cesarean should be scheduled at or after 39 weeks gestational age to avoid this complication of preterm delivery. If a patient would like to avoid a cesarean section but does not want to undergo a vaginal breech delivery, then an external cephalic version is an appropriate management plan. An external cephalic version (ECV) is a procedure where the fetus with a breech presentation is manipulated through the abdominal wall to change the presenting part to vertex. Studies indicate that if an ECV is not performed, 80% of breech presentations will persist at term versus only 30% if a successful version is performed. ECV has an average success rate of about 60%; it is most successful in parous women with an unengaged breech and a normal amount of amniotic fluid (all conditions that exist in the patient described). A trial of labor for a pregnant woman with a fetus in the breech presentation is appropriate if the fetus is frank breech, has a flexed head, has a normal amount of amniotic fluid, and has an estimated weight between 2500 and 3800 g. In addition, the pelvis should be adequate as assessed with x-ray pelvimetry or a history of delivery of a previous baby of bigger size. A fetus with a hyperextended, or "stargazer," head has a higher risk of spinal cord injury during vaginal breech delivery; therefore delivery should be by cesarean delivery. The best course of management in this case is external cephalic version.

89. The answer is d. (*Cunningham, pp 373–387, 537, 539, 889–890.*) Postterm or prolonged pregnancies are those pregnancies that have gone beyond 42 completed weeks of gestation. In general, obstetricians do not allow pregnancies to persist after 42 weeks because of the significantly increased incidence of perinatal morbidity and mortality. If a patient has a ripe cervix, it is reasonable to induce the patient at 41 weeks because the chance of having a successful vaginal delivery is very high. On the other hand, if the patient has an unripe cervix, it is generally recommended that she continue with the pregnancy. Alternatively, a patient can be induced at 41 weeks with an unripe cervix if cervical ripening agents are used. If a patient waits until 42 weeks and still has an unripe cervix, then admission with administration of cervical ripening agents prior to Pitocin induction is recommended to improve the likelihood of a successful vaginal delivery. The Bishop score is a way to determine the favorability of the cervix to induction. The elements of the Bishop score include effacement, dilation, station, consistency, and position of the cervix (see table). Points are assigned for each element, then totaled to give the Bishop's score. Induction to active labor is usually successful with a Bishop score of 9 or greater. In the scenario described here, the patient has a Bishop score of 4, which is unfavorable for induction. Therefore, expectant management is a reasonable management plan to try to give the cervix time to ripen to avoid a cesarean section. It is not recommended to perform an elective section without a trial of labor because of the risks of major surgery.

BISHOP SCORE

Points	Dilation	Effacement	Station	Consistency	Position
0	Closed	0–30%	−3	Firm	Posterior
1	1–2 cm	40–50%	−2	Medium	Midposition
2	3–4 cm	60–70%	−1, 0	Soft	Anterior
3	≥5 cm	≥80%	+1, +2	—	—

90. The answer is c. (*Cunningham, pp 374–382, 882–890.*) As discussed in question 89, patients at 41 to 42 weeks gestation with good dating criteria and a favorable cervix should undergo induction of labor. If the cervix is unfavorable, fetal well-being should be assessed prior to allowing the pregnancy to continue. Patient self-assessment by measurement of fetal kick counts, nonstress testing, contraction stress testing, and fetal biophysical profile may be used to assess fetal well-being. The biophysical profile allows assessment of the fetal heart rate tracing and the amniotic fluid level, which in this case is the next best step in the management of this patient. Induction of labor is recommended at 42 weeks regardless of the favorability of the cervix because of the increased risk of perinatal morbidity after that gestational age. As noted above, it is not recommended to perform an elective section without a trial of labor because of the risks of major surgery.

91. The answer is b. (*Cunningham, pp 536–542, 882–890. ACOG, Practice Bulletin 10.*) Patients with oligohydramnios at term should be delivered. If there is no contraindication to vaginal delivery, the patient should be induced. The patient with an unfavorable cervix may undergo cervical ripening after assessment of fetal well-being. If fetal testing is reassuring, the unfavorable cervix can be ripened with a variety of mechanical and pharmacologic agents prior to initiating Pitocin. Pharmacologic agents include prostaglandin E_2 preparations available as a vaginal/cervical gel (Preperdil) or vaginal insert (Cervidil). Misoprostil, a synthetic PGE_1 analogue, has been used off-label for preinduction cervical ripening and induction. It can be administered via the oral or vaginal route. Mechanical ripening of the cervix can be achieved with laminaria, which is a hygroscopic dilator that is placed in the cervical canal and absorbs water from the surrounding cervical tissue. Pitocin is not considered a cervical ripening agent but a labor-inducing agent. In patients with oligohydramnios, cervical ripening should be performed in the hospital under continuous fetal monitoring.

92. The answer is a. (*ACOG, Technical Bulletin 207.*) A fetal heart rate tracing indicating tachycardia, decreased or absent variability, and persistent late decelerations is indicative of fetal metabolic acidosis and hypoxia. Prompt intervention and delivery is indicated. There is no indication for administering $MgSO_4$ since the patient is not preeclamptic; her blood pressure is not elevated. Since imminent delivery of the fetus is indicated by the nonreassuring fetal heart rate pattern, there is no role for administering cervical ripening agents or Pitocin.

93. The answer is e. (*Cunningham, pp 374–385. ACOG, Practice Bulletin 9.*) Maternal perception of decreased fetal movement has preceded fetal death in utero. Therefore, kick counts have been employed as a method of antepartum assessment. The optimal number of fetal movements that should be perceived per hour has not been determined. However, studies indicate that the perception of 10 distinct movements in a period of up to 2 h is reassuring. Since this patient is experiencing only one movement per hour, and this movement is decreased from her previous baseline, further antepartum testing is indicated. A nonstress test is the preferred modality, because a contraction stress test involves giving a preterm pregnancy uterine contractions. Delivery is not indicated until nonreassuring fetal status can be documented.

94. The answer is b. (*ACOG, Practice Bulletin 9.*) The biophysical profile (BPP) consists of five components:

1. Nonstress test
2. Fetal breathing movements—one or more episodes of fetal breathing movements of 30 s or more within 30 min
3. Fetal movement—three or more discrete body or limb movements within 30 min
4. Fetal tone—one or more episodes of extension of a fetal extremity with return to flexion, or opening or closing of a hand
5. Determination of amniotic fluid volume—a single vertical pocket of amniotic fluid exceeding 2 cm

Each of these components is assigned a score of 2 (normal) or 0 (abnormal or absent). In the modified BPP, only the NST and determination of amniotic fluid volume are assessed.

95. The answer is c. *(ACOG, Practice Bulletin 9. Cunningham, pp 381–382.)* A BPP score of 8 or 10 is normal. A score of 0 to 2 dictates imminent delivery, because fetal asphyxia is probable. Scores of 4 to 6 require repeat testing and delivery if persistent.

96. The answer is b. *(Cunningham, p 208.)* The expected date of delivery can be estimated by using Naegele's rule. To do this, count back 3 months and then add 7 days to the date of the first day of the last normal menstrual period.

97. The answer is e. *(Cunningham, p 205.)* At 11 weeks of gestation the uterus is still within the pelvis and should not be palpable above the symphysis pubis. A uterus that is palpable midway between the symphysis pubis and the umbilicus is 14 to 16 weeks in size. The fetal heart tones are audible in most patients at 10 weeks. If no fetal heart tones are audible by Doppler auscultation and the patient is 10 weeks or more, an ultrasound of the pregnancy should be ordered. Molar pregnancy, twin gestation, incorrect dates, and uterine fibroids are all possible diagnoses when the uterus is large for dates. Dilation and curettage are not indicated before evaluation of the patient with ultrasonography for gestational age and fetal viability. Although the patient is of advanced maternal age, genetic amniocentesis should not be performed without first knowing the gestational age and viability of the pregnancy.

98. The answer is e. *(Cunningham, pp 607–617.)* The desire for sterilization is not an indication for an elective repeat cesarean section. The morbidity of repeat cesarean section is greater than that of vaginal birth with postpartum tubal ligation. The risk of uterine rupture in a woman who undergoes a trial of labor and has had one prior cesarean section is approximately 0.6%. With a history of two prior cesarean sections, the risk of uterine rupture is about 1.8%. The risk of uterine rupture in someone who has had a classical or T-shaped uterine incision is 4 to 6%. The success rate for a trial of labor is generally about 60 to 80% Success rates are higher when the original cesarean section was performed for breech rather than dystocia. Induction of labor should not be performed without an obstetrical indication (e.g., preeclampsia); some studies suggest that high doses of oxytocin infusion increase a patient's risk of uterine rupture.

99. The answer is e. (*Cunningham, pp 763–765, 781–785, 794.*) Hypertension is diagnosed in pregnancy when the resting blood pressure is 140/90 or greater. The patient may have a history of chronic hypertension. Gestational hypertension is diagnosed if the patient develops hypertension without proteinuria during the pregnancy. Preeclampsia is diagnosed when the hypertension is associated with proteinuria of greater than 300 mg in a 24 hour collection or persistent 1+ proteinuria in random urine sampling. The cure for gestational hypertension and preeclampsia is delivery. Select preterm patients may be managed conservatively at home or in the hospital depending upon the severity of the hypertension. Biophysical profile testing is useful when following the patient conservatively. Although bed rest may transiently improve elevated blood pressure, a patient at full term should be delivered. Based on the severity of this patient's blood pressure and the 4+ proteinuria, she has severe preeclamsia and she should be delivered. Since this patient's fetus is breech, cesarean delivery rather than induction of labor is the next best step in the management of this patient. Diuretics should not be used in the management of preeclampsia, as they deplete the maternal intravascular volume and may compromise placental perfusion.

100. The answer is b. (*Cunningham, p 224.*) Lower back pain is a common symptom of pregnancy and is reported by about 50% of pregnant women. It is caused by stress placed on the lower spine and associated muscles and ligaments by the gravid uterus, especially in late pregnancy. The pain can be exacerbated with excessive bending and lifting. In addition, obesity predisposes the patient to lower back pain in pregnancy. Treatment options include heat, massage, and analgesia. This patient has no evidence of labor since she is lacking regular uterine contractions and cervical change. Without any urinary symptoms or a urinalysis suggestive of infection, cystitis is unlikely. The diagnosis of chorioamnionitis does not fit since the patient has intact membranes, no fever, and a nontender uterus. Round ligament pain is characterized by sharp groin pain.

101–105. The answers are 101-a, 102-e, 103-b, 104-c, 105-d. (*Reece, pp 813–815, Cunningham, pp 446–456.*) Fetal heart rate tracings are obtained in most pregnancies in the United States through the use of electronic fetal monitoring equipment. Accurate interpretation of these tracings with resultant action to expedite delivery in fetuses threatened by hypoxemia has certainly improved neonatal outcome, although it has had very little effect on the overall incidence of cerebral palsy, which seems most often to have its etiology remote from the time of labor. Tracing **a** shows a classic hyperstimulation pattern, with a tonic contraction lasting several minutes with distinctly raised intrauterine pressure and a consequent fall in fetal heart rate. Despite the increased pressure, there remains good beat-to-beat variability, which suggests that the fetus is withstanding the stress. Tracing **b** shows fetal heart rate accelerations occurring spontaneously both before and after contractions, with good beat-to-beat variability, and is representative of a very healthy fetus. Tracing **c** shows variable decelerations with a late component in which the classic V-shaped picture of a variable deceleration is maintained, but the first deceleration on the left shows a prolonged recovery of several minutes before reaching the original baseline. Such compound decelerations are not as ominous as classic late decelerations, but they bear careful scrutiny. Tracing **d** shows late decelerations following two consecutive contractions. While the decrement in fetal heart rate is not great, it is seen in both contractions. The baseline variability is significantly reduced. This pattern is caused by uteroplacental insufficiency.

Obstetrical Complications of Pregnancy

Questions

DIRECTIONS: Each item below contains a question followed by suggested responses. Select the **one best** response to each question.

106. A 29-year-old G3P2 presents to the emergency center with complaints of abdominal discomfort for 2 weeks. A pregnancy test is positive and an ultrasound of the abdomen and pelvis reveals a viable 16-week gestation located behind a normal-appearing $10 \times 6 \times 5.5$ cm uterus. Both ovaries appear normal. No free fluid is noted. Which of the following is the most likely cause of these findings?

a. Ectopic ovarian tissue
b. Fistula between the peritoneum and uterine cavity
c. Primary peritoneal implantation of the fertilized ovum
d. Tubal abortion
e. Uterine rupture of prior cesarean section scar

107. A 32-year-old G2P1 at 28 weeks gestation presents to labor and delivery with the complaint of vaginal bleeding. She denies any contraction and states that the baby is moving normally. On ultrasound the placenta is anteriorly located and completely covers the internal cervial os. Which of the following would increase her risk for hysterectomy?

a. Desire for sterilization
b. Development of disseminated intravascular coagulopathy
c. Placenta accreta
d. Prior vaginal delivery
e. Smoking

108. A patient at 17 weeks gestation is diagnosed as having an intrauterine fetal demise. She returns to your office 5 weeks later and has not had a miscarriage, although she has had some occasional spotting. This patient is at increased risk for which of the following?

a. Septic abortion
b. Recurrent abortion
c. Consumptive coagulopathy with hypofibrinogenemia
d. Future infertility
e. Ectopic pregnancies

109. A 24-year-old presents at 30 weeks with a fundal height of 50 cm. Which of the following statements concerning polyhydramnios is true?

a. Acute polyhydramnios always leads to labor prior to 28 weeks
b. The incidence of associated malformations is approximately 3%
c. Maternal edema, especially of the lower extremities and vulva, is rare
d. Esophageal atresia is accompanied by polyhydramnios in nearly 10% of cases
e. Complications include placental abruption, uterine dysfunction, and postpartum hemorrhage

110. A 20-year-old gravida 1 at 32 weeks presents for her routine OB visit. She has no medical problems. She is noted to have a blood pressure of 150/96, and her urine dip shows 1+ protein. She complains of a constant headache and vision changes that are not relieved with rest or a pain reliever. The patient is sent to the hospital for further management. At the hospital her blood pressure is 158/98 and she is noted to have tonic-clonic seizure. Which of the following is indicated in the management of this patient?

a. Low-dose aspirin
b. Dilantin (phenytoin)
c. Antihypertensive therapy
d. Magnesium sulfate
e. Cesarean delivery

111. During routine ultrasound surveillance of a twin pregnancy, twin A weighs 1200 g and twin B weighs 750 g. Hydramnios is noted around twin A, while twin B has oligohydramnios. Which statement concerning the ultrasound findings in this twin pregnancy is true?

a. The donor twin develops hydramnios more often than does the recipient twin
b. Gross differences may be observed between donor and recipient placentas
c. The donor twin usually suffers from a hemolytic anemia
d. The donor twin is more likely to develop widespread thromboses
e. The donor twin often develops polycythemia

112. A 32-year-old G5P1 presents for her first prenatal visit. A complete obstetrical, gynecological, and medical history and physical exam is done. Which of the following would be an indication for elective cerclage placement?

a. Three spontaneous first-trimester abortions
b. Twin pregnancy
c. Three second-trimester pregnancy losses without evidence of labor or abruption
d. History of loop electrosurgical excision procedure for cervical dysplasia
e. Cervical length of 35 mm by ultrasound at 18 weeks

DIRECTIONS: Each group of questions below consists of lettered options followed by a set of numbered items. For each numbered item, select the **one** lettered option with which it is **most** closely associated. Each lettered option may be used once, more than once, or not at all.

Questions 113–117

Match each description with the correct type of abortion.

a. Complete abortion
b. Incomplete abortion
c. Threatened abortion
d. Missed abortion
e. Inevitable abortion

113. Uterine bleeding at 12 weeks gestation accompanied by cervical dilation without passage of tissue.

114. Passage of some but not all placental tissue through the cervix at 9 weeks gestation.

115. Fetal death at 15 weeks gestation without expulsion of any fetal or maternal tissue for at least 8 weeks.

116. Uterine bleeding at 7 weeks gestation without any cervical dilation.

117. Expulsion of all fetal and placental tissue from the uterine cavity at 10 weeks gestation.

DIRECTIONS: Each item below contains a question followed by suggested responses. Select the one best response to each question.

118. A 19-year-old primigravida is expecting her first child; she is 12 weeks pregnant by dates. She has vaginal bleeding and an enlarged-for-dates uterus. In addition, no fetal heart sounds are heard. The ultrasound shown below is obtained. Which of the following is true regarding the patient's diagnosis?

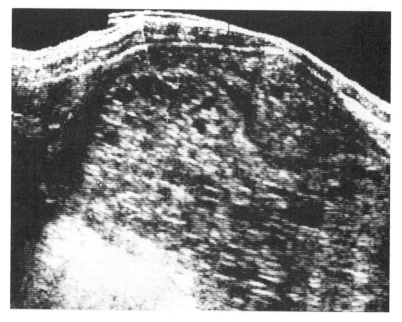

a. The most common chromosomal makeup of a partial or incomplete mole is 46,XX, of paternal origin
b. Older maternal age is not a risk factor for hydatidiform mole
c. Partial or incomplete hydatidiform mole has a higher risk of developing into choriocarcinoma than complete mole
d. Vaginal bleeding is a common symptom of hydatidiform mole
e. Hysterectomy is contraindicated as primary therapy for molar pregnancy in women who have completed childbearing

119. A 20-year-old G1P0 presents to your clinic for follow-up for a suction dilation and curettage for an incomplete abortion. She is asymptomatic without any vaginal bleeding, fever, or chills. Her exam is normal. The pathology report reveals trophoblastic proliferation and hydropic degeneration with the absence of vasculature; no fetal tissue is identified. A chest x-ray is negative for any evidence of metastatic disease. Which of the following is the best next step in her management?

a. Weekly hCG titers
b. Hysterectomy
c. Single-agent chemotherapy
d. Combination chemotherapy
e. Radiation therapy

120. A 22-year-old G1P0 presents to your clinic for follow-up of evacuation of a complete hydatiform mole. She is asymptomatic and her exam is normal. Which of the following would be an indication to start single-agent chemotherapy?

a. A rise in hCG titers
b. A plateau of hCG titers for 1 week
c. Return of hCG titer to normal at 6 weeks after evacuation
d. Appearance of liver metastasis
e. Appearance of brain metastasis

121. A 32-year-old G3P3 presents with abdominal pain. Her last menstrual period was 6 weeks ago, and a pregnancy test is positive. The specimen shown below is obtained at laparotomy. Which of the following is the most likely diagnosis?

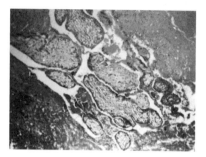

a. Incomplete abortion
b. Missed abortion
c. Hydatidiform mole
d. Tubal ectopic pregnancy
e. Ovarian pregnancy

122. A 19-year-old woman comes to the emergency room and reports that she fainted at work earlier in the day. She has mild vaginal bleeding. Her abdomen is diffusely tender and distended. In addition, she complains of shoulder and abdominal pain. Her temperature is 97.6°F, pulse rate is 120/min, and blood pressure is 80/42 mmHg. To confirm the diagnosis suggested by the available clinical data, which of the following is the best diagnostic procedure?

a. Pregnancy test
b. Posterior colpotomy
c. Dilation and curettage
d. Culdocentesis
e. Laparoscopy

123. An 18-year-old G2P1 presents to the emergency department with abdominal pain and vaginal bleeding for the past day. Her last menstrual period was 7 weeks ago. On exam she is afebrile with normal blood pressure and pulse. Her abdomen is tender in the left lower quadrant with voluntary guarding. On pelvic exam, she has a small anteverted uterus, no adnexal masses, mild left andexal tenderness, and mild cervical motion tenderness. Labs reveal a normal white count, hemoglobin of 10.5, and a quantitative beta hCG of 2342. Ultrasound reveals a $10 \times 5 \times 6$ cm uterus with a normal-appearing 1-cm stripe and no gestation sac or fetal pole. A 2.8-cm complex andexal mass is noted on the left. In the treatment of this patient, laparoscopic salpingostomy has what advantage over salpingectomy via laparotomy?

a. Decreased hospital stays
b. Lower fertility rate
c. Lower repeat ectopic pregnancy rate
d. Comparable persistent ectopic tissue rate
e. Greater scar formation

124. A 27-year-old has just had an ectopic pregnancy. Which of the following events would be most likely to predispose to ectopic pregnancy?

a. Previous cervical conization
b. Pelvic inflammatory disease (PID)
c. Use of a contraceptive uterine device (IUD)
d. Induction of ovulation
e. Exposure in utero to diethylstilbestrol (DES)

125. An 18-year-old G1 at 8 weeks gestation complains of nausea and vomiting over the past week occurring on a daily basis. Nausea and emesis are a common symptom in early pregnancy. Which of the following signs or symptoms would indicate a more serious diagnosis of hyperemesis gravidarum?

a. Hypothyroidism
b. Hypokalemia
c. Weight gain
d. Proteinuria
e. Diarrhea

126. A 32-year-old G2P0101 presents to labor and delivery at 34 weeks of gestation, complaining of regular uterine contractions about every 5 min for the past several hours. She has also noticed the passage of a clear fluid per vagina. A nurse places the patient on an external fetal monitor and calls you to evaluate her status. The external fetal monitor demonstrates a reactive fetal heart rate tracing, with regular uterine contractions occurring about every 3 to 4 min. On sterile speculum exam, the cervix is visually closed. A sample of pooled amniotic fluid seen in the vaginal vault is fern- and nitrazine-positive. The patient has a temperature of 102°F, P = 102, and her fundus is tender to deep palpation. Her admission blood work comes back indicating a WBC of 19,000. The patient is very concerned because she had previously delivered a baby at 35 weeks who suffered from respiratory distress syndrome. You perform a bedside sonogram, which indicates oligohydramnios and a fetus whose size is appropriate for gestational age and with a cephalic presentation. Which of the following is the most appropriate next step in the management of this patient?

a. Administer betamethasone
b. Administer tocolytics
c. Place a cervical cerclage
d. Administer antibiotics
e. Perform emergent cesarean section

127. A 30-year-old G1P0 with a twin gestation at 25 weeks presents to labor and delivery complaining of irregular uterine contractions and back pain. She reports an increase in the amount of her vaginal discharge, but denies any rupture of membranes. She reports that earlier in the day she had some very light vaginal bleeding, which has now resolved. She says that the babies have been active and moving as much as usual. She thinks that she may be feeling cramping because she may have overdone it with too much activity and lifting as she is trying to fix up the nursery to get it ready for the babies. She denies any change in her bowel or urine habits. She reports having had regular prenatal care during the pregnancy and denies any prior problems or complications. On arrival to L and D, she is placed on an external fetal monitor, which indicates uterine contractions every 2 to 4 min. She is afebrile and her vital signs are all normal. Her gravid uterus is nontender. The nurses call you to evaluate the patient. Which of the following is the most appropriate first step in the evaluation of vaginal bleeding in this patient?

a. Vaginal exam to determine cervical dilation
b. Ultrasound to check placental location
c. Urine culture to check for urinary tract infection
d. Labwork to evaluate for disseminated intravascular coagulopathy
e. Apt test to determine if blood is from the fetus

128. A 30-year-old gravida 1 with twin gestation at 28 weeks is being evaluated for vaginal bleeding and uterine contractions. A bedside ultrasound examination indicates that both fetuses are in the cephalic presentation and rules out the presence of a placenta previa. Fetal heart rate tracing is reactive on both twins, and the uterine contractions are every 2 to 3 minutes and last 60 seconds. A sterile speculum exam is then performed, and a vaginal swab is obtained to perform a fern test on the vaginal discharge. The fern and nitrazine tests are negative. A subsequent digital exam indicates that the cervix is 2 to 3 centimers dilated and 50% effaced, and the presenting part is at −3 station. Tocolysis with magnesium sulfate is initiated and intravenous antibiotics are started for group B streptococcus prophylaxis. Betamethasone, a corticosteroid, is also administered. Which of the following statements regarding the use of betamethasone in the treatment of preterm labor is true?

a. Betamethasone enhances the tocolytic effect of magnesium sulfate and decreases the risk of preterm delivery
b. Betamethasone has been shown to decrease intraamniotic infections
c. Betamethasone promotes fetal lung maturity and decreases the risk of respiratory distress syndrome
d. The anti-inflammatory effect of betamethasone decreases the risk of GBS sepsis in the newborn
e. Betamethasone is the only corticosteroid proven to cross the placenta

129. A maternal fetal medicine specialist is consulted and performs an in-depth sonogram on a 30-year-old gravida 1 at 28 weeks with a twin gestation. The sonogram indicates that the fetuses are both male, and the placenta appears to be diamniotic and monochorionic. Twin B is noted to have oligohydramnios and to be much smaller than twin A. Which of the following would be a finding associated with twin A?

a. Congestive heart failure
b. Anemia
c. Hypovolemia
d. Hypotension
e. Low amniotic fluid level

130. A 30-year-old G1 at 28 weeks gestation with a twin pregnancy is admitted to the hospital for preterm labor with regular painful contractions every 2 minutes. She is 3 cm dilated with membranes intact and a small amount of bloody show. Ultrasound reveals growth restriction of twin A and oligohydramnios, otherwise normal anatomy. Twin B has normal anatomy and has appropriate-for-gestational-age weight. Which of the following is a contraindication to the use of indocin as a tocolytic in this patient?

a. Twin gestation
b. Gestational age greater than 26 weeks
c. Vaginal bleeding
d. Oligohydramnios
e. Fetal growth restriction

131. A healthy 42-year-old G2P1001 presents to labor and delivery at 30 weeks gestation complaining of a small amount of bright red blood per vagina earlier in the day. The bleeding occurred shortly after intercourse. It started off as spotting and then progressed to a light bleeding. By the time the patient arrived at L and D, the bleeding had completely resolved. The patient denies any regular uterine contractions, but admits to occasional abdominal cramping. She reports the presence of good fetal movements. She denies any complications during the pregnancy. She reported a normal ultrasound done at 14 weeks of gestation. Her obstetrical history is significant for a previous low transverse cesarean section at term for a fetus that was footling breech. She wants to have an elective repeat cesarean section with a tubal ligation for delivery of this baby when she gets to term. Which of the following can be ruled out as a cause for her vaginal bleeding?

a. Cervicitis
b. Preterm labor
c. Placental abruption
d. Placenta previa
e. Subserous pedunculated uterine fibroid
f. Uterine rupture

132. A 34-year-old G2P1 at 31 weeks gestation presents to labor and delivery with complaints of vaginal bleeding earlier in the day that resolved on its own. She denies any leakage of fluid or uterine contractions. She reports good fetal movement. In her last pregnancy, she had a low transverse cesarean delivery for breech presentation at term. She denies any medical problems. Her vital signs are normal and electronic external monitoring reveals a reactive fetal heart rate tracing and no uterine contractions. Which of the following is the most appropriate next step in the management of this patient?

a. Send her home, since the bleeding has completely resolved and she is experiencing good fetal movements
b. Perform a sterile digital exam
c. Perform an amniocentesis to rule out infection
d. Perform a sterile speculum exam
e. Perform an ultrasound exam

133. A 34-year-old G2P1 at 31 weeks gestation with a known placenta previa presents to the hospital with vaginal bleeding. On assessment, she has normal vital signs and the fetal heart rate tracing is 140 beats per minute with accelerations and no decelerations. No uterine contractions are demonstrated on external tocometer. Heavy vaginal bleeding is noted. Which of the following is the best next step in the management of this patient?

a. Administer intramuscular terbutaline
b. Administer methylergonovine
c. Admit and stabilize the patient
d. Perform cesarean delivery

134. A 34-year-old G2P1 at 31 weeks gestation with a known placenta previa is admitted to the hospital for vaginal bleeding. The patient continues to bleed heavily and you observe persistent late decelerations on the fetal heart monitor with loss of variability in the baseline. Her blood pressure and pulse are normal. You explain to the patient that she needs to be delivered. The patient is delivered by cesarean section under general anesthesia. The baby and placenta are easily delivered, but the uterus is noted to be boggy and atonic despite intravenous infusion of Pitocin. Which of the following is contraindicated in this patient for the treatment of uterine atony?

a. Methylergonovine (Methergine) administered intramuscularly
b. Prostaglandin $F_{2\alpha}$ (Hemabate) suppositories
c. Misoprostil (Cytotec) suppositories
d. Terbutaline administered intravenously
e. Prostaglandin E_2 suppositories

135. A 20-year-old G1P0 at 30 weeks gestation with a known placenta previa is delivered by cesarean section under general anesthesia for vaginal bleeding and nonreassuring fetal heart rate tracing. The baby is easily delivered, but the placenta is adherent to the uterus and cannot be completely removed, and heavy uterine bleeding is noted. Which of the following is the best next step in the management of this patient?

a. Administer methylergonovine (Methergine) intramuscularly
b. Administer misoprostil (Cytotec) suppositories per rectum
c. Administer prostaglandin $F_{2\alpha}$ (Hemabate) intramuscularly
d. Perform hysterectomy
e. Close the uterine incision and perform curettage

136. A 40-year-old G2P1001 presents to your office for a routine OB visit at 30 weeks gestational age. Her first pregnancy was delivered 10 years ago and was uncomplicated. She had a normal vaginal delivery at 40 weeks and the baby weighed 7 lb. During this present pregnancy, she has not had any complications, and she reports no significant medical history. She is a non-smoker and has gained about 25 lb to date. Despite being of advanced maternal age, she declined any screening or diagnostic testing for Down syndrome. Her blood pressure range has been 100–120/60–70. During her exam, you note that her fundal height measures only 25 cm. Which of the following is a possible explanation for this patient's decreased fundal height?

a. Multiple gestation
b. Hydramnios
c. Fetal growth restriction
d. The presence of fibroid tumors in the uterus

137. A 38-year-old G4P3 at 33 weeks gestation is noted to have a fundal height of 29 centimeters on routine obstetrical visit. An ultrasound is performed by the maternal fetal medicine specialist. The estimated fetal weight is determined to be in the fifth percentile for the estimated gestational age. The biparietal diameter and abdominal circumference are concordant in size. Which of the following is associated with symmetric growth restriction?

a. Nutritional deficiencies
b. Chromosome abnormalities
c. Hypertension
d. Uteroplacental insufficiency

138. A 37-year-old G4P2 presents to your office for new OB visit at 8 weeks. In a prior pregnancy, the fetus had multiple congenital anomalies consistent with trisomy 18, and the baby died shortly after birth. The mother is worried that the current pregnancy will end the same way, and she wants testing performed to see whether this baby is affected. Which of the following can be used for chromosome analysis of the fetus?

a. Biophysical profile
b. Chorionic villus sampling
c. Fetal umbilical Doppler velocimetry
d. Maternal serum screen
e. Nuchal translucency

139. A 26-year-old G1 at 37 weeks presents to the hospital in active labor. She has no medical problems and has a normal prenatal course except for fetal growth restriction. She undergoes an uncomplicated vaginal delivery of a female infant weighing 1950 g. The infant is at risk for which of the following complications?

a. Hyperglycemia
b. Fever
c. Hypertension
d. Anemia
e. Hypoxia

140. A 38-year-old G1P1 comes to see you for her first prenatal visit at 10 weeks gestational age. She had a previous term vaginal delivery without any complications. You detect fetal heart tones at this visit, and her uterine size is consistent with dates. You also draw her prenatal labs at this visit and tell her to follow up in 4 weeks for a return OB visit. Two weeks later, the results of the patient's prenatal labs come back. Her blood type is A−, with an anti-D antibody titer of 1:4. Which of the following is the most appropriate next step in the management of this patient?

a. Schedule an amniocentesis for amniotic fluid bilirubin at 16 weeks
b. Repeat the titer in 4 weeks
c. Repeat the titer at 28 weeks
d. Schedule PUBS to determine fetal hematocrit at 20 weeks
e. Schedule PUBS as soon as possible to determine fetal blood type

141. A 23-year-old G3P1011 at 6 weeks presents for routine prenatal care. She had a cesarean delivery 3 years ago for breech presentation after a failed external cephalic version. Her daughter is Rh negative. She also had an elective termination of pregnancy 1 year ago. She is Rh-negative and is found to have a positive anti-D titer of 1:8 on routine prenatal labs. Failure to administer RhoGam at which time is the most likely cause of her sensitization?

a. After elective termination
b. At the time of cesarean delivery
c. At the time of external cephalic version
d. Within 3 days of delivering an Rh− fetus

142. A 27-year-old G2P1 at 29 weeks gestational age who is being followed for Rh isoimmunization presents for her OB visit. The fundal height is noted to be 33 centimeters. An ultrasound reveals fetal asites and a pericardial effusion. Which of the following can be another finding in fetal hydrops?

a. Oliohydramnios
b. Hydrocephaleus
c. Hydronephrosis
d. Subcutaneous edema

143. A 39-year-old G1P0 at 39 weeks gestational age is sent to labor and delivery from her obstetrician's office because of a blood pressure reading of 150/100 obtained during a routine OB visit. Her baseline blood pressures during the pregnancy were 100–120/60–70. On arrival to labor and delivery, the patient denies any headache, visual changes, nausea, vomiting, or abdominal pain. The heart rate strip is reactive and the tocodynamometer indicates irregular uterine contractions. The patient's cervix is 3 cm dilated. Her repeat BP is 160/90. Hematocrit is 34.0, platelets are 160,000, SGOT is 22, SGPT is 15, and urinalysis is negative for protein. Which of the following is the most likely diagnosis?

a. Preeclampsia
b. Chronic hypertension
c. Chronic hypertension with superimposed preeclampsia
d. Eclampsia
e. Pregnancy-induced hypertension (gestational hypertension)

144. A 20-year-old G1 at 36 weeks is being monitored for preeclampsia; she rings the bell for the nurse because she is developing a headache and feels funny. As you and the nurse enter the room, you witness the patient undergoing a tonic-clonic seizure. You secure the patient's airway, and within a few minutes the seizure is over. The patient's blood pressure monitor indicates a pressure of 160/110. Which of the following medications is recommended for the prevention of a recurrent eclamptic seizure?

a. Hydralzine
b. Magnesium sulfate
c. Labetalol
d. Pitocin
e. Nifedipine

145. You are doing postpartum rounds on a 22-year-old G1P1 who vaginally delivered an infant male at 36 weeks after an induction for severe preeclampsia. During her labor she required hydralazine to control her blood pressures. She is on magnesium sulfate for seizure prophylaxis. Her vital signs are blood pressure 154/98, pulse 93, respiratory rate 24, and temperature 99.2°F. She has adequate urine output at > 40cc/h. On examination, she is oriented to time and place, but she is somnolent and her speech is slurred. She has good movement and strength of her extremities, but her deep tendon reflexes are absent. Which of the following is the most likely cause of her symptoms?

a. Adverse reaction to hydralazine
b. Hypertensive stroke
c. Magnesium toxicity
d. Sinus venous thrombosis
e. Transient ischemic attack

Obstetrical Complications of Pregnancy

Answers

106. The answer is d. (*Cunningham, pp 256–257, 265–266.*) Almost all cases of abdominal pregnancy follow early rupture or abortion of a tubal pregnancy. Women with abdominal pregnancy are likely to be uncomfortable but with vague gastrointestinal symptoms such as nausea, vomiting, flatulence, constipation, and diarrhea. Fetal survival is precarious with a perinatal loss of 75%. Fetal malformations and deformities such as craniofacial asymmetry, limb deficiencies, and joint abnormalities are present in 20% of fetuses. Expectant management carries the risk of sudden life-threatening hemorrhage and is rarely if ever indicated if the diagnosis of abdominal pregnancy is made. Surgery is the usual treatment of abdominal pregnancy, but massive hemorrhage may ensue with separation and removal of the placenta. In general the fetus should be delivered, the cord severed close to the placenta, and the abdomen closed. Leaving the placenta in situ can cause infectious abscess formation, adhesions, and intestinal obstruction. The use of methotrexate to hasten placental involution is controversial. Maternal mortality is increased substantively compared with normal pregnancy.

107. The answer is c. (*Cunningham, pp 831–833.*) Prior cesarean delivery and placenta previa, especially an anteriorly located placenta, increase your risk of placenta accreta, increta, and percreta. Placenta accreta, increta, or percreta are treated with hysterectomy. Advancing maternal age, multiparity, prior cesarean delivery, and smoking are associated with previa. Painless bleeding is the most common symptom, and is rarely fatal. Vaginal examination to evaluate for placenta previa is never permissible unless the women is in the operating room prepared for immediate cesarean delivery, because even the most gentle exam can cause torrential hemorrhage. These "double setup" exams are rarely necessary because ultrasound is usually readily available to make the diagnosis of placenta previa. Cesarean delivery is necessary in practically all cases of previa. Because of the poor contractile nature of the lower uterine segment, uncontrollable hemorrhage may follow removal of the placenta. Hysterectomy may be indicated if conservative methods to control hemorrhage fail. Resuscitation with blood products is the treatment of disseminated intravascular coagulopathy (DIC), not hysterectomy. Sterilization itself is not an indication for hysterectomy at the time of cesarean delivery, because the complications of surgery are much increased with a cesarean hysterectomy.

108. The answer is c. (*Gleicher, p 1153.*) In modern clinical medicine, once the diagnosis of fetal demise has been made, the products of conception are removed. If, however, the gestational age is over 14 weeks and the fetal death occurred 5 weeks ago, coagulation abnormalities may be seen. Septic abortions were more frequently seen during the era of illegal abortions, although occasionally sepsis can occur if there is incomplete evacuation of the products of conception in either a therapeutic or spontaneous abortion.

109. The answer is e. (*Rodeck, pp 865–873.*) Polyhydramnios is an excessive quantity of amniotic fluid. The frequency of diagnosis varies, but polyhydramnios sufficient to cause clinical symptoms probably occurs in 1 of 1000 pregnancies, exclusive of twins. The incidence of associated malformations is about 20%, with CNS and GI abnormalities being particularly common. For example, polyhydramnios accompanies about half of cases of anencephaly and nearly all cases of esophageal atresia. Edema of the lower extremities, vulva, and abdominal wall results from compression of major venous systems. Acute hydramnios tends to occur early in pregnancy and, as a rule, leads to labor before the twenty-eighth week. The most frequent maternal complications are placental abruption, uterine dysfunction, and postpartum hemorrhage.

110. The answer is d. (*ACOG Practice Bulletin No. 33.*) This patient has eclampsia. She requires delivery. Magnesium sulfate is given for seizure prophylaxis. Antihypertensive therapy is usually initiated for systolic blood pressure >160 or diastolic blood pressure >110. Preeclampsia is a syndrome of hypertension and proteinuria that can be associated with a other signs and symptoms such as visual disturbances, headaches, epigastric pain, and laboratory abnormalities such as hemolysis, elevated liver enzyme, and low platelets (HELLP syndrome). Criteria for the diagnosis of preeclampsia includes blood pressure of 140 mmHg systolic or higher or

90 mmHg or higher that occurs after 20 weeks of gestation in a woman with previously normal blood pressure. Proteinuria is defined as urinary excretion of 300 mg or higher on a 24-h urine specimen. The diagnosis of severe preeclampsia is made if one or more of the following criteria is present: blood pressure 160 mmHg systolic or higher or 110 mmHg diastolic or higher, proteinuria of 5 g or more on a 24-h urine collection or 3+ or greater on random urine samples, oliguria of less than 500 mL in 24 h, cerebral or visual disturbances, pulmonary edema or cyanosis, epigastric or right upper quadrant pain, impaired liver function, thrombocytopenia, or fetal growth restriction. The incidence of preeclampsia is 5 to 8% and primarily occurs in first pregnancies. Risk factors include preeclampsia in previous pregnancy, chronic hypertension, pregestational diabetes, multifetal gestations, vascular and connective tissue disease, nephropathy, antiphospholipid syndrome, obesity, older age, and African American race. Eclampsia is the presence of new-onset grand mal seizures in a woman with preeclampsia. Women with eclampsia should be stabilized quickly; magnesium sulfate should be started to prevent further seizures; and antihypertensives should be used to control blood pressure. The patient should be delivered in a timely fashion, and the method of delivery should depend on factors such as gestational age, fetal presentation, and cervical exam. Cesarean delivery is not always necessary. Magnesium sulfate has been shown in randomized control trials to be better than phenytoin or diazepam at preventing seizures. Low-dose aspirin and calcium supplementation have not been shown to be beneficial in preventing preeclampsia.

111. The answer is b. (*Cunningham, pp 929–932.*) In the twin-to-twin transfusion syndrome, the donor twin is always anemic, owing not to a hemolytic process but to the direct transfer of blood to the recipient twin, who becomes polycythemic. The recipient may suffer thromboses secondary to hypertransfusion and subsequent hemoconcentration. Although the donor placenta is usually pale and somewhat atrophied, that of the recipient is congested and enlarged. Hydramnios can develop in either twin, but is more frequent in the recipient because of circulatory overload. When hydramnios occurs in the donor, it is due to congestive heart failure caused by severe anemia.

112. The answer is c. (*ACOG, Practice Bulletin No. 48.*) The diagnosis of cervical insufficiency or incompetence is based on the presence of painless cervical dilation with a history of pregnancy loss in the second trimester or early-third-trimester preterm delivery. A patient with a history of three or more midtrimester pregnancy losses or early preterm deliveries is a candidate for a cerclage. Cerclage is not indicated for the prevention of first-trimester losses. Cerclage has not been shown to improve the preterm delivery rate or neonatal outcome in twin gestations. A simple punch biopsy or loop electrosurgical excision procedure of the cervix is unlikely to disrupt functional structure of the cervix and prophylactic cerclage is not warranted. Serial transvaginal ultrasound evaluation of cervical length can be considered in women with a history of second and early-third-trimester deliveries. A cervical length less than 25 millimeters or funneling of more than 25% or both is associated with an increased risk of preterm delivery.

113–117. The answers are 113-e, 114-b, 115-d, 116-c, 117-a. *(Scott, pp 143–146.)* Bleeding occurs in about 30 to 40% of human gestations before 20 weeks of pregnancy, with about half of these pregnancies ending in spontaneous abortion. A threatened abortion takes place when this uterine bleeding occurs without any cervical dilation or effacement. In a patient bleeding during the first half of pregnancy, the diagnosis of inevitable abortion is strengthened if the bleeding is profuse and associated with uterine cramping pains. If cervical dilation has occurred, with or without rupture of membranes, the abortion is inevitable. If only a portion of the products of conception has been expelled and the cervix remains dilated, a diagnosis of incomplete abortion is made. However, if all fetal and placental tissue has been expelled, the cervix is closed, bleeding from the canal is minimal or decreasing, and uterine cramps have ceased, a diagnosis of complete abortion can be made. The diagnosis of missed abortion is suspected when the uterus fails to continue to enlarge with or without uterine bleeding or spotting. A missed abortion is one in which fetal death occurs before 20 weeks gestation without expulsion of any fetal or maternal tissue for at least 8 weeks thereafter. When a fetus is retained in the uterus beyond 5 weeks after fetal death, consumptive coagulability with hypofibrogenemia may occur. This is uncommon, however, in gestations of less than 14 weeks in duration.

118. The answer is d. *(Fleisher, pp 732–735. Ransom, 2000, pp 511–515.)* The history, clinical picture, and ultrasound of the woman in the question are characteristic of hydatidiform mole. The most common initial symptoms include an enlarged-for-dates uterus and continuous or intermittent bleeding in the first two trimesters. Other symptoms include hypertension, proteinuria, and hyperthyroidism. Hydatidiform mole is 10 times as common in the Far East as in North America, and it occurs more frequently in women over 45 years of age. A tissue sample would show a villus with hydropic changes and no vessels. Grossly, these lesions appear as small, clear clusters of grapelike vesicles, the passage of which confirms the diagnosis. Hysterectomy may be considered as primary therapy for molar pregnancy in women who have completed childbearing.

119. The answer is a. (*Rock, pp 1631–1632.*) The condition of women who have hydatidiform moles but no evidence of metastatic disease should be followed routinely by hCG titers after uterine evacuation. Most authorities agree that prophylactic chemotherapy should not be employed in the routine management of women having hydatidiform moles because 85 to 90% of affected patients will require no further treatment. For a young woman in whom preservation of reproductive function is important, surgery is not routinely indicated.

120. The answer is a. (*Stenchever, pp 455–456.*) Single-agent chemotherapy is usually instituted if levels of hCG remain elevated 8 weeks after evacuation of a hydatidiform mole. Approximately 50% of the patients who have persistently high hCG titers will develop malignant sequelae. If hCG titers rise or reach a plateau for 2 to 3 successive weeks following molar evacuation, a single-agent chemotherapy should be instituted, provided that the trophoblastic disease has not metastasized to the liver or brain. The presence of such metastases usually requires initiation of combination chemotherapy.

121. The answer is d. (*Scott, pp 155–168.*) The photomicrograph shows villi within a tubular structure; the villi are easily identified by the presence of cytotrophoblasts. The diagnosis is tubal ectopic pregnancy. Molar pregnancy, incomplete abortion, and missed abortion can also be associated with the presence of villi, but specimens from these disorders would not be obtained at laparotomy.

122. The answer is d. (*Rock, pp 121–122.*) The clinical history presented in this question is classic for a ruptured tubal pregnancy accompanied by hemoperitoneum. Dilation and curettage would not permit rapid enough diagnosis, and the results obtained by this procedure are variable. Posterior colpotomy requires an operating room, surgical anesthesia, and an experienced operator with a scrubbed and gowned associate. Refined optic and electronic systems have improved the accuracy of laparoscopy, but this new equipment is not always available, and the procedure requires an operating room and, usually, surgical anesthesia. Culdocentesis is a rapid, nonsurgical method to confirm the presence of unclotted intraabdominal blood from a ruptured tubal pregnancy. Culdocentesis, however, is also not perfect, and a negative culdocentesis should not be used as the sole criterion for whether or not to operate on a patient.

123. The answer is a. (*Speroff, p 1163.*) Conservative laparoscopic treatment of ectopic pregnancy is now commonplace, although not yet universal. With increasing sophistication of techniques and fiberoptics, many microsurgical procedures can be done through the laparoscope. Recent studies suggest that the fertility rates for laparoscopy and laparotomy are comparable, as are the implications of repeat ectopic pregnancies. Certainly laparoscopy, because of its small incision, results in fewer breakdowns and shorter hospital stays, but the incidence of complications due to retained ectopic tissue is higher.

124. The answer is b. (*Stenchever, pp 452–457.*) Any factor delaying transit of the ovum through the fallopian tube may predispose a patient to ectopic pregnancy. The major predisposing factor in the development of ectopic pregnancy is pelvic inflammatory disease. However, any operative procedure on the fallopian tubes may increase a patient's risk. It appears that tubal sterilizations with laparoscopic fulguration have a higher rate of ectopic pregnancy than tubal ligations performed with clips or rings. Women who have had one ectopic pregnancy are at increased risk of having a second. DES exposure, induction of ovulation, and IUD use increase the possibility of ectopic pregnancy.

125. The answer is b. (*Reece, pp 1112–1113.*) Hyperemesis gravidarum is intractable vomiting of pregnancy and is associated with disturbed nutrition. Early signs of the disorder include weight loss (up to 5% of body weight) and ketonuria. Electrolyte abnormalities can also be present. Because vomiting causes potassium loss, electrocardiographic evidence of potassium depletion, such as inverted T waves and prolonged QT and PR intervals, is usually a later finding. Jaundice also is a later finding and is probably due to fatty infiltration of the liver; occasionally, acute hepatic necrosis occurs. Metabolic acidosis is rare. Hypokalemic nephropathy with isosthenuria may occur late. Hypoproteinemia also may result, caused by poor diet as well as by albuminuria. Patients who have hyperemesis gravidarum are best treated (if the disease is early in its course) with parenteral fluids and electrolytes, sedation, rest, vitamins, and antiemetics if necessary. In some cases, isolation of the patient is necessary. Very slow reinstitution of oral feeding is permitted after dehydration and electrolyte disturbances are corrected. Therapeutic abortion may be necessary in rare instances; however, the disease usually improves spontaneously as pregnancy progresses.

126. The answer is d. (*ACOG, Practice Bulletin 1. Cunningham, pp 864–873.*) This patient with premature rupture of membranes (PROM) has a physical exam consistent with an intrauterine infection or chorioamnionitis. Chorioamnionitis can be diagnosed clinically by the presence of maternal fever, tachycardia, and uterine tenderness. Leukocyte counts are a nonspecific indicator of infection because they can be elevated with labor and the use of corticosteroids. When chorioamnionitis is diagnosed, fetal and maternal morbidity increases and delivery is indicated regardless of the fetus's gestational age. In the case described, antibiotics need to be administered to avoid neonatal sepsis. Ampicillin is the drug of choice to treat group B streptococcal infection. Since the fetal heart rate is reactive, there is no indication for cesarean section. Augmentation with Pitocin should be instituted as indicated. There is no role for tocolysis in the setting of chorioamnionitis, since delivery is the goal. There is also no role for the administration of steroids, since delivery is imminent. In addition, steroids are indicated at 32 weeks gestational age or less only with PROM. A cerclage (cervical stitch) would be placed in a previable pregnancy where an incompetent cervix is diagnosed in the absence of ruptured membranes.

127. The answer is b. (*Cunningham, pp 867–872. Beckmann, pp 306–307.*) The concern with this patient who presents with a twin gestation and symptoms of bleeding, cramping, and increased vaginal discharge is preterm labor. Intravenous hydration is appropriate because dehydration can be a cause of premature contractions and uterine irritability. Urinary infections can be associated with uterine contractions, and therefore a urinalysis and urine culture should be obtained. Infection caused by group B streptococci can be associated with preterm labor, so a culture to detect this organism should be obtained. Before performing a digital exam on this patient to determine her cervical status, an ultrasound should be performed to rule out placenta previa in light of the history of vaginal bleeding.

128. The answer is c. (*Cunningham, pp 867–873.*) The patient is in preterm labor, because she has a dilated and effaced cervix in the presence of regular uterine contractions. Therefore, treatment is aimed at delaying delivery to allow continued fetal growth and maturity. The administration of tocolytic therapy to treat the preterm contractions is indicated. In addition, from 24 to 34 weeks, management also includes the administration of steroids such as betamethasone to promote fetal lung maturity. Respiratory distress syndrome (RDS) is a sequela of preterm neonates and occurs less often in infants given betamethasone in utero. If delivery seems likely, intravenous antibiotics are administered to prevent possible neonatal sepsis. If the patient's contractions subside and there is no evidence of infection, then the antibiotics can be discontinued. It is advantageous to obtain a neonatology consult on any patient who appears to be in preterm labor so the parents know what to expect if they give birth to preterm infants. There is no need to prepare for a cesarean section in this patient. Attempts are made to stop the labor first. If the patient continues to progress, then a vaginal delivery is preferred since the twins do not have a malpresentation.

129. The answer is a. (*Cunningham, pp 928–932. Beckmann, pp 271–272.*) In twin gestations where monochorionic placentas exist, twin-to-twin transfusion syndrome can occur. In this syndrome, there are vascular communications or anastomoses between the twins. There is blood flow or transfusion from one twin to another. The donor twin becomes anemic and may suffer growth retardation and oligohydramnios. The recipient twin may develop hydramnios, hypervolemia, hypertension, polycythemia, and congestive heart failure.

130. The answer is d. (*Cunningham, pp 870–871, 821–822.*) Indomethacin would not be an appropriate tocolytic agent in this patient. Indocin is a prostaglandin synthetase inhibitor that can decrease fetal urine production and cause oligohydramnios. Since twin B already has oligohydramnios secondary to twin-to-twin transfusion syndrome, it is best to avoid this therapy.

Nifedipine is used for tocolysis and is thought to work by preventing entry of calcium into muscle cells. It can be associated with hypotension, so blood pressure must be followed carefully. Ritodrine and terbutaline are tocolytic agents that are β-adrenergic agents. They work by increasing cAMP in cells, which decreases free calcium. These agents can be associated with tachycardia, hypotension, and pulmonary edema. Magnesium sulfate is a tocolytic agent that works by competing with calcium for entry into cells. At high levels, it can cause respiratory and cardiac depression.

131. The answer is e. (*Cunningham, pp 239, 614–615, 811–819, 962–963. Beckmann, pp 285–292.*) During pregnancy, if placental implantation occurs over or in contact with a myoma, then there is an increased risk of placental abruption, preterm labor, and postpartum hemorrhage. A subserous pedunculated fibroid is attached to the uterus by a stalk and grows outward into the abdominal cavity; therefore, there is no vaginal bleeding associated with such a fibroid. Cervical inflammation (cervicitis) can render the cervix friable and able to bleed easily, especially after intercourse. Placental abruption occurs when there is a premature separation of the placenta from the uterine wall. While vaginal bleeding can be observed, the hemorrhage can be completely concealed, with the blood being trapped between the detached placenta and the uterine wall. Labor can be associated with vaginal bleeding due to cervical dilation. Placenta previa occurs when the placenta is located over or in close proximity to the internal os of the cervix. When the lower uterine segment is formed or cervical dilation occurs in the presence of placenta previa, a certain degree of spontaneous placental separation and hemorrhage from disrupted blood vessels will occur. Uterine rupture most commonly occurs as a result of a separation of a previous cesarean scar. Most of the bleeding is into the abdominal cavity, but vaginal bleeding can be observed as well.

132. The answer is e. (*Cunningham, pp 820–822.*) Any patient who gives a history of vaginal bleeding in the third trimester should undergo an ultrasound exam as the first step in evaluation to rule out the presence of a placenta previa. A digital or speculum exam performed in the presence of a placenta previa can precipitate a hemorrhage. There is no indication to work the patient up for infection in the case described here; therefore, an amniocentesis is not indicated. She should not be sent home even though the bleeding has resolved. She first needs to undergo an ultrasound and should be monitored for uterine contractions and further bleeding prior to being discharged.

133. The answer is c. (*Cunningham, pp 819–823.*) In this patient who is starting to hemorrhage from a placenta previa, steps should be taken to stabilize the patient and prepare for possible emergent cesarean section. The patient is not contracting, and therefore there is no role for tocolysis. In addition, terbutaline should never be used in a patient who is actively bleeding because it is associated with maternal tachycardia and vasodilation. The actively bleeding patient should be resuscitated with intravenous fluids while blood is being cross-matched for possible transfusion. A Foley catheter should be placed because urinary output is a reflection of the patient's volume status. Finally, anesthesia should be notified because the patient may require imminent delivery.

134. The answer is d. (*Decherney, pp 538–539. Cunningham, p 827. Beckmann, pp 174–175.*) Methylergonovine, prostaglandin $F_{2\alpha}$, prostaglandin E_1 (Misoprostil), and prostaglandin E_2 are all uretotonic agents than can be used in situations where there is a postpartum hemorrhage due to uterine atony. Terbutaline would be contraindicated in this situation because it is a tocolytic that is used to promote uterine relaxation.

135. The answer is d. (*Cunningham, pp 821. Beckmann, pp 286–289.*) Women who have a placenta previa have about a 10% risk of also having a placenta accreta. The risk of placenta accreta is even greater in women who have a history of a previous cesarean section (estimated to be between 14 and 24%). The incidence of placenta accreta continues to increase as the numbers of prior cesarean sections increase. If a placenta accreta indeed exists, a hysterectomy is indicated.

136. The answer is c. (*Beckmann, pp 85–86, 279. Cunningham, pp 900–902.*) In a normal singleton pregnancy from about 15 to 36 weeks, the number of weeks of gestation should approximate the fundal height measurement. A fundal height measurement that is 2 to 3 cm less than expected, or small for dates, suggests the possibility that the patient's dates are incorrect, that oligohydramnios is present, or that the fetus has growth restriction or has undergone demise. The presence of fibroid tumors would enlarge the uterus and can be a cause of increased fundal height, or a uterus that is large for dates.

137. The answer is b. (*Cunningham, pp 895–904. Beckmann, pp 279–282.*) Intrauterine growth restriction (IUGR) is diagnosed when the estimated weight of the fetus falls below the tenth percentile for a given age. By the use of ultrasonography, IUGR can be classified as either symmetric or asymmetric. In asymmetric IUGR, the abdominal circumference is low, but the biparietal diameter may be at or near normal. In cases of symmetric IUGR, all fetal structures (including both head and body size) are proportionately diminished in size. Fetal infections, chromosome abnormalities, and congenital anomalies usually result in symmetric IUGR. Asymmetric IUGR is seen in cases where fetal access to nutrients is compromised, such as with severe maternal nutritional deficiencies or hypertension.

138. The answer is b. (*Beckmann, pp 280–281. Cunningham, pp 328–331, 902.*) Fetal tissue for chromosome analysis can be obtained via amniocentesis, chorionic villus sampling (CVS), percutaneous umbilical blood sampling, or direct biopsy of fetal muscle or skin. Amniocentesis involves obtaining a sample of amniotic fluid, which contains fetal fibroblasts. Chorionic villus sampling involves taking a biopsy of the placenta. In the case of PUBS, the umbilical vein is punctured under direct ultrasound guidance near the placental origin and blood is obtained for genetic analysis. Doppler velocimetry is an ultrasound technique used to examine blood flow through the umbilical artery. IUGR has been associated with abnormal umbilical artery Doppler velocimetry. Therefore, this technique is used with other modalities such as BPP and NSTS to monitor fetal well-being.

139. The answer is e. (*Cunningham, p 904. Beckmann, pp 281–282.*) Fetuses that are growth-restricted often have difficulty transitioning to the extrauterine environment. Therefore, it is critical that neonatologists be present at such deliveries. Growth-restricted fetuses more commonly pass meconium; therefore aspiration is a concern at the time of delivery. In addition, growth-restricted fetuses compensate for poor placental oxygen transfer by having a polychemia that can then result in multiorgan thrombosis at or after birth. At the time of delivery, such infants may suffer from hypoxia due to placental insufficiency. Infants with IUGR have less subcutaneous fat deposition; therefore, hypothermia and hypoglycemia are a potential concern.

140. The answer is b. (*Beckmann, pp 166–169. Decherney, pp 295–299. Cunningham, pp 668–671.*) During the first prenatal visit, all pregnant women are screened for the ABO blood group and the Rh group, which includes the D antigen. If the woman is Rh-negative, antibody screening is performed. If the antibody D titer is positive, the woman is considered sensitized because she has produced antibodies against the D antigen. Sensitization occurs as a result of exposure to blood from an Rh+ fetus in a prior pregnancy. A fetus that is Rh+ possesses red blood cells that express the D antigen. Therefore, the maternal anti-D antibodies can cross the placenta and cause fetal hemolysis. Once the antibody screen is positive for isoimmunization, the titer should be followed at regular intervals (about every 4 weeks). A titer of 1:16 or greater is usually indicative of the possibility of severe hemolytic disease of the fetus. Once the critical titer is reached, further evaluation is done by amniotic fluid assessment or analysis of fetal blood via PUBS. In the presence of fetal hemolysis, the amniotic fluid contains elevated levels of bilirubin that can be determined via spectrophotometric analysis. Cordocentesis, or percutaneous umbilical blood sampling, involves obtaining a blood sample from the umbilical cord under ultrasound guidance. The fetal blood sample can then be analyzed for Hct and determination of fetal blood type. Cordocentesis also allows the fetus with anemia to undergo a blood transfusion.

141. The answer is a. (*ACOG, Practice Bulletin 4. Beckmann, pp 166–170.*) To prevent maternal Rh sensitization, pregnant women who are Rh− should receive RhoGam or Rh immune globulin (antibody to the D antigen) in the following situations: after a spontaneous or induced abortion, after an ectopic pregnancy, at the time of an amniocentesis/CVS/PUBS, at 28 weeks gestational age, within 3 days of a delivery of an Rh+ fetus, at the time of external cephalic version, with second- or third-trimester antenatal bleeding, and in the setting of abdominal trauma.

142. The answer is d. (*Cunningham, p 666.*) Fetal hydrops occurs as a result of excessive and prolonged hemolysis due to isoimmunization. Characteristics of fetal hydrops include abnormal fluid in two or more sites such as the thorax, abdomen, and skin. The placenta is also markedly erythematous, enlarged, and boggy. In addition, massive hepatomegaly and splenomegaly may be present.

143. The answer is e. (*Cunningham, pp 761–808.*) Hypertension in pregnancy is defined as blood pressure of 140/90 mmHg or greater on at least two separate occasions that are 6 h or more apart. The presence of edema is no longer used as a diagnostic criteria because it is so prevalent in normal pregnant women. A rise in systolic blood pressure of 30 mmHg and a rise in diastolic blood pressure of 15 mmHg is no longer used, because women meeting this criteria are not likely to suffer adverse pregnancy outcomes if their absolute blood pressure is below 140/90 mmHg. In gestational hypertension, maternal blood pressure reaches 140/90 or greater for the first time during pregnancy, and proteinuria is not present. In preeclampsia, blood pressure increases to 140/90 after 20 weeks gestation and proteinuria is present (300 mg in 24 h or 1+ protein or greater on dipstick). Eclampsia is present when women with preeclampsia develop seizures. Chronic hypertension exists when a woman has a blood pressure of 140/90 or greater prior to the pregnancy or before 20 weeks gestation. A woman with hypertension who develops preeclampsia is described as having chronic hypertension with superimposed preeclampsia.

144. The answer is b. (*Beckmann, pp 265–267. Cunningham, pp 781–797.*) Women who have suffered an eclamptic seizure need to have their blood pressure controlled with antihypertensive medications if the diastolic is increased above 105 to 110 mmHg. The purpose of antihypertensive therapy is to avoid a maternal stroke. Hydralazine, nifedipine, and labetalol are commonly used in acute hypertensive crises. Magnesium sulfate is administered as a loading dose and then as a continuous infusion to prevent further seizures. Steps to effect a vaginal delivery should then be undertaken. To avoid maternal risks from surgery, cesarean section should be avoided. In the case presented here, the bradycardia seen in the fetus is transient and is due to the maternal hypoxia that has occurred with the seizure. Delivery during a bradycardic episode would impose unnecessary risk for the fetus and should be avoided. In the case presented here, the patient has a ripe cervix and labor should be induced with amniotomy and Pitocin. A Foley catheter should be placed to keep track of maternal renal function.

145. The answer is c. (*Cunningham, p 870. Beckmann, p 265.*) The therapeutic range of serum magnesium to prevent seizures is 4 to 7 mg/dL. At levels between 8 and 12 mg/dL, patellar reflexes are lost. At 10 to 12 mg/dL, somnolence and slurred speech commonly occur. Muscle paralysis and respiratory difficulty occur at 15 to 17 mg/dL, and cardiac arrest occurs at levels greater than 30 mg/dL.

Medical and Surgical Complications of Pregnancy

Questions

DIRECTIONS: Each item below contains a question followed by suggested responses. Select the **one best** response to each question.

146. A 33-year-old G3P2 at 30 weeks gestation has an infection in pregnancy. Which of the following is a reactivation and therefore not a risk to the fetus?

a. Group B coxsackievirus
b. Rubella virus
c. Chickenpox virus
d. Shingles
e. Herpesvirus type 2

147. A 22-year-old G1 at 14 weeks gestation presents to your office with a history of recent exposure to her 3-year-old nephew who had a rubella viral infection. In which time period does maternal infection with rubella virus carry the greatest risk for congenital rubella syndrome in the fetus?

a. Preconception
b. First trimester
c. Second trimester
d. Third trimester
e. Postpartum

148. A pregnant woman is discovered to be an asymptomatic carrier of *Neisseria gonorrhoeae*. A year ago, she was treated with penicillin for a gonococcal infection and developed a severe allergic reaction. Which of the following is the treatment of choice at this time?

a. Tetracycline
b. Ampicillin
c. Spectinomycin
d. Chloramphenicol
e. Penicillin

149. A 22-year-old has just been diagnosed with toxoplasmosis. You try to determine what her risk factors were. The highest risk association is which of the following?

a. Eating raw meat
b. Eating raw fish
c. Having a dog
d. Being English
e. Having viral infections in early pregnancy

150. A 17-year-old woman at 22 weeks gestation presents to the emergency center with a 3-day history of nausea, vomiting, and abdominal pain. The pain started in the middle of the abdomen and is now located along her right side. She is noted to have a temperature of 101.2°F. She denies any past medical problems or surgeries. How does pregnancy alter the diagnosis and treatment of the disease?

a. Due to anatomical and physiological changes in pregnancy, diagnosis is easier to make
b. Surgical treatment should be delayed since the patient is pregnant
c. Fetal outcome is improved with delayed diagnosis
d. The incidence is unchanged in pregnancy

151. A 24-year-old woman appears at 8 weeks of pregnancy and reveals a history of pulmonary embolism 7 years ago during her first pregnancy. She was treated with intravenous heparin followed by several months of oral warfarin (Coumadin) and has had no further evidence of thromboembolic disease for more than 6 years. Which of the following statements about her current condition is true?

a. Having no evidence of disease for more than 5 years means that the risk of thromboembolism is not greater than normal
b. Impedance plethysmography is not a useful study to evaluate for deep-venous thrombosis in pregnancy
c. Doppler ultrasonography is not a useful technique to evaluate for deep-venous thrombosis in pregnancy
d. The patient should be placed on low-dose heparin therapy throughout pregnancy and puerperium
e. The patient is at highest risk for recurrent thromboembolism during the second trimester of pregnancy

152. A 29-year-old G3P2 black woman in the thirty-third week of gestation is admitted to the emergency room because of acute abdominal pain that has been increasing during the past 24 h. The pain is severe and is radiating from the epigastrium to the back. The patient has vomited a few times and has not eaten or had a bowel movement since the pain started. On examination, you observe an acutely ill patient lying on the bed with her knees drawn up. Her blood pressure is 100/70 mmHg, her pulse is 110/min, and her temperature is 38.8°C (100.8°F). On palpation, the abdomen is somewhat distended and tender, mainly in the epigastric area, and the uterine fundus reaches 31 cm above the symphysis. Hypotonic bowel sounds are noted. Fetal monitoring reveals a normal pattern of fetal heart rate (FHR) without uterine contractions. On ultrasonography, the fetus is in vertex presentation and appropriate in size for gestational age; fetal breathing and trunk movements are noted, and the volume of amniotic fluid is normal. The placenta is located on the anterior uterine wall and of grade 2 to 3. Laboratory values show mild leukocytosis (12,000 cells per mL); a hematocrit of 43; mildly elevated serum glutamic-oxaloacetic transaminase (SGOT), serum glutamic-pyruvic transaminase (SGPT), and bilirubin; and serum amylase of 180 U/dL. Urinalysis is normal. Which of the following is the most likely diagnosis?

a. Acute degeneration of uterine leiomyoma
b. Acute cholecystitis
c. Acute pancreatitis
d. Acute appendicitis
e. Severe preeclamptic toxemia

153. An 18-year-old has asymptomatic bacteriuria (ASB) at her first prenatal visit at 15 weeks gestation. Which of the following statements is true?

a. The prevalence of ASB during pregnancy may be as great as 30%
b. There is a decreased incidence of ASB in multiparas with sickle cell trait
c. Fifteen percent of women develop a urinary tract infection after an initial negative urine culture
d. Twenty to thirty percent of women with ASB subsequently develop an acute symptomatic urinary infection during that pregnancy
e. One percent of women with ASB have pyelographic evidence of chronic infection or congenital abnormalities of the urinary tract

154. A 20-year-old female at 34 weeks of gestation develops a lower urinary tract infection. Which of the following is the best choice for treatment?

a. Cephalosporin
b. Tetracycline
c. Sulfonamide
d. Nitrofurantoin

155. A 30-year-old class D diabetic is concerned about pregnancy. She can be assured that which of the following risks is the same for her as for the general population?

a. Preeclampsia and eclampsia
b. Infection
c. Fetal cystic fibrosis
d. Postpartum hemorrhage after vaginal delivery
e. Hydramnios

156. You are called in to evaluate the heart of a 19-year-old primigravida at term. Listening carefully to the heart, you determine that there is a split S_1, normal S_2, S_3 easily audible with a 2/6 systolic ejection murmur greater during inspiration, and a soft diastolic murmur. You immediately recognize which of the following?

a. The presence of the S_3 is abnormal
b. The systolic ejection murmur is unusual in a pregnant woman at term
c. Diastolic murmurs are rare in pregnant women
d. The combination of a prominent S_3 and soft diastolic murmur is a significant abnormality
e. All findings recorded are normal changes in pregnancy

157. A 21-year-old has a positive purified protein derivative (PPD) and is about to be treated for tuberculosis. She can be reassured that her risk of which of the following is minimal?

a. A flulike syndrome caused by rifampin
b. A peripheral neuropathy caused by isoniazid
c. Optic neuritis caused by INH
d. Ototoxicity as a side effect of streptomycin
e. A positive antinuclear antibody (ANA) titer with INH therapy

158. A 33-year-old woman at 10 weeks presents for her first prenatal exam. Routine labs are drawn and her hepatitis B surface antigen is positive. Liver function tests are normal and her hepatitis B core and surface antibody tests are negative. Which of the following is the best way to prevent neonatal infection?

a. Provide immune globulin to the mother
b. Provide hepatitis B vaccine to the mother
c. Perform a cesarean delivery at term
d. Provide hepatitis B vaccine to the neonate
e. Provide immune globulin and the hepatitis B vaccine to the neonate

159. A 38-year-old G1P0 presents to the obstetrician's office at 37 weeks gestational age complaining of a rash on her abdomen that is becoming increasingly pruritic. The rash started on her abdomen, and the patient notes that it is starting to spread downward to her thighs. The patient reports no previous history of any skin disorders or problems. She denies any malaise or fever. On physical exam, she is afebrile and her physician notes that her abdomen, and most notably her stretch marks, are covered with red papules and plaques. No excoriations or bullae are present. The patient's face, arms, and legs are unaffected by the rash. Which of the following is this patient's most likely diagnosis?

a. Herpes gestationis
b. Pruritic urticarial papules and plaques of pregnancy
c. Prurigo gravidarum
d. Intrahepatic cholestasis of pregnancy
e. Impetigo herpetiformis

160. A 25-year-old G2P0 at 30 weeks gestation presents with the complaint of a new rash and itching on her abdomen over the last few weeks. She denies any constitutional symptoms or any new lotions, soaps, or detergents. On exam she is afebrile with a small, papular rash on her trunk and forearms. Excoriations from scratching are also noted. Which of the following is the recommended first-line treatment for this patient?

a. Delivery
b. Cholestyramine
c. Topical steroids and oral antihistamines
d. Oral steroids
e. Antibiotic therapy

161. A 23-year-old G3P2002 presents for a routine OB visit at 34 weeks. She reports a history of genital herpes for 5 years. She reports that she has had only two outbreaks during the pregnancy, but is very concerned about the possibility of transmitting this infection to her baby. Which of the following statements is accurate regarding how this patient should be counseled?

a. There is no risk of neonatal infection during a vaginal delivery if no lesions are present at the time the patient goes into labor
b. The patient should be scheduled for an elective cesarean section at 39 weeks of gestation to avoid neonatal infection
c. Starting at 36 weeks, weekly genital herpes cultures should be done
d. The herpes virus is commonly transmitted across the placenta in a patient with a history of herpes
e. Suppressive antiviral therapy can be started at 36 weeks to help prevent an outbreak from occurring at the time of delivery

162. A 28-year-old G1 presents to your office at 8 weeks gestation. She has a history of diabetes since the age of 14. She uses insulin and she denies any complications related to her diabetes. Which of the following is the most common birth defect associated with diabetes?

a. Anencephaly
b. Encephalocele
c. Meningomyelocele
d. Sacral agenesis
e. Ventricular septal defect

163. A 32-year-old G1 at 10 weeks gestation presents for her routine OB visit. She is worried about her pregnancy because she has a history of insulin-requiring diabetes since the age of 18. Prior to becoming pregnant, her endocrinologist diagnosed her with microalbumuria. She has had photolaser ablation of retinopathy in the past. Which diabetic complication may be worsened by pregnancy?

a. Benign retinopathy
b. Gastroparesis
c. Nephropathy
d. Neuropathy
e. Proliferative retinopathy

164. A 37-year-old G3P2 presents to your office for her first OB visit at 10 weeks gestation. She has a history of Graves' disease and has been maintained on propylthiouracil (PTU) as treatment for her hyperthyroidism. She is currently euthyroid but asks you if her condition poses any problems for the pregnancy. Which of the following statements should be included in your counseling session with the patient?

a. She may need to discontinue the use of the thioamide drug because it is commonly associated with leukopenia
b. Infants born to mothers on PTU who are euthyroid may develop a goiter and be clinically hypothyroid
c. Propylthiouracil does not cross the placenta
d. Pregnant hyperthyroid women, even when appropriately treated, have an increased risk of developing preeclampsia
e. Thyroid storm is a common complication in pregnant women with Graves' disease

165. A 40-year-old G3P2 obese patient at 37 weeks presents for her routine OB visit. She has gestational diabetes that is controlled with diet. She reports that her fasting and postprandial sugars have all been within the normal range. Her fetus has an estimated fetal weight of 6½ lb by Leopold's maneuvers. Which of the following is the best next step in her management?

a. Administration of insulin to prevent macrosomia
b. Cesarean delivery at 39 weeks to prevent shoulder dystocia
c. Induction of labor at 38 weeks
d. Kick counts and routine return OB visit in 1 week
e. Weekly biophysical profile

166. A 36-year-old G1P0 at 35 weeks gestation presents to your office complaining of a several-day history of generalized malaise, anorexia, nausea, and emesis. She has also been experiencing abdominal discomfort, which she attributes to indigestion. She has had a poor appetite and has lost several pounds since her last office visit 1 week ago. She denies any headache or visual changes. Her fetal movement has been good, and she denies any regular uterine contractions, vaginal bleeding, or rupture of membranes. This patient is on no medications except for a prenatal vitamin, and has no history of any medical problems. On physical exam, you notice that she is mildly jaundiced and appears to be a little confused. Her vital signs indicate a temperature of 100°F, pulse of 70, and BP of 100/62. She has no significant edema, and in fact appears very dehydrated. You send her to labor and delivery for IV hydration and additional evaluation. Once in labor and delivery, the patient is hooked up to an external fetal monitor, which indicates a fetal heart rate in the 160s that is nonreactive, but with good variability. Blood is drawn and the following results are obtained: WBC = 25,000, Hct = 42.0, platelets = 51,000, SGOT/PT = 287/350, glucose = 43, creatinine = 2.0, fibrinogen = 135, PT/PTT = 16/50 s, serum ammonia level = 90 mmol/L (nl = 11–35). Urinalysis is positive for 3+ protein and large ketones. Which of the following is the most likely diagnosis?

a. Hepatitis B
b. Acute fatty liver of pregnancy
c. Intrahepatic cholestasis of pregnancy
d. Severe preeclampsia
e. Hyperemesis gravidarum

167. A 27-year-old G1P0 at 34 weeks gestation presents to your office complaining of a 2-day history of nausea and emesis. She also complains of indigestion. She appears dehydrated and has lost several pounds since her last office visit 1 week ago. She denies any headache or visual changes. Her fetal movement has been good, and she denies any regular uterine contractions, vaginal bleeding, or rupture of membranes. This patient is on no medications except for a prenatal vitamin, and has no history of any medical problems. On physical exam, you notice that she is icteric sclera and skin. Her vital signs indicate a temperature of 99°F, pulse of 102, and BP of 130/84. She is sent to labor and delivery for IV hydration and additional evaluation. Once in labor and delivery, the patient is hooked up to an external fetal monitor, which indicates a fetal heart rate in the 160s with good variability, but nonreactive. Blood is drawn and the following results are obtained: WBC = 22,000, Hct = 40.0, platelets = 72,000, SGOT/PT = 334/386, glucose = 58, creatinine = 2.2, fibrinogen = 209, PT/PTT = 16/50 s, serum ammonia level = 65 mmol/L (nl = 11–35). Urinalysis is positive for 3+ protein and large ketones. Which of the following is the recommended treatment for this patient?

a. Immediate delivery
b. Cholecystectomy
c. Intravenous diphenhydramine
d. MgSO$_4$ therapy
e. Bed rest and supportive measures since this condition is self-limited

168. A 32-year-old G1P0 reports to your office for a routine OB visit at 14 weeks gestational age. Labs drawn at her first prenatal visit 4 weeks ago reveal a platelet count of 60,000. All her other labs were within normal limits. During the present visit, the patient has a blood pressure of 120/70. Her urine dip reveals the presence of trace protein. The patient denies any complaints. The only medication she is currently taking is a prenatal vitamin. On taking a more in-depth history you learn that, prior to pregnancy, your patient had a history of occasional nose and gum bleeds, but no serious bleeding episodes. She has considered herself to be a person who just bruises easily. Which of the following is the most likely diagnosis?

a. Alloimmune thrombocytopenia
b. Gestational thrombocytopenia
c. Immune thrombocytopenic purpura
d. HELLP syndrome
e. Pregnancy-induced hypertension

169. A 23-year-old G1P0 reports to your office for a routine OB visit at 28 weeks gestational age. Labs drawn at her prenatal visit 2 weeks ago reveal a 1-h glucose test of 128, hemoglobin of 10.8, and a platelet count of 80,000. All her other labs were within normal limits. During the present visit, the patient has a blood pressure of 120/70. Her urine dip is negative for protein, glucose, and blood. The patient denies any complaints. The only medication she is currently taking is a prenatal vitamin. She does report a history of epistaxis on occasion, but no other bleeding. Which of the following medical treatments should you recommend to treat the thrombocytopenia?

a. No treatment is necessary
b. Stop prenatal vitamins
c. Oral corticosteroid therapy
d. Intravenous immune globulin
e. Splenectomy

170. A 21-year-old G2P1 at 25 weeks gestation presents to the emergency room complaining of shortness of breath. She reports a history of asthma and states her peak expiratory flow rate (PEFR) with good control is usually around 400. During speaking the patient has to stop to catch her breath between words; her PEFR is 210. An arterial blood gas is drawn and oxygen therapy is initiated. She is afebrile and on physical exam expiratory wheezes are heard in all lung fields. Which of the following is the most appropriate next step in her management?

a. Antibiotics
b. Chest x-ray
c. Inhaled β-agonist
d. Intravenous corticosteroids
e. Theophylline

171. One of your obstetric patients presents to the office at 25 weeks complaining of severe left calf pain and swelling. The area of concern is slightly edematous, but no erythema is apparent. The patient demonstrates a positive Homan sign, and you are concerned that she may have a deep vein thrombosis. Which of the following diagnostic modalities should you order?

a. MRI
b. Computed tomographic scanning
c. Venography
d. Real-time ultrasonography

DIRECTIONS: Each group of questions below consists of lettered options followed by a set of numbered items. For each numbered item, select the **one** lettered option with which it is **most** closely associated. Each lettered option may be used once, more than once, or not at all.

Questions 172–180

For each description, select the most likely causative infectious agent.

a. Cytomegalovirus
b. Group B streptococcus
c. Hepatitis B
d. Herpes simplex
e. Influenza A
f. Parvovirus
g. Rubella virus
h. Rubeola
i. Toxoplasma gondii
j. Treponemal pallidum
k. Varicella zoster

172. A 20-year-old G1 patient delivers a live-born infant with cutaneous lesions, limb defects, cerebral cortical atrophy, and chorioretinitis. Her pregnancy was complicated by pneumonia.

173. A 34-year-old G2 at 36 weeks delivers a growth-restricted infant with cataracts, anemia, patent ductous arteriosus, and sensorineural deafness. She has a history of chronic hypertension, which was well controlled with methyldopa during pregnancy. She had a viral syndrome with rash in early pregnancy.

174. A 25-year-old G3 at 39 weeks delivers a small-for-gestational-age infant with chorioretinitis, intracranial calcifications, jaundice, hepatosplenomegaly, and anemia. The infant displays poor feeding and tone in the nursery. The patient denies eating any raw or undercooked meat and does not have any cats living at home with her. She works as a nurse in the pediatric intensive care unit at the local hospital.

175. A 23-year-old G1 with a history of a flulike illness, fever, myalgias, and lymphadenopathy during her pregnancy delivers a growth-restricted infant with seizures, intracranial calcifications, hepatosplenomegaly, jaundice, and anemia.

176. A 32-year-old G5 delivers a stillborn fetus at 34 weeks. The placenta is noted to be much larger than normal. The fetus appeared hydropic and had petechiae over much of the skin.

177. A 38-year-woman at 39 weeks delivers a 7-lb infant female without complications. At 2 weeks of life the infant develops fulminant liver failure and dies.

178. A 20-year-old woman who works as a kindergarten teacher presents for her routine visit at 32 weeks. Her fundal height measures 40 centimeters. An ultrasound reveals polyhydramnios, an appropriately grown fetus with ascites and scalp edema. The patient denies any recent illnesses, but some of the children at her school have been sick recently.

179. A 25-year-old female in her first pregnancy delivers a 6-lb male infant at 38 weeks. The infant develops fever, vesicular rash, poor feeding, and listlessness at 1 week of age.

180. A 22-year-old woman delivers a 7-lb male infant at 40 weeks without any complications. On day 3 of life, the infant develops respiratory distress and septic shock.

Medical and Surgical Complications of Pregnancy

Answers

146. The answer is d. *(Rodeck, p 858.)* A mild group B coxsackievirus infection of the mother during the antepartum period may give rise to a virulent infection in the newborn, sometimes resulting in a fatal encephalomyocarditis. A maternal rubella infection may cause neonatal hepatosplenomegaly, petechial rash, and jaundice; in addition, viral shedding may last for months or years. Herpes zoster, the causative agent of varicella (chickenpox), is an especially dangerous organism for the newborn. Varicella is rare in pregnancy, but if it occurs shortly before delivery, the viremia may spread to the fetus before protective maternal antibodies have had a chance to form. Congenital varicella can be fatal to the newborn; the increasing availability of zoster immunoglobulin, however, may allow clinicians to attack the infection before significant fetal viremia has developed. Shingles, which is a reactivation of varicella, would not likely have fetal effects because of already existing maternal IgG from the initial exposure. Herpesvirus can be acquired by the fetus as it passes down the genital tract and can cause a severe, often fatal herpes infection in the newborn.

147. The answer is b. *(Cunningham, p 1282.)* Rubella is one of the most teratogenic agents known. Risk of congenital rubella infection in the fetus is 80% when the mother has a rubella infection in the first trimester. This risk decreases to 25% by the end of the second trimester.

148. The answer is c. *(Gleicher, pp 647–652.)* Spectinomycin is the treatment of choice for pregnant women who have asymptomatic *N. gonorrhoeae* infections and who are allergic to penicillin. Erythromycin is another drug that is effective in treating asymptomatic gonorrhea. Although tetracycline is an effective alternative to penicillin, its use is generally contraindicated in pregnancy. Administration of chloramphenicol is not recommended to treat women, pregnant or not, who have cervical gonorrhea, and the use of ampicillin or penicillin analogues is contraindicated for penicillin-allergic patients.

149. The answer is a. (*Rodeck, pp 851–853.*) Toxoplasmosis, a protozoal infection caused by *Toxoplasma gondii,* can result from ingestion of raw or undercooked meat infected by the organism or from contact with infected cat feces. The French, because their diet includes raw meat, have a high incidence. The incidence of toxoplasmosis in pregnant women is estimated to be 1 in every 150 to 700 pregnancies. Infection early in pregnancy may cause abortion; later in pregnancy, the fetus may become infected. A small number of infected infants develop involvement of the central nervous system or the eye; most infants who have the disease, however, escape serious clinical problems.

150. The answer is d. (*Gleicher, pp 1512–1515.*) The incidence of appendicitis in pregnancy is 1 in 2000, the same as that in the nonpregnant population. The diagnosis is very difficult in pregnancy because leukocytosis, nausea, and vomiting are common in pregnancy and the upward displacement of the appendix by the uterus may cause appendicitis to simulate cholecystitis, pyelonephritis, gastritis, or degenerating myomas. Surgery is necessary even if the diagnosis is not certain. Delays in surgery due to difficulty in diagnosis as the appendix moves up are probably the cause of increasing maternal mortality with increasing gestational age. Premature birth and abortion account for a rate of fetal loss close to 15%.

151. The answer is d. (*Gleicher, pp 1540–1541.*) Patients with a history of thromboembolic disease in pregnancy are at high risk of developing it in subsequent pregnancies. Impedance plethysmography and Doppler ultrasonography are useful techniques even in pregnancy and should be done as baseline studies. Patients should be treated prophylactically with low-dose heparin therapy through the postpartum period as this is the time of highest risk of this disease.

152. The answer is c. (*Reece, pp 1142–1145.*) The most probable diagnosis in this case is acute pancreatitis. The pain caused by a myoma in degeneration is more localized to the uterine wall. Low-grade fever and mild leukocytosis may appear with a degenerating myoma, but liver function tests are usually normal. The other obstetric cause of epigastric pain, severe preeclamptic toxemia (PET), may exhibit disturbed liver function [sometimes associated with the HELLP syndrome (hemolysis, elevated liver enzymes, low platelets)], but this patient has only mild elevation of blood pressure and no proteinuria. Acute appendicitis in pregnancy is one of the more common nonobstetric causes of abdominal pain. Symptoms of acute appendicitis in pregnancy are similar to those in nonpregnant patients, but the pain is more vague and poorly localized and the point of maximal tenderness moves to the right upper quadrant with advancing gestation. Liver function tests are normal with acute appendicitis. Acute cholecystitis may cause fever, leukocytosis, and pain of the right upper quadrant with abnormal liver function tests, but amylase levels would be elevated only mildly, if at all, and pain would be less severe than described in this patient. The diagnosis that fits the clinical description and the laboratory findings is acute pancreatitis. This disorder may be more common during pregnancy, with an incidence of 1 in 100 to 1 in 10,000 pregnancies. Cholelithiasis, chronic alcoholism, infection, abdominal trauma, some medications, and pregnancy-induced hypertension are known predisposing factors. Patients with pancreatitis are usually in acute distress—the classic finding is a person who is rocking with knees drawn up and trunk flexed in agony. Fever, tachypnea, hypotension, ascites, and pleural effusion may be observed. Hypotonic bowel sounds, epigastric tenderness, and signs of peritonitis may be demonstrated on examination.

Leukocytosis, hemoconcentration, and abnormal liver function tests are common laboratory findings in acute pancreatitis. However, the most important laboratory finding is an elevation of serum amylase levels, which appears 12 to 24 h after onset of clinical disease. Values may exceed 200 U/dL (normal values are 50 to 160 U/dL). A useful diagnostic tool in the pregnant patient with only modest elevation of amylase values is the amylase-creatinine ratio. In patients with acute pancreatitis, the ratio of amylase clearance to creatinine clearance is always greater than 5 to 6%.

Treatment considerations for the pregnant patient with acute pancreatitis are similar to those in nonpregnant patients. Intravenous hydration, nasogastric suction, enteric rest, and correction of electrolyte imbalance and of hyperglycemia are the mainstays of therapy. Careful attention to tissue perfusion, volume expansion, and transfusions to maintain a stable cardiovascular performance are critical. Gradual recovery occurs over 5 to 6 days.

153. The answer is d. *(Reece, pp 1277–1280.)* The term *asymptomatic bacteriuria* is used to indicate persisting, actively multiplying bacteria within the urinary tract without symptoms of a urinary infection. The reported prevalence during pregnancy varies from 2% to as great as 12%. The highest incidence has been reported in black multiparas with sickle cell trait. In women who demonstrate ASB, the bacteriuria is typically present at the time of the first prenatal visit; after an initial negative culture of the urine, fewer than 1.5% acquire a urinary infection. Twenty to forty percent of women with ASB develop an acute infection during that pregnancy. Postpartum urologic investigation has often shown pyelographic evidence of chronic infection, obstructive lesions, or congenital abnormalities of the urinary tract.

154. The answer is a. *(Reece, pp 1277–1280.)* Although quite effective, sulfonamides should be avoided during the last few weeks of pregnancy because they competitively inhibit the binding of bilirubin to albumin, which increases the risk of neonatal hyperbilirubinemia. Nitrofurantoin may not be tolerated in pregnancy because of the effect of nausea. It should also be avoided in late pregnancy because of the risk of hemolysis due to deficiency of erythrocyte phosphate dehydrogenase in the newborn. Tetracyclines are contraindicated during pregnancy because of dental staining in the fetus. Thus, the drugs of choice for treatment of UTI in pregnancy are ampicillin and the cephalosporins.

155. The answer is c. *(Reece, pp 1055–1084.)* Maternal diabetes mellitus can affect a pregnant woman and her fetus in many ways. The development of preeclampsia or eclampsia is about 4 times as likely as among nondiabetic women. Infection is also more likely not only to occur but to be severe. The incidences of fetal macrosomia or death and of dystocia are increased, and hydramnios is common. The likelihood of postpartum hemorrhage after vaginal delivery and the frequency of cesarean section are both increased in diabetic women. The incidence of fetal genetic disorders such as cystic fibrosis is unaffected by diabetes.

156. The answer is e. *(Gleicher, pp 27–31.)* Numerous changes occur in the cardiovascular system during pregnancy. Heart rate increases by about 10 to 15/min. Blood volume and cardiac output increase significantly. Many cardiac sounds that would be abnormal in a nonpregnant state are normal during pregnancy. All the findings listed in the question are normal. Ninety percent of pregnant women have systolic ejection murmurs. In approximately 20% of women, a soft diastolic murmur can be heard.

157. The answer is c. (*James, pp 547–548, 623.*) Rifampin has occasionally been known to cause a flulike syndrome, abdominal pain, acute renal failure, and thrombocytopenia. It may also resemble hepatitis and can cause orange urine, sweat, and tears. INH has been associated with hepatitis, hypersensitivity reactions, and peripheral neuropathies. The neuropathy can be prevented by the administration of pyridoxine, especially in the pregnant patient, where pyridoxine requirements are increased. INH may also cause a rash, a fever, and a lupuslike syndrome with a positive ANA titer. Streptomycin has a potential for ototoxicity in both the mother and the fetus. The most commonly seen fetal side effects include minor vestibular impairment, auditory impairment, or both. Cases of severe and bilateral hearing loss and marked vestibular abnormalities have been reported with streptomycin use. Optic neuritis is a well-described side effect of ethambutol, although it is rare at the usual prescribed doses.

158. The answer is e. (*Cunningham, p 1131.*) Infection of the newborn whose mother chronically carries the hepatitis B virus can usually be prevented by the administration of hepatitis B immune globulin very soon after birth, followed promptly by the hepatitis B vaccine.

159. The answer is b. (*Cunningham, pp 1126–1127, 1250–1253.*) Pruritic urticarial papules and plaques of pregnancy (PUPPP) is the most common dermatologic condition of pregnancy. It is more common in nulliparous women and occurs most often in the second and third trimesters of pregnancy. PUPPP is characterized by erythematous papules and plaques that are intensely pruritic and appear first on the abdomen. The lesions then commonly spread to the buttocks, thighs, and extremities with sparing of the face. Herpes gestationis is a blistering skin eruption that occurs more commonly in multiparous patients in the second or third trimester of pregnancy. The presence of vesicles and bullae help differentiate this skin condition from PUPPP. Prurigo gestationis is a very rare dermatosis of pregnancy that is characterized by small, pruritic excoriated lesions that occur between 25 and 30 weeks. The lesions first appear on the trunk and forearms and can spread throughout the body as well. In cases of intrahepatic cholestasis of pregnancy, bile acids are cleared incompletely and accumulate in the dermis, which causes intense itching. These patients develop pruritus in late pregnancy; there are no characteristic skin changes or rashes except in women who develop excoriations from scratching. Impetigo herpetiformis is a rare pustular eruption that forms along the margins of erythematous patches. This skin condition usually occurs in late pregnancy. The skin lesions usually begin at points of flexure and extend peripherally; mucous membranes are commonly involved. Patients with impetigo herpetiformis usually do not have intense pruritus, but more commonly have systemic symptoms of nausea, vomiting, diarrhea, chills, and fever.

160. The answer is c. (*Cunningham, pp 1127, 1252–1253.*) The first-line treatment for prurigo gestationis and papular dermatitis is oral antihistamines and topical corticosteroids. If these treatments do not give relief, oral steroids should be administered. The rash will resolve quickly following delivery, but delivery would not be the first-line treatment. Cholestyramine is often used in cases of cholestasis of pregnancy to lower serum bile salts and decrease pruritus. There is no role for antibiotic therapy in the treatment since no bacterial etiology has been identified.

161. The answer is e. (*ACOG, Practice Bulletin 8. Cunningham, pp 1307–1310.*) A maternal HSV infection can be passed to the fetus via vertical transmission. If a pregnant woman with a history of herpes has no lesions present at the time she goes into labor, vaginal delivery is permitted. If lesions are present at the time of labor, then there is a 3 to 5% risk of transmitting the infection to the fetus, and cesarean delivery is recommended. Viral shedding can occur without the presence of a lesion. It is not recommended that a patient with a history of herpes be scheduled for an elective cesarean section. It is not recommended that weekly genital viral cultures be performed because such cultures do not predict whether a patient will be shedding the virus at the time of delivery. For patients at or beyond 36 weeks gestation, daily suppressive therapy with an antiviral medication such as acyclovir can be used to try to decrease the risk of viral shedding and outbreaks and the likelihood of a cesarean section.

162. The answer is e. (*Cunningham, pp 198, 1177.*) The incidence of major malformations in women with diabetes is 5 to 10%. It is believed that they are a consequence of poorly controlled diabetes and higher glycosylated hemoglobin values in the preconception and early pregnancy period. The most common single organ system anomalies are cardiac (38%), musculoskeletal (15%), and central nervous system (10%). Sacral agenesis is a rare malformation seen commonly in severely diabetic women.

163. The answer is e. (*Cunningham, pp 1180–1182.*) The incidence of renal failure is almost 30% in type 1 diabetics and 4 to 20% in type 2 diabetics. Pregnancy has not been found to exacerbate or modify diabetic nephropathy. Diabetic neuropathy and gastroparesis may complicate some pregnancies, but pregnancy does not affect the overall disease process. Proliferative retinopathy is the one diabetic complication that pregnancy is thought to worsen.

164. The answer is b. (*ACOG, Practice Bulletin 32. Cunningham, pp 1192–1194.*) Hyperthyroidism in pregnancy is treated with thioamides, namely, propylthiouracil (PTU) and methimazole. These medications block thyroid hormone synthesis. Both cross the placenta, and fetal hypothyroidism and goiter have been associated with maternal thioamide treatment for Graves' disease. Transient leukopenia occurs in about 10% of patients taking thioamide drugs, but does not necessitate stopping the medication. Women who remain hyperthyroid despite therapy have a higher incidence of preeclampsia and heart failure. Thyroid storm occurs only rarely in untreated women with Graves' disease. This emergent medical condition involves thyrotoxicosis, which is characterized by fever, tachycardia, altered mental status, vomiting, diarrhea, and cardiac arrythmia. The treatment of thyroid storm involves administering multiple medications to suppress thyroid function.

165. The answer is d. (*Cunningham, pp 1175–1176. ACOG, Practice Bulletin 30.*) In general, women with gestational diabetes who do not require insulin seldom need early delivery or other interventions. There is no consensus on whether antepartum fetal testing is necessary in women with well-controlled gestational diabetes. Antepartum fetal testing is recommended for women with preexisting DM and those who require insulin therapy. There is no good evidence to support routine delivery before 40 weeks when glucose control is good and no other complications supervene. Cesarean delivery may be considered in women with gestational diabetes if the estimated fetal weight is 4500 grams or more. Insulin therapy is indicated if diet cannot keep fasting glucose below 105 and 2-h values below 120.

166. The answer is b. (*Cunningham, pp 1127–1129.*) Acute fatty liver of pregnancy is a rare complication of pregnancy. Estimates of its incidence range from 1 in 7,000 to 1 in 15,000 pregnancies. This disorder is usually fatal for both mother and baby. Recently it has been suggested that recessively inherited mitochondrial abnormalities of fatty acid oxidation predispose a woman to fatty liver in pregnancy. This disorder usually manifests itself late in pregnancy and is more common in nulliparous women. Typically, a patient will present with a several-day or -week history of general malaise, anorexia, nausea, emesis, and jaundice. Liver enzymes are usually not elevated above 500. Indications of liver failure are present, manifested by elevated PT/PTT, bilirubin, and ammonia levels. In addition, there is marked hypoglycemia. Low fibrinogen and platelet levels occur secondary to a consumptive coagulopathy. In cases of viral hepatitis, serum transaminase levels are usually much higher and marked hypoglycemia or elevated serum ammonia levels would not be seen. Sometimes the HELLP syndrome can initially be difficult to differentiate from acute fatty liver, but in this case the patient has a normal blood pressure. In addition, hepatic failure is not characteristic of severe preeclampsia. Hyperemesis gravidarum is characterized by nausea and vomiting unresponsive to simple therapy. It usually occurs early in the first trimester and resolves by about 16 weeks. In some cases, there can be a transient hepatic dysfunction. Intrahepatic cholestasis of pregnancy is characterized by pruritus and/or icterus. Some women develop cholestasis in the third trimester secondary to estrogen-induced changes. There is an accumulation of serum bile salts, which causes the pruritus. Liver enzymes are seldom elevated above 250 U/L.

167. The answer is a. (*Cunningham, pp 1127–1129.*) Acute fatty liver resolves spontaneously after delivery. Delayed diagnosis and movement toward delivery can result in risk of coma and death from severe hepatic failure. In addition, procrastination can result in severe hemorrhage and renal failure. Bed rest and supportive therapy would be the treatment for viral hepatitis. Benadryl treatment would apply to therapy for cholestasis of pregnancy. MgSO$_4$ therapy would be applicable to cases of the HELLP syndrome.

168. The answer is c. (*ACOG, Practice Bulletin 6.*) Immune thrombocytopenic purpura (ITP) typically occurs in the second or third decade of life and is more common in women than in men. The diagnosis of ITP is one of exclusion, because there are no pathognomonic signs, symptoms, or diagnostic tests. Traditionally, ITP is associated with a persistent platelet count of less than 100,000 in the absence of splenomegaly. Most women have a history of easy bruising and nose and gum bleeds that precede pregnancy. If the platelet count is maintained above 20,000, hemorrhagic episodes rarely occur. In cases of ITP, the patient produces IgG antiplatelet antibodies that increase platelet consumption in the spleen and in other sites. Gestational thrombocytopenia occurs in up to 8% of pregnancies. Affected women are usually asymptomatic, have no prior history of bleeding, and usually maintain platelet counts above 70,000. In gestational thrombocytopenia, platelet counts usually return to normal in about 3 months. The cause of gestational thrombocytopenia has not been clearly elucidated. HELLP syndrome of severe preeclampsia is associated with thrombocytopenia, but this condition occurs in the third trimester and is associated with hypertension. In neonatal alloimmune thrombocytopenia, there is a maternal alloimmunization to fetal platelet antigens. The mother is healthy and has a normal platelet count, but produces antibodies that cross the placenta and destroy fetal/neonatal platelets.

169. The answer is a. (*ACOG, Practice Bulletin 6.*) Asymptomatic pregnant women with platelet counts above 50,000 do not need to be treated, because the count is sufficient to prevent bleeding complications. For severely low platelet counts, therapy can include prednisone, intravenous immune globulin, and splenectomy.

170. The answer is c. (*Cunningham, pp 1060–1064.*) Inhaled β-agonists are the primary treatment for an acute asthma exacerbation. Intravenous steroids should be given if the exacerbation is severe, if the patient is currently taking oral steroids, or if the response to bronchodilator therapy is incomplete or poor. Antibiotics are used for patients with fever, leukocytosis, or evidence of infection. A febrile patient should have a chest x-ray to rule out pneumonia. Methylxanthines are not used for acute asthma exacerbations.

171. The answer is d. (*Cunningham, pp 1079–1081.*) Noninvasive modalities are currently the preferred tests for diagnosing venous thromboemboli. Venography is still the gold standard, but it is not commonly used because it is cumbersome to perform and expensive and has serious complications. Real-time ultrasonography or color Doppler ultrasound is the procedure of choice to detect proximal deep vein thrombosis. MRI and CT scanning are used in specific cases when ultrasound findings are equivocal.

172–180. The answers are 172-k, 173-g, 174-a, 175-i, 176-j, 177-c, 178-f, 179-d, 180-b. *(Cunningham, pp 1130–1131, 1276–1293, 1307–1310.)* Maternal infection with viruses and bacteria during pregnancy can cause an array of fetal effects from none to congenital malformations and death. Rubeola (measles) virus does not appear to have any teratogenic effect on the fetus. Maternal infection with varicella-zoster during the first half of pregnancy can cause malformations such as cutaneous and bony defects, chorioretinitis, cerebral cortical atrophy, and hydronephrosis. Adults with varicella infection fare much worse than children; about 10% will develop a pneumonitis, and some of these will require ventilatory support. Influenza does not cause any fetal effects. Rubella is one of the most teratogenic agents known. Fetal manifestations of infection correlate with time of maternal infection and fetal organ development. It includes one or more of the following: eye lesions, cardiac disease, sensorineural deafness, CNS defects, growth restriction, thrombocytopenia, anemia, liver dysfunction, interstitial pneumonitis, and osseous changes. Cytomegalovirus in the mother is usually asymptomatic, but 15% of adults will have a mononucleosis-like syndrome. Maternal immunity does not prevent recurrence or congenital infection. Congenital infection includes low birth weight, microcephaly, intracranial calcifications, chorioretinitis, mental and motor retardation, sensorineural deficits, heptosplenomegaly, jaundice, anemia, and thrombocytopenic purpura. The virus is shed in the secretions of affected individuals. *Toxoplasmosis gondii* is transmitted by eating infected raw or undercooked meat and contact with infected cat feces. Maternal immunity appears to protect against fetal infection, and up to one-third of American women are immune prior to pregnancy. Acute infection in the mother is often subclinical, but symptoms can include fatique, lymphadenopathy, and myalgias. Fetal infection is more common when disease is acquired later in pregnancy (60% in third trimester versus 10% in first trimester). Congenital disease consists of low birth weight, hepatosplenomegaly, jaundice, anemia, neurological disease with seizures, intracranial calcifications, and mental retardation. In the past, syphyllis accounted for about one-third of all stillbirths. Transplacental infection can occur with any stage of syphilis, but the highest incidence of congenital infection occurs in women with primary or secondary disease. The fetal and neonatal effects include hepato-splenomegaly, edema, ascites, hydrops, petechiae or purpuric skin lesions, osteochondritis, lymphadenopathy, rhinitis, pneumonia, myocarditis, and nephrosis. The placenta is enlarged, sometimes weighing as much as the fetus. Transplacental transfer of hepatitis B from the mother to fetus occurs with acute hepatitis, not chronic seropositivity. Acute infection in first trimester infects 10% of fetuses, and in third trimester 80 to 90% are affected. Perinatal transmission occurs by ingestion of infected material during delivery or exposure subsequent to birth in mothers who are chronic carriers. Some infected infants may be asymptomatic, and others develop fulminant hepatic disease. Administration of hepatitis B immune globulin after birth, followed by the vaccine, can prevent disease in infants born to mothers who are chronic carriers. Parvovirus is trophic for eryth-roid cells and can cause fetal anemia. Maternal infection can lead to fetal hydrops, abortion, or stillbirth. In suspectible adults 20 to 30% will ac-quire disease during school outbreaks. If a pregnant woman has diagnosis confirmed with IgM antibodies, ultrasound is done for fetal surveillance. If hydrops is diagnosed fetal transfusion can be offered. One-third of fetuses will have spontaneous resolution of hydrops, and 85% of fetuses who receive transfusion will survive. Neonatal herpes infection has three forms: disseminated with involvement of major organs; localized, with involvement confined to the central nervous system; and asymptomatic. A 50% risk of neonatal infection occurs with primary maternal infection, but only 4 to 5% risk with recurrent outbreaks. Postnatal infection can occur through contact with oral and skin lesions. Neonatal infection pre-sentation is nonspecific, with signs and symptoms such as irritability, lethargy, fever, and poor feeding. Less than 50% of infants do not have skin lesions. Early-onset group B streptococcus disease occurs within 1 week of birth. Signs of the disease include respiratory distress, apnea, and shock. Late-onset disease usually occurs after 7 days and manifests as meningitis.

Normal and Abnormal Labor and Delivery

Questions

DIRECTIONS: Each item below contains a question followed by suggested responses. Select the **one best** response to each question.

181. A 20-year-old G1 at 38 weeks gestation presents with regular painful contractions every 3 to 4 min lasting 60 seconds. On pelvic exam she is 3 cm dilated and 90% effaced; an amniotomy is performed and clear fluid is noted. The patient receives epidural analgesia for pain management. The fetal heart rate tracing is reactive. One hour later on repeat exam her cervix is 5 cm dilated and 100% effaced. Which of the following is the best next step in her management?

a. Begin pushing
b. Initiate Pitocin augmentation for protracted labor
c. No intervention; labor is progressing normally
d. Perform cesarean delivery for inadequate cervical effacement
e. Stop epidural infusion to enhance contractions and cervical change

182. A 30-year-old G2P0 at 39 weeks is admitted in active labor with spontaneous rupture of membranes occurring 2 h prior to admission. The patient noted clear fluid at the time. On exam her cervix is 4 cm dilated and completely effaced. The fetal head is at 0 station and the fetal heart rate tracing is reactive. Two hours later on repeat exam her cervix is 5 cm dilated and the fetal head is at +1 station. Early decelerations are noted on the fetal heart rate tracing. Which of the following is the best next step in her labor management?

a. Administer terbutaline
b. Initiate amnioinfusion
c. Initiate Pitocin augmentation
d. Perform cesarean delivery for arrest of descent

183. A 32-year-old G3P2 at 39 weeks gestation with an epidural has been pushing for 30 minutes with good descent. The presenting fetal head is left occiput anterior with less than 45° of rotation with a station of +3 of 5. The fetal heart rate has been in the 90s for the past 5 min and the delivery is expedited with forceps. Which of the following best describes the type of forceps delivery performed?

a. Outlet forceps
b. Low forceps
c. Midforceps
d. High forceps

184. A 27-year-old G2P1 at 38 weeks gestation was admitted in active labor at 6 cm dilated; spontaneous rupture of membranes occurred prior to admission. Currently, the fetal heart rate tracing is reactive. Which of the following labor abnormalities would increase neonatal morbidity?

a. Prolonged latent phase
b. Protracted descent
c. Secondary arrest of dilation
d. Protracted active-phase dilation

185. A 38-year-old G6P4 is brought to the hospital by ambulance for vaginal bleeding at 34 weeks. She undergoes an emergency cesarean delivery for fetal bradycardia under general anesthesia. In the recovery room 4 h after her surgery the patient develops respiratory distress and tachycardia. Lung exam reveals rhonchi and rales in the right lower lobe. Oxygen therapy is initiated and chest x-ray is ordered. Which of the following is most likely to have contributed to her condition?

a. Fasting during labor
b. Antacid medications prior to anesthesia
c. Endotracheal intubation
d. Extubation with the patient in the lateral recumbent position with her head lowered
e. Extubation with the patient in the semierect position (semi-Fowler's)

186. A 23-year-old G1 at 38 weeks gestation presents in active labor at 6 cm dilated with ruptured membranes. On cervical exam the fetal nose, eyes, and lips can be palpated. The fetal heart rate tracing is 140 beats per minute with accelerations and no decelerations. The patient's pelvis is adequate. Which of the following is the most appropriate management for this patient?

a. Perform immediate cesarean section without labor
b. Allow spontaneous labor with vaginal delivery
c. Perform forceps rotation in the second stage of labor to convert mentum posterior to mentum anterior and to allow vaginal delivery
d. Allow patient to labor spontaneously until complete cervical dilation is achieved and then perform an internal podalic version with breech extraction
e. Attempt manual conversion of the face to vertex in the second stage of labor

187. A 32-year-old G3P2 at 39 weeks gestation presented to the hospital with ruptured membranes and 4 cm dilated. She has a history of two prior vaginal deliveries, with her largest child weighing 3800 g at birth. Over the next 2 h she progresses to 7 cm dilated. Two hours later she remains 7 cm dilated. The estimated fetal weight by ultrasound is 3200 g. Which of the following labor abnormalities best describes this patient?

a. Prolonged latent phase
b. Protracted active-phase dilation
c. Hypertonic dysfunction
d. Secondary arrest of dilation
e. Primary dysfunction

188. You are following a 38-year-old G2P1 at 39 weeks in labor. She has had one prior vaginal delivery of a 3800-g infant. One week ago, the estimated fetal weight was 3200 g by ultrasound. Over the past 3 h her cervical exam remains unchanged at 6 cm. Fetal heart rate tracing is reactive. An intrauterine pressure catheter reveals two contractions in 10 min with an amplitude of 40 mmHg each. Which of the following is the best management for this patient?

a. Ambulation
b. Sedation
c. Administration of oxytocin
d. Cesarean section
e. Expectant

189. A primipara is in labor and an episiotomy is about to be cut. Compared with a midline episiotomy, which of the following is an advantage of mediolateral episiotomy?

a. Ease of repair
b. Fewer breakdowns
c. Less blood loss
d. Less dyspareunia
e. Less extension of the incision

190. A 27-year-old woman (gravida 3, para 2) comes to the delivery floor at 37 weeks gestation. She has had no prenatal care. She complains that, on bending down to pick up her 2-year-old child, she experienced sudden, severe back pain that now has persisted for 2 h. Approximately 30 min ago she noted bright red blood coming from her vagina. By the time she arrives at the delivery floor, she is contracting strongly every 3 min; the uterus is quite firm even between contractions. By abdominal palpation, the fetus is vertex with the head deeply engaged. Fetal heart rate is 130/min. The fundus is 38 cm above the symphysis. Blood for clotting is drawn, and a clot forms in 4 min. Clotting studies are sent to the laboratory. Which of the following actions can wait until the patient is stabilized?

a. Stabilizing maternal circulation
b. Attaching a fetal electronic monitor
c. Inserting an intrauterine pressure catheter
d. Administering oxytocin
e. Preparing for cesarean section

DIRECTIONS: Each group of questions below consists of lettered options followed by a set of numbered items. For each numbered item, select the **one** lettered option with which it is **most** closely associated. Each lettered option may be used once, more than once, or not at all.

Questions 191–193

For each clinical description, select the most appropriate procedure.

a. External version
b. Internal version
c. Midforceps rotation
d. Low transverse cesarean section
e. Classic cesarean section

191. A 24-year-old primigravid woman, at term, has been in labor for 16 h and has been dilated to 9 cm for 3 h. The fetal vertex is in the right occiput posterior position, at +1 station, and molded. There have been mild late decelerations for the past 30 min. Twenty minutes ago the fetal scalp pH was 7.27; it is now 7.20.

192. You have just delivered an infant weighing 2.5 kg (5.5 lb) at 39 weeks gestation. Because the uterus still feels large, you do a vaginal examination. A second set of membranes is bulging through a fully dilated cervix, and you feel a small part presenting in the sac. A fetal heart is auscultated at 60/min.

193. A 24-year-old woman (gravida 3, para 2) is at 40 weeks gestation. The fetus is in the transverse lie presentation.

Questions 194–196

Select the appropriate treatment for each clinical situation.
a. Epidural block
b. Meperidine (Demerol) 100 mg intramuscularly
c. Oxytocin intravenously
d. Midforceps delivery
e. Cesarean section

194. A multiparous woman has had painful uterine contractions every 2 to 4 min for the past 17 h. The cervix is dilated to 2 to 3 cm and effaced 50%; it has not changed since admission.

195. A nulliparous woman is in active labor (cervical dilation 5 cm with complete effacement, vertex at 0 station); the labor curve shows protracted progression without descent following the administration of an epidural block. An intrauterine pressure catheter shows contractions every 4 to 5 min, peaking at 40 mmHg.

196. A nulliparous woman has had arrest of descent for the past 2 h and arrest of dilation for the past 3 h. The cervix is dilated to 7 cm and the vertex is at +1 station. Monitoring shows a normal pattern and adequate contractions. Fetal weight is estimated at 7.5 lb.

Questions 197–200

Match each description with the most appropriate type of obstetric anesthesia.

a. Paracervical block
b. Pudendal block
c. Spinal block
d. Epidural block

197. Appears to lengthen the second stage of labor

198. Is frequently associated with fetal bradycardia

199. May be complicated by profound hypotension

200. May be associated with increased need for augmentation of labor with oxytocin and for instrument-assisted delivery

DIRECTIONS: Each item below contains a question followed by suggested responses. Select the **one best** response to each question.

201. A 23-year-old G1 at 40 weeks gestation presents to the hospital with the complaint of contractions. She states they are occurring every 4 to 8 min and each lasts approximately 1 min. She reports good fetal movement and denies any leakage of fluid or vaginal bleeding. The nurse places an external tocometer and fetal monitor and reports that the patient is having contractions every 2 to 10 minutes. The nurse states that the contractions are mild to palpation. On exam the cervix is 2 cm dilated, 50% effaced, and the vertex is at −1 station. The patient had the same cervical exam in your office last week. The fetal heart rate tracing is 140 beats per minute with accelerations and no decelerations. Which of the following stages of labor is this patient in?

a. Active labor
b. Latent labor
c. False labor
d. Stage 1 of labor
e. Stage 2 of labor

202. A 19-year-old G1 at 40 weeks gestation presents to the hospital with the complaint of contractions. She states they are very painful and occurring every 3 to 5 minutes. She reports good fetal movement and denies any leakage of fluid or vaginal bleeding. The nurse places an external tocometer and fetal monitor and reports that the patient is having contractions every 4 to 12 minutes. The nurse states that the contractions are mild to moderate to palpation. On exam the cervix is 1 cm dilated, 60% effaced, and the vertex is at −1 station. The patient had the same cervical exam in your office last week. The fetal heart rate tracing is 140 beats per minute with accelerations and no decelerations. Which of the following is the most appropriate next step in the management of this patient?

a. Send her home
b. Admit her for an epidural for pain control
c. Rupture membranes
d. Administer terbutaline
e. Augment labor with Pitocin

203. A 38-year-old G3P2 at 40 weeks gestation presents to labor and delivery with gross rupture of membranes occurring 1 h prior to arrival. The patient is having contraction every 3 to 4 min on the external tocometer, and each contraction lasts 60 s. The fetal heart rate tracing is 120 beats per minute with accelerations and no decelerations. The patient has a history of rapid vaginal deliveries, and her largest baby was 3200 g. On cervical exam she is 5 cm dilated and completely effaced, with the vertex at −2 station. The estimated fetal weight is 3300 g. The patient is in a lot of pain and requesting medication. Which of the following is the most appropriate method of pain control for this patient?

a. Intramuscular Demerol
b. Pudendal block
c. Local block
d. Epidural block
e. General anesthesia

204. You are following a 22-year-old G2P1 at 39 weeks during her labor. She is given an epidural for pain management. Three hours after administrating the pain medication, the patient's cervical exam is unchanged. Her contractions are now every 2 to 3 min, lasting 60 s. The fetal heart rate tracing is 120 beats per minute with accelerations and early decelerations. Which of the following is the best next step in management of this patient?

a. Place a fetal scalp electrode
b. Rebolus the patient's epidural
c. Place an intrauterine pressure catheter (IUPC)
d. Prepare for a cesarean section secondary to a diagnosis of secondary arrest of labor
e. Administer Pitocin for augmentation of labor

205. A 25-year-old G3P2 at 39 weeks is admitted in labor at 5 cm dilated. The fetal heart rate tracing is reactive. Two hours later she is reexamined and her cervix is unchanged at 5 cm dilated. An intrauterine pressure catheter (IUPC) is placed and the patient is noted to have 280 Montevideo units by the IUPC. After an additional 2 h of labor the patient is noted to still be 5 cm dilated. The fetal heart rate tracing remains reactive. Which of the following is the best next step in the management of this labor?

a. Perform a cesarean section
b. Continue to wait and observe the patient
c. Augment labor with Pitocin
d. Attempt delivery via vacuum extraction
e. Perform an operative delivery with forceps

206. A 29-year-old G2P1 at 40 weeks is in active labor. Her cervix is 5 cm dilated, completely effaced, and the vertex is at 0 station. She is on oxytocin to augment her labor and she has just received an epidural for pain management. The nurse calls you to the room because the fetal heart rate has been in the 70s for the past 3 min. The contraction pattern is noted to be every 3 min, each lasting 60 s, with return to normal tone in between contractions. The patient's vital signs are blood pressure 90/40, pulse 105, respiratory rate 18, and temperature 97.6°F. On repeat cervical exam the vertex is well applied to the cervix and the patient remains 5 cm dilated and at 0 station, and no vaginal bleeding is noted. Which of the following is the most likely cause for the deceleration?

a. Cord prolapse
b. Epidural analgesia
c. Pitocin
d. Placental abruption
e. Uterine hyperstimulation

207. You are delivering a 26-year-old G3P2002 at 40 weeks. She has a history of two previous uncomplicated vaginal deliveries and has had no complications this pregnancy. After 15 min of pushing, the baby's head delivers spontaneously, but then retracts back against the perineum. As you apply gentle downward traction to the head, the baby's anterior shoulder fails to deliver. Which of the following is the best next step in the management of this patient?

a. Call for help
b. Cut a symphysiotomy
c. Instruct the nurse to apply fundal pressure
d. Perform a Zavanelli maneuver

208. You are delivering a 33-year-old G3P2 and encounter a shoulder dystocia. After performing the appropriate maneuvers, the baby finally delivers, and the pediatricians attending the delivery note that the right arm is hanging limply to the baby's side with the forearm extended and internally rotated. Which of the following is the baby's most likely diagnosis?

a. Erb palsy
b. Klumpke's paralysis
c. Humeral fracture
d. Clavicular fracture

209. A 41-year-old G1P0 at 39 weeks, who has been completely dilated and pushing for 3 h, has an epidural in place and remains undelivered. She is exhausted and crying and tells you that she can no longer push. Her temperature is 101°F. The fetal heart rate is in the 190s with decreased variability. The patient's membranes have been ruptured for over 24 h, and she has been receiving intravenous ampicillin for a history of colonization with group B strep bacteria. The patient's cervix is completely dilated and effaced and the fetal head is in the direct OA position and is visible at the introitus between pushes. Extensive caput is noted, but the fetal bones are at the +3 station. Which of the following is the most appropriate next step in the management of this patient?

a. Deliver the patient by cesarean section
b. Encourage the patient to continue to push after a short rest
c. Attempt operative delivery with forceps
d. Rebolus the patient's epidural
e. Cut a fourth-degree episiotomy

210. A 28-year-old G1 at 38 weeks had a normal progression of her labor. She has an epidural and has been pushing for 2 hours. The fetal head is direct occiput anterior at +3 station. The fetal heart rate tracing is 150 beats per minute with variable decelerations. With the patient's last push the fetal heart rate had a prolonged deceleration to the 80s for 3 min. You recommend forceps to assist the delivery due to the nonreassuring fetal heart rate tracing. Compared to the use of the vacuum extractor, forceps are associated with an increased risk of which of the following neonatal complications?

a. Cephalohematoma
b. Retinal hemorrhage
c. Jaundice
d. Intracranial hemorrhage
e. Corneal abrasions

211. You are going to perform a forceps-assisted vaginal delivery on a 20-year-old G1 at 40 weeks for maternal exhaustion. The patient has been pushing for 3 h with an epidural for pain management. The fetal head is molded with a large caput. The position is direct occiput anterior and the head is visible at the introitus between pushes. Which of the following is the most appropriate forceps to use for this delivery?

a. Kielland
b. Piper
c. Simpson
d. Zavanelli

212. A 20-year-old G1 at 41 weeks has been pushing for 2½ h. The fetal head is at the introitus and beginning to crown. It is necessary to cut an episiotomy. The tear extends through the sphincter of the rectum, but the rectal mucosa is intact. How should you classify this type of episiotomy?

a. First-degree
b. Second-degree
c. Third-degree
d. Fourth-degree

213. A 16-year-old G1P0 at 38 weeks gestation comes to the labor and delivery suite for the second time during the same weekend that you are on call. She initially presented to labor and delivery at 2:00 P.M. Saturday afternoon complaining of regular uterine contractions. Her cervix was 1 cm dilated, 50% effaced with the vertex at −1 station, and she was sent home after walking for 2 h in the hospital without any cervical change. It is now Sunday night at 8:00 P.M., and the patient returns to L and D with increasing pain. She is exhausted because she did not sleep the night before because her contractions kept waking her up. The patient is placed on the external fetal monitor. Her contractions are occurring every 2 to 3 min. You reexamine the patient and determine that her cervix is unchanged. Which of the following is the best next step in the management of this patient?

a. Perform artificial rupture of membranes to initiate labor
b. Administer an epidural
c. Administer Pitocin to augment labor
d. Achieve cervical ripening with prostaglandin gel
e. Administer 10 mg intramuscular morphine
f. Perform a cesarean section

214. A 25-year-old G1P0 patient at 41 weeks presents to labor and delivery complaining of gross rupture of membranes and painful uterine contractions every 2 to 3 min. On digital exam, her cervix is 3 cm dilated and completely effaced with fetal feet palpable through the cervix. The estimated weight of the fetus is about 6 lb, and the fetal heart rate tracing is reactive. Which of the following is the best method to achieve delivery?

a. Deliver the fetus vaginally by breech extraction
b. Deliver the baby vaginally after external cephalic version
c. Perform an emergent cesarean section
d. Perform an internal podalic version

215. A 25-year-old G1 at 37 weeks presents to labor and delivery with gross rutpure of membranes. The fluid is noted to be clear and the patient is noted to have regular painful contractions every 2 to 3 min lasting for 60 s each. The fetal heart rate tracing is reactive. On cervical exam she is noted to be 4 cm dilated, 90% effaced with the presenting part a −3 station. The presenting part is soft and felt to be the fetal buttock. A quick bedside ultrasound reveals a breech presentation with both hips flexed and knees extended. What type of breech presentation is described?

a. Frank
b. Incomplete, single footling
c. Complete
d. Double footling

Normal and Abnormal Labor and Delivery

Answers

181. The answer is c. (*Cunningham, pp 420–424, 484.*) Patient has normal and adequate labor; no intervention is needed at this time. The patient is not completely dilated, so pushing is not warranted and it can cause cervical lacerations and swelling. Epidural analgesia has not been shown to affect active labor, so stopping it will not make labor progress more quickly.

182. The answer is c. (*Cunningham, pp 498–500.*) The patient has a protracted active phase of labor (cervical dilation <1.2 cm/h) Either expectant management or Pitocin augmentation may be used for treatment. There is no arrest of descent at this time, and cesarean delivery is not warranted. Amnioinfusion is not indicated for early decelerations. It may decrease the need for cesarean delivery in patients with variable or prolonged decelerations. Terbutaline would cause uterine relaxation and is not indicated.

183. The answer is b. (*Hankins, pp 129–130, 137–138.*) In the late 1980s and early 1990s, the classic definitions of forceps deliveries were slightly altered to conform with obstetric reality and the need for realistic definitions of procedures vis-à-vis both medical and legal guidelines and standards. Outlet forceps delivery requires a visible scalp, the fetal skull on the pelvic floor, the sagittal suture in essentially OA position, and the fetal head on the perineum. A rotation can occur, but only up to 45°. A low forceps delivery requires a station of at least +2, but not on the pelvic floor. Rotation can be more than 45°. Midforceps delivery is from a station above +2, but with an engaged head. High forceps delivery, for which there are no modern indications, would reflect a head not engaged.

184. The answer is c. (*Cunningham, pp 498–502.*) Three significant advances in the treatment of uterine dysfunction have reduced the risk of perinatal morbidity and mortality: (1) the avoidance of undue prolongation of labor; (2) the use of intravenous oxytocin in the treatment of some patterns of uterine dysfunction; and (3) the liberal use of cesarean section (rather than midforceps) to effect delivery when oxytocin fails. Prolonged latent phase is not associated with increased risk of perinatal morbidity (PNM) or low Apgar scores and should be treated by therapeutic rest. Protraction disorders have a higher rate of PNM and low Apgar scores, but not if spontaneous labor follows the abnormality. Arrest disorders are associated with significantly higher rates of PNM following either spontaneous or instrument-assisted delivery.

185. The answer is e. (*Cunningham, pp 488–491, Dewan, pp 3–5.*) Aspiration pneumonitis is the most common cause of anesthetic-related death in obstetrics. Its occurrence may be minimized by reducing both the volume and acidity of gastric contents, which is often difficult in the patient in labor whose stomach is extremely slow to empty. All obstetric patients should be intubated for general anesthesia by a skilled professional. Extubation must be accomplished only after the patient is fully conscious and recumbent with her head turned to the side and lowered below the level of her chest. A woman who aspirates may develop evidence for respiratory distress immediately to several hours after the incident. Decreased oxygen saturation, along with tachypnea, bronchospasm, rhonchi, rales, atelectasis, cyanosis, tachycardia, and hypotension, can develop. Intubation should be done by skilled personnel with cricoid pressure (Sellick maneuver).

186. The answer is b. (*Cunningham, pp 506–508.*) In the event of a face presentation, successful vaginal delivery will occur the majority of the time with an adequate pelvis. Spontaneous internal rotation during labor is required to bring the chin to the anterior position, which allows the neck to pass beneath the pubis. Therefore, the patient is allowed to labor spontaneously; a cesarean section is employed for failure to progress or for fetal distress. Manual conversion to vertex, forceps rotation, and internal version are no longer employed in obstetrics to deliver the face presentation because of undue trauma to both the mother and the fetus.

187. The answer is d. (*Scott, pp 438–444.*) The labor portrayed is characteristic of a secondary arrest of dilation. The woman has entered the active phase of labor, as she previously progressed from 4 to 7 cm in less than 2 hours and then remains 7 cm over an additional 2 hours. The multiparous woman normally progresses at a rate of at least 1.5 cm/h (and the nullipara at least 1.2 cm/h) in the active phase. Dilation at a slower rate is a protraction disorder. Primary dysfunction, prolonged latent phase, and hypertonic dysfunction occur prior to the active phase. The best evidence available indicates that this labor is hypotonic. Since the ultrasound indicates a fetus without obvious abnormalities, and since the patient's previous infants were larger than this one, we assume the absence of cephalopelvic disproportion (CPD). Oxytocin is the treatment of choice. If CPD were suspected, then the treatment preferred by many obstetricians would be cesarean section.

188. The answer is c. (*Scott, pp 438–444.*) The best evidence available indicates that this labor is hypotonic. Since the ultrasound indicates a fetus without obvious abnormalities, and since the patient's previous infants were larger than this one, we assume the absence of cephalopelvic disproportion (CPD). Oxytocin is the treatment of choice. If CPD were suspected, then the treatment preferred by many obstetricians would be cesarean section.

189. The answer is e. (*Hankins, pp 106–122.*) Midline episiotomies are easier to fix and have a smaller incidence of surgical breakdown, less pain, and lower blood loss. The incidence of dyspareunia is somewhat less. However, the incidence of extensions of the incision to include the rectum is considerably higher than with mediolateral episiotomies. Regardless of technique, attention to hemostasis and anatomic restoration is the key element of a technically appropriate repair.

190. The answer is d. (*Cunningham, pp 817–819.*) The patient described in the question presents with a classic history for abruption—that is, the sudden onset of abdominal pain accompanied by bleeding. Physical examination reveals a firm, tender uterus with frequent contractions, which confirms the diagnosis. The fact that a clot forms within 4 min suggests that coagulopathy is not present. Because abruption is often accompanied by hemorrhaging, it is important that appropriate fluids (i.e., lactated Ringer solution and whole blood) be administered immediately to stabilize the mother's circulation. Cesarean section may be necessary in the case of a severe abruption, but only when fetal distress is evident or delivery is unlikely to be accomplished vaginally. Internal monitoring equipment should provide an early warning that the fetus is compromised. The internal uterine catheter provides pressure recordings, which are important if oxytocin stimulation is necessary. Generally, however, patients with abruptio placentae are contracting vigorously and do not need oxytocin.

191–193. The answers are 191-d, 192-b, 193-a. (*Cunningham, pp 498–500.*) A woman who has been dilated 9 cm for 3 h is experiencing a secondary arrest in labor. The deteriorating fetal condition (as evidenced, for example, by late decelerations and falling scalp pH) dictates immediate delivery. A forceps rotation would be inappropriate because the cervix is not fully dilated. Cesarean section would be the safest and most expeditious method. Classic cesarean section is rarely used now because of greater blood loss and a higher incidence in subsequent pregnancies of rupture of the scar prior to labor. The best procedure would be a low transverse cesarean section. According to some studies, 25% of twins are diagnosed at the time of delivery. Although sonography or radiography can diagnose multiple gestation early in pregnancy, these methods are not used routinely in all medical centers. The second twin is probably the only remaining situation where internal version is permissible. Although some obstetricians might perform a cesarean section for a second twin presenting as a footling or shoulder, fetal bradycardia dictates that immediate delivery be done, and internal podalic version is the quickest procedure. A transverse lie is undeliverable vaginally. One treatment option is to do nothing and hope that the lie will be longitudinal by the time labor commences. The only other appropriate maneuver would be to perform an external cephalic version. This maneuver should be done in the hospital, with monitoring of the fetal heart. If the version is successful and the cervix is ripe, it might be best to take advantage of the favorable vertex position by rupturing the membranes at that point and inducing labor.

194. The answer is b. (*Cunningham, pp 452, 498–500.*) The multiparous patient is in prolonged latent phase, characterized by painful uterine contractions without significant progression in cervical dilation. Prolongation of the latent phase is defined as 20 h in nulliparous and 14 h in multiparous. The diagnosis of this category of uterine dysfunction is difficult and is made in many cases only in retrospect. Only rarely is there need to resort to oxytocic agents or to cesarean section. The recommended management is meperidine (Demerol) 100 mg intramuscularly; this will allow most patients to rest and wake up in active labor. About 10% of patients will wake up without contractions and the diagnosis of false labor will be made. Only about 5% of patients will wake up after meperidine in the same state of contractions without progression. Epidural block may lead to abnormal labor patterns and to delay of descent of the presenting part.

195. The answer is c. (*Cunningham, pp 452, 498–500.*) This protracted labor is associated with hypotonic uterine dysfunction, a condition that may have been exacerbated by the epidural block. If not contraindicated by other factors (e.g., uterine scar), augmentation of labor by intravenous oxytocin is the treatment of choice in this situation.

196. The answer is e. (*Cunningham, pp 452, 498–500.*) The patient with arrest of descent and secondary arrest of dilation has adequate uterine contractions. Thus there is no reason to attempt to augment these contractions by oxytocin. The small-framed mother and the relatively large fetus may suggest cephalopelvic disproportion (CPD). Arrest disorders, common in CPD, and the absence of head engagement despite cervical dilation also support this diagnosis. The safest way to deliver such a baby would be cesarean section. Early decelerations occur before the onset of the contraction and represent a vagal response to increased intracranial pressure from uterine pressure on the fetal head.

197–200. The answers are 197-d, 198-a, 199-c, 200-d. (*Cunningham, 22/e, pp 477–489.*) Pudendal block is perhaps the most common form of anesthesia used for vaginal delivery. It provides adequate pain relief for episiotomy, spontaneous delivery, forceps delivery, or vacuum extraction. The success of a pudendal block depends on a clear understanding of the anatomy of the pudendal nerve and its surroundings. Complications (vaginal hematomas, retropsoas, or pelvic abscesses) are quite rare. Paracervical block was a popular form of anesthesia for the first stage of labor until it was implicated in several fetal deaths. It has been shown that paracervical block was associated with fetal bradycardia in 25 to 35% of cases, probably the response to rapid uptake of the drug from the highly vascular paracervical space with a resultant reduction of uteroplacental blood flow. Death in some cases was related to direct injection of the local anesthetic into the fetus. Low spinal anesthesia (saddle block) provides prompt and adequate relief for spontaneous and instrument-assisted delivery. The local anesthetic is injected at the level of the L4–L5 interspace with the patient sitting. Although this method is intended to anesthetize the saddle area, the level of anesthesia may sometimes reach as high as T10. Hypotension and a decrease in uteroplacental perfusion are common results of the profound sympathetic blockade caused by spinal anesthesia. Epidural anesthesia provides effective pain relief for the first and second stages of labor and for delivery. It may be associated with late decelerations suggestive of utero-placental insufficiency in as many as 20% of cases, but the frequency of this complication may be reduced by prehydration of the mother and by avoiding the supine position. Epidural block appears to lengthen the second stage of labor and is associated with an increased need for augmentation of labor with oxytocin and for instrument-assisted delivery. In experienced hands, however, epidural anesthesia has an excellent safety record.

201–202. The answers are 201-c, 202-a. *(Beckmann, pp 103, 122–123.)* This patient is most likely experiencing false labor, or Braxton-Hicks contractions. False labor is characterized by contractions that are irregular in timing and duration and that are located in the lower abdomen and do not result in any cervical dilation. In the case of true labor, the uterine contractions occur at regular intervals and tend to become increasingly more intense with time. In true labor, the contractions tend to be felt in the patient's back as well as lower abdomen, and cervical change occurs over time. Active labor occurs when the cervix has reached about 4 cm and there are regular uterine contractions that rapidly dilate the cervix with time. The first stage of labor is the interval between the onset of labor and full cervical dilation. The second stage of labor begins with complete cervical dilation and ends with the delivery of the infant. The latent phase of labor is part of the first stage of labor; it encompasses cervical effacement and early dilation. Since this patient is not in true labor, the best plan of management is to send her home.

203. The answer is d. *(Cunningham, pp 477–491.)* The most appropriate modality for pain control in this patient is administration of an epidural block. An epidural block provides relief from the pain of uterine contractions and delivery. It is accomplished by injecting a local anesthetic agent into the epidural space at the level of the lumbar intervertebral space. An indwelling catheter can be left in place to provide continuous infusion of an anesthetic agent throughout labor and delivery via a volumetric pump. When delivery is imminent, as in the case of this patient, a rapidly acting agent can be administered through the epidural catheter to effect perineal anesthesia. In this patient, intramuscular narcotics such as Demerol or morphine would not be preferred because these agents can cause respiratory depression in the newborn if delivery is imminent. A pudendal block involves local infiltration of the pudendal nerve, which provides anesthesia to the perineum for delivery but no pain relief for uterine contractions. A local block refers to infusing a local anesthetic to the area of an episiotomy. The inhalation of anesthetic gases (general anesthesia) is reserved primarily for situations involving emergent cesarean sections and difficult deliveries. All anesthetic agents that depress the maternal CNS cross the placenta and affect the fetus. In addition, a major complication of general anesthesia is maternal aspiration, which can result in fatal aspiration pneumonitis.

204. The answer is c. (*Cunningham, pp 498–500. Beckmann, pp 116–118.*) Arrest of labor cannot be diagnosed during the first stage of labor until the cervix has reached 4 cm dilation and until adequate uterine contractions (both in frequency and intensity) have been documented. The actual pressure within the uterus cannot be measured via an external tocodynamometer; an intrauterine pressure catheter needs to be placed. It is generally accepted that 200 Montevideo units (number of contractions in 10 min × average contraction intensity in mmHg) are required for normal labor progress. A fetal scalp electrode would need to be placed in cases where the fetal heart rate tracing is difficult to monitor externally. A cesarean section would need to be performed once arrest of labor is diagnosed. Augmentation with Pitocin would be indicated if inadequate uterine contractions are diagnosed via the IUPC. The epidural would need to be rebolused if the patient requires additional pain relief.

205. The answer is a. (*Cunningham, pp 498–500, 519–520. Beckmann, p 127.*) The patient is having adequate uterine contractions as determined by the intrauterine pressure catheter. Therefore, augmentation with Pitocin is not indicated. The patent's diagnosis is secondary arrest of labor, which requires cesarean section. In the active phase of labor, a multiparous patient should undergo dilation of the cervix at a rate of at least 1.5 cm/h if uterine contractions are adequate. There is no indication for the use of vacuum or forceps in this patient because the patient's cervix is not completely dilated and the head is unengaged. Assisted vaginal delivery with vacuum or forceps is indicated when the patient is completely dilated, to augment maternal pushing when maternal expulsive efforts are insufficient to deliver the fetus. It is not recommended to continue to allow the patient to labor if dystocia is diagnosed, because uterine rupture is a potential complication.

206. The answer is b. (*Cunningham, pp 484–485. Beckmann, pp 141–142.*) Prolonged fetal heart rate decelerations are isolated decelerations lasting 2 min or longer, but less than 10 min from onset to return to baseline.

Epidural analgesia is a very common cause of fetal heart rate decelerations because it can be associated with maternal hypotension and decreased placental perfusion. Therefore, maternal blood pressure should always be noted in cases of fetal heart rate decelerations. If maternal blood pressure is abnormally low, ephedrine can be given to correct the hypotension. Because an umbilical cord prolapse can be associated with decelerations, the patient should undergo a cervical exam. In addition, the Pitocin infusion should be stopped because hyperstimulation of the uterus can be a cause of fetal hypoxia. The patient should be turned to the left lateral position to decrease uterine pressure on the great vessels and enhance uteroplacental flow. Supplemental oxygen should be given to the patient in an attempt to increase oxygen to the fetus. Only if the heart rate deceleration persists is a cesarean section performed.

207. The correct answer is a. (*Cunningham, p 517.*) In this clinical scenario, a shoulder dystocia is encountered. A shoulder dystocia occurs when the fetal shoulders fail to spontaneously deliver secondary to impaction of the anterior shoulder against the pubic bone after delivery of the head has occurred. Shoulder dystocia is an obstetric emergency and one should always call for help when such a situation is encountered. A generous episiotomy should always be made to allow the obstetrician to have adequate room to perform a number of manipulations to try to relieve the dystocia. Such maneuvers include the following: suprapubic pressure, McRobert's maneuver (flexing maternal legs upon the abdomen), Wood's corkscrew maneuver (rotating the posterior shoulder), and delivery of the posterior shoulder. There is no role for fundal pressure because this action further impacts the shoulder against the pubic bone and makes the situation worse.

208. The correct answer is a. (*Cunningham, pp 513–514. Beckmann, p 298.*) Shoulder dystocias can be associated with significant fetal morbidity including brachial plexus palsies, clavicular fractures, and humeral fractures. Fractures of the clavicle and humerus usually heal rapidly and are clinically insignificant. Injury to the brachial plexus may be localized to the upper or lower roots. In Erb (or Erb-Duchenne) palsy, the upper roots of the brachial plexus are injured (C5–6), resulting in paralysis of the shoulder and arm muscles; the arm hangs limply to the side and is extended and internally rotated. In the case of Klumpke's paralysis, the lower nerves of the brachial plexus are affected (C7–T1) and the hand is paralyzed.

209. The correct answer is c. (*ACOG, Practice Bulletin 17.*) Indications for an operative vaginal delivery with a vacuum extractor or forceps occur in situations where the fetal head is engaged, the cervix is completely dilated, and there is a prolonged second stage, suspicion of potential fetal compromise, or need to shorten the second stage for maternal benefit. In this situation, all the indications for operative delivery apply. This patient has been pushing for 3 h, which is the definition for prolonged second stage of labor in a nulliparous patient with an epidural. In addition, potential maternal and fetal compromise exists since the patient has the clinical picture of chorioamnionitis and the fetal heart rate is nonreassuring. It is best to avoid cesarean section since it would take more time to achieve and since the patient is infected.

210. The correct answer is e. (*ACOG, Practice Bulletin 17.*) Corneal abrasions and ocular trauma are more common with forceps versus the vacuum unless the vacuum is inadvertently placed over the eye. Vacuum deliveries have a higher rate of neonatal cephalohematomas, retinal hemorrhages, intracranial hemorrhages, and jaundice.

211. The answer is c. (*Beckmann, pp 321–322.*) The Simpson forceps are commonly used in low or outlet forceps deliveries. Kielland forceps are used for midforceps deliveries that involve rotation of the fetal head. Piper forceps are designed to deliver the aftercoming head during a vaginal breech delivery.

212. The answer is c. (*Beckmann, pp 109–112.*) A first-degree tear involves the vaginal mucosa or perineal skin, but not the underlying tissue. In a second-degree episiotomy, the underlying subcutaneous tissue is also involved, but not the rectal sphincter or rectal mucosa. In a third-degree tear, the rectal sphincter is affected. A fourth-degree episiotomy involves a tear that extends into the rectal mucosa.

213. The answer is e. (*Cunningham, p 500.*) This patient is either experiencing prolonged latent labor or is in false labor. The latent phase of labor begins with the onset of regular uterine contractions and is accompanied by progressive but slow cervical dilation. The latent phase ends when the cervical dilation rate reaches about 1.2 cm/h in nulliparous patients and 1.5 cm/h in multiparous patients; this normally occurs when the cervix is about 3 to 4 cm dilated. In nulliparous patients, the latent phase of labor usually lasts less than 20 h (in multiparous patients, it lasts less than 14 h). To correct prolonged latent labor, it is generally recommended that a strong sedative such as morphine be administered to the patient. This is preferred over augmentation with Pitocin or performing an amniotomy, because 10% of patients will actually have been in false labor and these patients will stop contracting after administration of morphine. If a patient truly is in labor, then, after the sedative wears off, she will have undergone cervical change and will have benefited from the rest in terms of having additional energy to proceed with labor. An epidural would not be recommended because the patient may be in false labor. There is no role for cervical ripening in this patient because of the fact that she might be in false labor and can go home and wait for natural cervical ripening if her uterine contractions resolve with a therapeutic rest with morphine.

214–215. The answers are 214-c, 215-a. (*Cunningham, pp 568–579.*) The patient described here has a fetus in the double footling breech presentation. In cases of frank breech presentations, the lower extremities are flexed at the hips and extended at the knees so that the feet lie in close proximity to the head and the fetal buttocks is the presenting part. With a complete breech presentation, one or both knees are flexed. In the case of an incomplete breech presentation, single footling, one hip is not flexed and one foot or knee is lowermost in the birth canal. Because of the risk of a prolapsed cord, it is generally recommended that fetuses with footling breech presentations undergo delivery by cesarean section. External cephalic version is a procedure whereby the presentation of the fetus is changed from breech to cephalic by manipulating the fetus externally through the abdominal wall. It is not indicated in this patient because the membranes are ruptured and the risk of cord prolapse is great. In addition, this procedure generally requires that the uterus be soft and relaxed, which is not the case with this patient in labor. Internal podalic version is a procedure used in the delivery of a second twin. It involves turning the fetus by inserting a hand into the uterus, grabbing both feet, and delivering the fetus by breech extraction.

The Puerperium, Lactation, and Immediate Care of the Newborn

Questions

DIRECTIONS: Each item contains a question followed by suggested responses. Select the **one best** response to each question.

216. A 34-year-old G3P2 delivers a baby by spontaneous vaginal delivery. She had scant prenatal care and no ultrasound, so she is anxious to know the sex of the baby. At first glance you notice female genitalia, but on closer exam the genitalia are ambiguous. Which of the following is the best next step in the evaluation of this infant?

a. Chromosomal analysis
b. Evaluation at 1 month of age
c. Pelvic ultrasound
d. Thorough physical examination
e. Laparotomy for gonadectomy

217. A 24-year-old primigravid woman, who is intent on breast-feeding, decides on a home delivery. Immediately after the birth of a 4.1-kg (9-lb) infant, the patient bleeds massively from extensive vaginal and cervical lacerations. She is brought to the nearest hospital in shock. Over 2 h, 9 units of blood are transfused, and the patient's blood pressure returns to a reasonable level. A hemoglobin value the next day is 7.5 g/dL, and 3 units of packed red blood cells are given. The most likely late sequela to consider in this woman is which of the following?

a. Hemochromatosis
b. Stein-Leventhal syndrome
c. Sheehan syndrome
d. Simmonds syndrome
e. Cushing syndrome

218. A 27-year-old G4P3 at 37 weeks presents to the hospital with heavy vaginal bleeding and painful uterine contractions. Quick bedside ultrasound reveals a fundal placenta. The patient's vital signs are blood pressure 140/92, pulse 118, respiratory rate 20, and temperature 98.6°F. The fetal heart rate tracing reveals tachycardia with decreased variability and a few late decelerations. An emergency cesarean section delivers a male infant with Apgar scores of 4 and 9. With delivery of the placenta, a large retroplacental clot is noted. The patient becomes hypotensive, and bleeding is noted from the wound edges and her IV catheter sites. She requires 12 units of packed red blood cells and fresh frozen plasma for resuscitation. After a short stay in the intensive care unit the patient recovers. When can long-term complications related to sequela of postpartum hemorrhage first be noted?

a. 6 h postpartum
b. 1 week postpartum
c. 1 month postpartum
d. 6 month postpartum
e. 1 year postpartum

219. On postoperative day 3 after an uncomplicated repeat cesarean delivery the patient develops a fever of 100.8°F. She has no complaints except for some fullness in her breasts. On exam she appears in no distress; lung and cardiac exams are normal. Her breast exam reveals full, firm breasts bilaterally slightly tender with no erythema or masses. She is not breast-feeding. The abdomen is soft with firm, nontender fundus at the umbilicus. The lochia appears normal and is nonodorous. Urinalysis and white blood cell count are normal. Which of the following is a characteristic of the cause of her puerperal fever?

a. Appears in less than 5% of postpartum women
b. Appears 3 to 4 days after the development of lacteal secretion
c. Is almost always painless
d. Fever rarely exceeds 37.8°C (99.8°F)
e. Is less severe and less common if lactation is suppressed

220. A 38-year-old G3P3 begins to breast-feed her 5-day-old infant. The baby latches on appropriately and begins to suckle. In the mother, which of the following is a response to suckling?

a. Decrease of oxytocin
b. Increase of prolactin-inhibiting factor
c. Increase of hypothalamic dopamine
d. Increase of hypothalamic prolactin
e. Increase of luteinizing hormone–releasing factor

221. On postpartum day 2 after a vaginal delivery, a 32-year-old G2P2 develops acute shortness of breath and chest pain. Her vital signs are blood pressure 120/80, pulse 130, respiratory rate 32, and temperature 99.8°F. She has new onset of a cough. She appears to be in mild distress. Lung exam reveals clear bases with no rales or rhonchi. The chest pain is reproducible with deep inspiration. Cardiac exam reveals tachycardia with 2/6 systolic ejection murmur. Pulse oximetry reveals an oxygen saturation of 88% on room air. Oxygen suppplementation is initiated, and an arterial blood gas reveals a PaO_2 of 60. Which of the following statements regarding this postpartum patient's condition is true?

a. It is a relatively uncommon phenomenon, with an incidence of about 1 in 5000
b. In most cases, the classic triad of hemoptysis, pleuritic chest pain, and dyspnea suggests the diagnosis
c. A mismatch in ventilation-perfusion scan is pathognomonic for diagnosis
d. The most common finding at physical examination is a pleuritic friction rub

222. A 26-year-old G1P1 is now postoperative day (POD) 6 after a low transverse cesarean delivery for arrest of active phase. On POD 2 the patient developed a fever of 102.2°F and was noted to have uterine tenderness and foul-smelling lochia. She was started on broad-spectrum antibiotic coverage for endometritis. The patient states she feels fine now and wants to go home, but continues to spike fevers each evening. Her lung, breast, and cardiac exams are normal. Her abdomen is nontender with firm, nontender uterus below the umbilicus. On pelvic exam her uterus is appropriately enlarged, but nontender. The adnexa are nontender without masses. Her lochia is normal. Her white blood cell count is 12 with a normal differential. Blood, sputum, and urine cultures are all negative for growth after 3 days. Her chest x-ray is negative. Which of the following statements is true regarding this patient's condition?

a. It usually involves both the iliofemoral and ovarian veins
b. Antimicrobial therapy is usually ineffective
c. Fever spikes are rare
d. Heparin therapy is always needed for resolution of fever
e. Vena caval thrombosis may accompany either ovarian or iliofemoral thrombophlebitis

223. A 24-year-old G1P1 presents for her routine postpartum visit 6 weeks after an uncomplicated vaginal delivery. She states that she is having problems sleeping and is feeling depressed over the past 2 to 3 weeks. She reveals that she cries on most days and feels anxious about taking care of her newborn son. She denies any weight loss or gain, but states she doesn't feel like eating or doing any of her normal activities. She denies suicidal or homocidal ideation. Which of the following is true regarding this patient's condition?

a. A history of depression is not a risk factor for developing postpartum depression
b. Prenatal preventive intervention for patients at high risk for postpartum depression is best managed alone by a mental health professional
c. Young, multiparous patients are at highest risk
d. Postpartum depression is a self-limiting process that lasts for a maximum of 3 months
e. About 10 to 12% of women develop postpartum depression

224. A 35-year-old G3P3 presents to your office 3 weeks after an uncomplicated vaginal delivery. She has been successfully breast-feeding. She complains of chills and a fever to 101°F at home. She states that she feels like she has the flu but denies any sick contacts. She has no medical problems or prior surgeries. The patient denies any medicine allergies. On exam she has a low-grade temperature of 100.4°F and generally appears in no distress. Head, ear, throat, lung, cardiac, abdominal, and pelvic exams are within normal limits. A triangular area of erythema is located in the upper outer quadrant of the left breast. The area is tender to palpation. No masses are felt and no axillary lymphadenopathy is noted. Which of the following is the best option for treatment of this patient?

a. Admission to the hospital for intravenous antibiotics
b. Antipyretic for symptomatic relief
c. Incision and drainage
d. Oral dicloxacillin for 7 to 10 days
e. Oral erythromycin for 7 to 10 days

225. A 22-year-old G1 at 34 weeks is tested for tuberculosis because her father, with whom she lives, was recently diagnosed with tuberculosis. Her skin test is positive and her chest x-ray reveals a granuloma in the upper left lobe. Which of the following is true concerning infants born to mothers with active tuberculosis?

a. The risk of active disease during the first year of life may approach 90% without prophylaxis
b. Bacille Calmette-Guérin (BCG) vaccination of the newborn infant without evidence of active disease is not appropriate
c. Future ability for tuberculin skin testing is lost after BCG administration to the newborn
d. Neonatal infection is most likely acquired by aspiration of infected amniotic fluid
e. Congenital infection is common despite therapy

226. A 21-year-old G1 at 40 weeks, who underwent induction of labor for severe preeclampsia, delivered a 3900-g male infant via vaginal delivery after pushing for 2½ hours. A second-degree midline laceration and side-wall laceration were repaired in the usual fashion under local analgesia. The estimated blood loss was 450 cc. Magnesium sulfate is continued post-partum for the seizure prophylaxis. Six hours after the delivery the patient has difficulty voiding. Which is the most likely cause of her problem?

a. Preeclampsia
b. Infusion of magnesium sulfate
c. Vulvar hematoma
d. Ureteral injury
e. Use of local analgesia for repair

227. A 20-year-old G5P3 has undergone a repeat cesarean delivery. She wants to breast-feed. Her past medical history is significant for bipolar disorder and breast reduction. She is receiving intravenous antibiotics for endometritis. Breast-feeding can be encouraged despite which of the following conditions?

a. Acute maternal hepatitis B
b. Maternal reduction mammoplasty with transplantation of the nipples
c. Maternal treatment with ampicillin
d. Maternal treatment with lithium carbonate
e. Maternal treatment with levofloxacin

228. A 32-year-old G2P2 develops fever and uterine tenderness 2 days after cesarean delivery for nonreassuring fetal heart tones. She is placed on intravenous penicillin and gentamicin for her infection. After 48 hours of antibiotics she remains febrile, and on exam she continues to have uterine tenderness. Which of the following bacteria is resistant to these antibiotics and is likely to be responsible for this woman's infection?

a. *Proteus mirabilis*
b. *Bacteroides fragilis*
c. *Escherichia coli*
d. α streptococci
e. Anaerobic streptococci

229. A 23-year-old G2P2 requires a cesarean delivery for arrest of active phase. During labor she develops chorioamnionitis and is started on ampicillin and gentamicin. The antibiotics are continued after the cesarean delivery. On postoperative day 3 the patient remains febrile and symptomatic with uterine fundal tenderness. No masses are appreciated by pelvic exam. She is successfully breast-feeding and her breast exam is normal. Which antibiotic should be initated to provide better coverage?

a. Cephalothin
b. Polymixin
c. Levofloxacin
d. Vancomycin
e. Clindamycin

230. A 21-year-old G2P2 calls her physician 7 days postpartum because she is concerned that she is still bleeding from the vagina. She describes the bleeding as light pink to bright red and less heavy than the first few days postdelivery. She denies fever or any cramping pain. On exam she is afebrile and has an appropriately sized nontender uterus. The vagina contains about 10 cc of old, dark blood. The cervix is closed. Which of the following is the most appropriate treatment?

a. Antibiotics for endometritis
b. High-dose oral estrogen for placental subinvolution
c. Oxytocin for uterine atony
d. Suction dilation and curettage for retained placenta
e. Reassurance

231. A 28-year-old G2P2 presents to the hospital 2 weeks after vaginal delivery with the complaint of heavy vaginal bleeding that soaks a sanitary napkin every hour. Her pulse is 89, blood pressure 120/76, and temperature 98.9°F. Her abdomen is nontender and her fundus is located above the symphysis pubis. On pelvic exam her vagina contained small blood clots and no active bleeding is noted from the cervix. Her uterus is about 12 to 14 weeks size and nontender. Her cervix is closed. An ultrasound reveals an 8-mm endometrial stripe. Her hemoglobin is 10.9, unchanged from the one at her vaginal delivery. Beta hCG is negative. Which of the following potential treatments would be contraindicated?

a. Methylergonovine maleate (Methergine)
b. Oxytocin injection (Pitocin)
c. Ergonovine maleate (Ergotrate)
d. Prostaglandins
e. Dilation and curettage

232. A 22-year-old G1P0 has just undergone a spontaneous vaginal delivery. As the placenta is being delivered, a red fleshy mass is noted to be protruding out from behind the placenta. Which of the following is the best next step in management of this patient?

a. Begin intravenous oxytocin infusion
b. Call for immediate assistance from other medical personnel
c. Continue to remove the placenta manually
d. Have the anesthesiologist administer magneium sulfate
e. Shove the placenta back into the uterus

233. Following a vaginal delivery, a woman develops a fever, lower abdominal pain, and uterine tenderness. She is alert, and her blood pressure and urine output are good. Large gram-positive rods suggestive of clostridia are seen in a smear of the cervix. Which of the following is most closely tied to a decision to proceed with hysterectomy?

a. Close observation for renal failure or hemolysis
b. Immediate radiographic examination for hydrosalpinx
c. High-dose antibiotic therapy
d. Fever of 103°C
e. Gas gangrene

234. Three days ago you delivered a 40-year-old G1P1 by cesarean section following arrest of descent after 2 hours of pushing. Labor was also significant for prolonged rupture of membranes. The patient had an epidural, which was removed the day following delivery. The nurse pages you to come see the patient on the postpartum floor because she has a fever of 102°F and is experiencing shaking chills. Her BP is 120/70 and her pulse is 120. She has been eating a regular diet without difficulty and had a normal bowel movement this morning. She is attempting to breast-feed, but says her milk has not come in yet. On physical exam, her breasts are mildly engorged and tender bilaterally. Her lungs are clear. Her abdomen is tender over the fundus, but no rebound is present. Her incision has some serous drainage at the right apex, but no erythema is noted. Her pelvic exam reveals uterine tenderness but no masses. Which of the following is the most likely diagnosis?

a. Pelvic abscess
b. Septic pelvic thrombophlebitis
c. Wound infection
d. Endometritis
e. Atelectasis

235. You are called to see a 37-year-old G4P4 for a fever to 101.8°F. She is postoperative day 3 after cesarean delivery for arrest of active-phase labor. She underwent a long induction for postdate pregnancy and had rupture of membranes for more than 18 hours. Her other vital signs include pulse 118, respiratory rate 16, and blood pressure 120/80. She complains of some incisional and abdominal pain, but is otherwise fine. HEENT, lung, breast, and cardiac exams are within normal limits. On abdominal exam she has uterine fundal tenderness. Her incision has mild erythema around the staple edges and serous drainage along the left side. Pelvic exam reveals a tender uterus, but no adnexal masses. Which of the following is the most appropriate antibiotic to treat this patient with initially?

a. Oral Bactrim
b. Oral dicloxacillin
c. Oral ciprofloxacin
d. Intravenous gentamicin
e. Intravenous cefotetan

236. A 34-year-old G1P1 who delivered her first baby 5 weeks ago calls your office and asks to speak with you. She tells you that she is feeling very overwhelmed and anxious. She feels that she cannot do anything right and feels sad throughout the day. She tells you that she finds herself crying all the time and is unable to sleep at night. Which of the following is the most likely diagnosis?

a. Postpartum depression
b. Maternity blues
c. Postpartum psychosis
d. Bipolar disease
e. Postpartum blues

237. You are doing postpartum rounds on a 23-year-old G1P1 who is postpartum day 2 after an uncomplicated vaginal delivery. As you walk in the room you note that she is crying. She states she can't seem to help it. She denies feeling sad or anxious. She has not been sleeping well due to getting up every 2 to 3 hours to breast-feed her new baby. Her past medical history is unremarkable. Which of the following is the most appropriate treatment recommendation?

a. Time and reassurance, because this condition is self-limited
b. Referral to psychiatry for counseling and antidepressant therapy
c. Referral to psychiatry for admission to a psychiatry ward and therapy with Haldol
d. A sleep aid
e. Referral to a psychiatrist who can administer electroconvulsive therapy

238. A 20-year-old G1P1 is postpartum day 2 after an uncomplicated vaginal delivery of a 6-lb 10-oz baby boy. She is trying to decide whether to have you perform a circumcision on her newborn. The boy is in the well-baby nursery and is doing very well. In counseling this patient, you tell her which of the following recommendations from the American Pediatric Association?

a. Circumcisions should be performed routinely because they decrease the incidence of male urinary tract infections
b. Circumcisions should be performed routinely because they decrease the incidence of penile cancer
c. Circumcisions should be performed routinely because they decrease the incidence of sexually transmitted diseases
d. Circumcisions should not be performed routinely because of insufficient data regarding risks and benefits
e. Circumcisions should not be performed routinely because it is a risky procedure and complications such as bleeding and infection are common

239. You are counseling a new mother and father on the risks and benefits of circumcision for their 1-day-old son. The parents ask if you will use analgesia during the circumcision. What do you tell them regarding the recommendations for administering pain medicine for circumcisions?

a. Analgesia is not recommended because there is no evidence that newborns undergoing circumcision experience pain
b. Analgesia is not recommended because it is unsafe in newborns
c. Analgesia in the form of oral Tylenol is the pain medicine of choice recommended for circumcisions
d. Analgesia in the form of a penile block is recommended
e. The administration of sugar orally during the procedure will keep the neonate preoccupied and happy

240. A patient was induced for being postterm at 42³⁄₇ weeks. Immediately following the delivery, you examine the baby with the pediatricians and note the following on physical exam: a small amount of cartilage in the earlobe, occasional creases over the anterior two-thirds of the soles of the feet, 4-mm breast nodule diameter, fine and fuzzy scalp hair, and a scrotum with some but not extensive rugae. Based on this physical exam, what is the approximate gestational age of this male infant?

a. 33 weeks
b. 36 weeks
c. 38 weeks
d. 42 weeks

241. A 40-year-old G4P5 at 39 weeks gestation has progressed rapidly in labor with a reassuring fetal heart rate pattern. She has had an uncomplicated pregnancy with normal prenatal labs including an amniocentesis for advanced maternal age. The patient begins the second stage of labor and after 15 min of pushing starts to demonstrate deep variable heart rate accelerations. You suspect that she may have a fetus with a nuchal cord. You expediently deliver the baby by low-outlet forceps and hand the baby over to the neonatologists called to attend the delivery. As soon as the baby is handed off to the pediatric team, it lets out a strong spontaneous cry. The infant is pink with slightly blue extremities that are actively moving and kicking. The heart rate is noted to be 110 on auscultation. What Apgar score should the pediatricians assign to this baby at 1 min of life?

a. 10
b. 9
c. 8
d. 7
e. 6

242. A 32-year-old G2P1 at 41 weeks is undergoing an induction of oligo-hydramnios. During the course of her labor the fetal heart rate tracing demonstrates severe variable decelerations that do not respond to oxygen, fluid, or amnioinfusion. The patient's cervix is dilated to 4 cm. A low transverse cesarean delivery is performed for nonreassuring fetal heart tones. After delivery of the fetus you send a cord gas, which comes back with the following arterial blood values: pH 7.29, P_{CO_2} 50, and P_{O_2} 20. What condition does the cord blood gas indicate?

a. Normal fetal status
b. Fetal acidemia
c. Fetal hypoxia
d. Fetal asphyxia
e. Fetal metabolic acidosis

243. You are asked to assist in the well-born nursery with neonatal care. Which of the following is a part of routine care in a healthy infant?

a. Administration of ceftriaxone cream to the eyes for prophylaxis for gonorrhea and chlamydia
b. Administration of vitamin A to prevent bleeding problems
c. Administration of hepatitis B vaccination for routine immunization
d. Cool-water bath to remove vernix
e. Placement of a computer chip in left buttock for identification purposes

244. You are making rounds on a 29-year-old G1P1 who underwent an uncomplicated vaginal delivery at term on the previous day. The patient is still very confused about whether she wants to breast-feed. She is a very busy lawyer and is planning on going back to work in 4 weeks, and she does not think that she has the time and dedication that breast-feeding requires. She asks you what you think is best for her to do. Which of the following is an accurate statement regarding breast-feeding?

a. Breast-feeding decreases the time to return of normal menstrual cycles
b. Breast-feeding is associated with a decreased incidence of sudden infant death syndrome
c. Breast-feeding is a poor source of nutrients for required infant growth
d. Breast-feeding is associated with an increased incidence of childhood obesity
e. Breast-feeding is associated with a decreased incidence of childhood attention deficit disorder

245. A 22-year-old G1P1 who is postpartum day 2 and is bottle-feeding complains that her breasts are very engorged and tender. She wants you to give her something to make the engorgement go away. Which of the following is recommended to relieve her symptoms?

a. Breast binder
b. Bromocriptine
c. Estrogen-containing contraceptive pills
d. Pump her breasts
e. Use oral antibiotics

246. A 36-year-old G1P1 comes to see you for a routine postpartum exam 6 weeks after an uncomplicated vaginal delivery. She is currently nursing her baby without any major problems and wants to continue to do so for at least 9 months. She is ready to resume sexual activity and wants to know what her options are for birth control. She does not have any medical problems. She is a nonsmoker and is not taking any medications except for her prenatal vitamins. Which of the following methods may decrease her milk supply?

a. Intrauterine device
b. Progestin only pill
c. Depo-Provera
d. Combination oral contraceptives
e. Foam and condoms

247. A 30-year-old G3P3 who is 8 weeks postpartum and regularly breast-feeding calls you and is very concerned because she is having pain with intercourse secondary to vaginal dryness. Which of the following should you recommend to help her with this problem?

a. Instruct her to stop breast-feeding
b. Apply hydrocortisone cream to the perineum
c. Apply testosterone cream to the vulva and vagina
d. Apply estrogen cream to the vagina and vulva
e. Apply petroleum jelly to the perineum

248. A 25-year-old G1P1 comes to see you 6 weeks after an uncomplicated vaginal delivery for a routine postpartum exam. She denies any problems and has been breast-feeding her newborn without any difficulties since leaving the hospital. During the bimanual exam, you note that her uterus is irregular, firm, nontender, and about a 15-week size. Which of the following is the most likely etiology for this enlarged uterus?

a. Subinvolution of the uterus
b. The uterus is appropriate size for 6 weeks postpartum
c. Fibroid uterus
d. Adenomyosis
e. Endometritis

249. A 39-year-old G3P3 comes to see you on day 5 after a second repeat cesarean delivery. She is concerned because her incision has become very red and tender and pus started draining from a small opening in the incision this morning. She has been experiencing general malaise and reports a fever of 102°F. Physical exam indicates that the Pfannenstiel incision is indeed erythematous and is open about 1 cm at the left corner, and is draining a small amount of purulent liquid. There is tenderness along the wound edges. Which of the following is the best next step in the management of this patient?

a. Apply Steri-Strips to close the wound
b. Administer antifungal medication
c. Probe the fascia
d. Take the patient to the OR for debridement and closure of the skin

250. A 30-year-old G3P3 is postoperative day 4 after a repeat cesarean delivery. During the surgery she received 2 units of packed red blood cells for a hemorrhage related to uterine atony. She is to be discharged home today. She complains of some yellowish drainage from her incision and redness that just started earlier in the day. She states that she feels feverish. She is breast-feeding. Her past medical history is significant for type 2 diabetes mellitus and chronic hypertension. She weighs 110 kg. Her vital signs are temperature 100.1°F, pulse 69, respiratory rate 18, and blood pressure is 143/92. Breast, lung, and cardiac exams are normal. Her midline vertical skin incision is erythematous and has a foul-smelling purulent discharge from the lower segment of the wound. It is tender to touch. The uterine fundus is not tender. Which of the following is not a risk factor for her condition?

a. Diabetes
b. Corticosteroid therapy
c. Preoperative antibiotic administration
d. Anemia
e. Obesity

The Puerperium, Lactation, and Immediate Care of the Newborn

Answers

216. The answer is d. (*Speroff, pp 350–354.*) Ambiguous genitalia at birth is a medical emergency, not only for psychological reasons for the parents but also because hirsute female infants with congenital adrenal hyperplasia (CAH) may die if undiagnosed. CAH is an autosomally inherited disease of adrenal failure that causes hyponatremia and hyperkalemia because of lack of mineralocorticoids. A thorough physical examination is the best initial evaluation. While it will not give the definitive diagnosis of the sex, it can provide clues. Are the gonads palpable in the inguinal canal? Are the labia fused? Is there a vagina or pouch. Is there hyper- or hypotension, or signs of dehydration. Karyotype, electrolyte analysis, blood or urine assays for progesterone, 17α-hydroxyprogesterone, and serum androgens such as dehydroepiandrosterone sulfate are essential to the workup. Pelvic ultrasound or MRI can detect ovaries or undescended testes, but that is not the first step in management. Laparotomy or laparoscopy is sometimes necessary for ectopic gonadectomy after puberty has occurred.

217–218. The answers are 217-c, 218-b. (*Cunningham, pp 825–826.*) A disadvantage of home delivery is the lack of facilities to control postpartum hemorrhage. The woman described in the question delivered a large baby, suffered multiple soft tissue injuries, and went into shock, needing 9 units of blood by the time she reached the hospital. Sheehan syndrome seems a likely possibility in this woman. This syndrome of anterior pituitary necrosis related to obstetric hemorrhage can be diagnosed by 1 week postpartum, as lactation fails to commence normally. Although many modern women choose hormonal therapy to prevent lactation, the woman described in the question was intent on breast-feeding and so would not have received suppressant. She therefore could have been expected to begin lactation at the usual time. Other symptoms of Sheehan syndrome include amenorrhea, atrophy of the breasts, and loss of thyroid and adrenal function. The other presented choices for late sequelae are rather far-fetched. Hemochromatosis would not be expected to occur in this healthy young woman, especially since she did not receive prolonged transfusions. Cushing, Simmonds, and Stein-Leventhal syndromes are not known to be related to postpartum hemorrhage. It is important to note that home delivery is not a predisposing factor to postpartum hemorrhage.

219. The answer is e. (*James, pp 766–770.*) Puerperal fever from breast engorgement is relatively uncommon, affecting 13 to 18% of postpartum women. It appears 24 to 48 h following initiation of lacteal secretion and ranges from 38 to 39°C (100.4 to 102.2°F). Pain is an early and common symptom. Treatment consists of breast support, ice packs, and pain relievers. The incidence and severity of breast engorgement are lower if treatment is given for suppression of lactation.

220. The answer is d. (*Cunningham, pp 699–704.*) The normal sequence of events triggered by suckling is as follows: through a response of the central nervous system, dopamine is decreased in the hypothalamus. Dopamine suppression decreases production of prolactin-inhibiting factor (PIF), which normally travels through a portal system to the pituitary gland; because PIF production is decreased, production of prolactin by the pituitary is increased. At this time, the pituitary also releases oxytocin, which causes milk to be expressed from the alveoli into the lactiferous ducts. Suckling suppresses the production of luteinizing hormone–releasing factor and, as a result, acts as a mild contraceptive (because the midcycle surge of luteinizing hormone does not occur).

221. The answer is a. (*Cunningham, pp 1084–1088.*) The reported incidence of postpartum pulmonary embolism (PE) is 1 in 2700 to 1 in 7000. The classic triad—hemoptysis, pleuritic chest pain, and dyspnea—appears in only 20% of cases. The most common sign on physical examination is tachypnea (>16 breaths/min). Ventilation-perfusion scans with large perfusion defects and ventilation mismatches support the putative diagnosis of PE, but this finding can also be seen with atelectasis or other disorders of lung aeration. To confirm the diagnosis in doubtful cases, there may be a need for pulmonary angiography. Conversely, a normal ventilation-perfusion scan suggests that massive PE is not the etiology of the clinical symptoms.

222. The answer is e. *(Cunningham, pp 718–719.)* Septic thrombophlebitis may involve either the iliofemoral or the ovarian vein but rarely involves both sites in the same patient. Vena caval thrombosis may follow either ovarian or iliofemoral phlebitis. The clinical presentation is that of a pelvic infection with pain and fever. Following antimicrobial therapy, clinical symptoms usually resolve, but fever spikes may continue. Commonly, patients do not appear clinically ill. The diagnosis is made by computerized tomography (CT) or by magnetic resonance imaging (MRI). Before these diagnostic modalities were available, the heparin challenge test was advocated—lysis of fever after intravenous administration of heparin was accepted as diagnostic for pelvic thrombophlebitis. It seems, however, that the course of clinical symptoms is not changed significantly by administration of heparin.

223. The answer is e. *(Cunningham, pp 705–706.)* Patients at high risk for postpartum depression often have histories of depression or postpartum depression. They are more likely to be primiparous or older; they may have had a long interval between pregnancies or an unplanned pregnancy or be without a supportive partner. Prenatal intervention must include the obstetric team, with family or peer support when possible. Postpartum depression is variable in duration, but occasionally will not resolve without hospitalization, therapy, or medication.

224. The answer is d. *(Ransom, 2000, pp 172–174.)* Puerperal mastitis may be subacute, but is often characterized by chills, fever, and tachycardia. If undiagnosed, it may progress to suppurative mastitis with abscess formation that requires drainage. The most common offending organism is *Staphylococcus aureus,* which is probably transmitted from the infant's nose and throat. A culture of the breast milk should be done prior to initiation of antibiotic therapy. Dicloxacillin, a penicillinase-resistant antibiotic, is the initial treatment of choice. In penicillin-allergic patients, erythromycin is recommended. Treatment should last for 7 to 10 days. If a mass is palpable, an abscess should be suspected. Incision and drainage is recommended for a breast abscess. The patient should continue to breast-feed on the affected breast; if it is too painful she may pump. After antibiotic therapy is initiated the patient should be reevaluated to ensure improvement.

225. The answer is c. (*Cunningham, pp 1064–1066.*) The goal of management in the infant born to a mother with active tuberculosis is prevention of early neonatal infection. Congenital infection, acquired either by a hematogenous route or by aspiration of infected amniotic fluid, is rare. Most neonatal infections are acquired by postpartum maternal contact. The risk of active disease during the first year of life may approach 50% if prophylaxis is not instituted. BCG vaccination and daily isonicotinic acid hydrazide (isoniazid, INH) therapy are both acceptable means of therapy. BCG vaccination may be easier because it requires only one injection; however, the ability to perform future tuberculin skin testing is lost.

226. The answer is c. (*Cunningham, pp 836–837.*) An inability to void often leads to the diagnosis of a vulvar hematoma. Such hematomas are often large enough to apply pressure on the urethra. Pain from urethral lacerations is another reason women have difficulty voiding after delivery. Both epidural anesthesia, which can cause urinary retention, and oxytocin, which has an antidiuretic effect, can lead to an overdistended bladder and an inability to void. In this case an indwelling catheter should be inserted and left in for at least 24 h to allow recovery of normal bladder tone and sensation. Preeclampsia often leads to edema, which generally leads to diuresis postpartum.

227. The answer is c. (*James, pp 766–770.*) There are very few contraindications to breast-feeding. In acute viral infections, such as hepatitis B, there is the possibility of transmitting the virus in the milk. Most medications taken by the mother enter into breast milk, usually in concentrations similar to or less than those in maternal plasma. Breast-feeding is inadvisable when the mother is being treated with antimitotic drugs, tetracyclines, diagnostic or therapeutic radioactive substances, or lithium carbonate. Acute puerperal mastitis may be managed quite successfully while the mother continues to breast-feed. Reduction mammoplasty with autotransplantation of the nipple simply makes breast-feeding impossible.

228–229. The answers are 228-b, 229-e. (*Gleicher, pp 584–594.*) Infections caused by *B. fragilis,* a gram-negative anaerobic bacillus, are a significant obstetric problem. Not only is the organism resistant to many commonly used antibiotics (including penicillin and gentamicin), but it is difficult to isolate, culture, and identify as well. The high incidence of gynecologic and obstetric

B. fragilis infections may be due to the pathogen's predominance among the anaerobic bacteria of the lower bowel. Although the other organisms listed in the question can also cause postpartum infection, they are sensitive to antibiotic therapy with penicillin and gentamicin. Clindamycin is the most effective antibiotic for treating women who have bacteroidosis. Clindamycin should be used for the treatment of infections after cesarean delivery. Chloramphenicol and tetracycline are alternative choices for antibiotic therapy in nonpregnant women; however, tetracycline-resistant strains of *B. fragilis* may be emerging. Lincomycin and erythromycin can also be effective in the management of affected women. Tetracyclines and flouroquinolones should be avoided in breast-feeding women.

230. The answer is e. (*Cunningham, p 696.*) Bloody lochia can persist for up to 2 weeks without indicating an underlying pathology; however, if bleeding continues beyond 2 weeks, it may indicate placental site subinvolution, retention of small placental fragments, or both. At this point, appropriate diagnostic and therapeutic measures should be initiated. The physician should first estimate the blood loss and then perform a pelvic examination in search of uterine subinvolution or tenderness. Excessive bleeding or tenderness should lead the physician to suspect retained placental fragments or endometritis. A larger than expected but otherwise asymptomatic uterus supports the diagnosis of subinvolution.

231. The answer is e. (*Cunningham, p 698.*) Uterine hemorrhage after the first postpartum week is most often the result of retained placental fragments or subinvolution of the placental site. Curettage may do more harm than benefit by stimulating increased bleeding. Initial therapy should be aimed at decreasing the bleeding by stimulating uterine contractions with the use of Pitocin, Methergine, or Ergotrate. Prostaglandins could also be used in this setting.

232. The answer is b. (*Hankins, pp 273–279.*) This patient has a uterine inversion. Summon assistance immediately, including an anesthesiologist. Ensure that the patient has adequate IV access and that blood is available if needed. If attached, the placenta is not removed until the infusion systems are operational, fluids are being given, and anesthesia (preferably halothane) has been administered. To remove the placenta before this time increases hemorrhage. As soon as the uterus is restored to its normal configuration, the anesthetic agent used to provide relaxation is stopped and simultaneously oxytocin is started to contract the uterus.

233. The answer is e. (*Cunningham, pp 713–715, 996.*) Clostridia can be seen in 5 to 10% of pelvic cultures. When the organism is found, appropriate antibiotic therapy (e.g., with penicillin) and close observation for gas gangrene, hemolysis, and renal failure are in order. Presumed identification on the basis of Gram stain alone or the presence of mild infection without signs of sepsis or extrauterine involvement is not reason enough to proceed to hysterectomy.

234. The answer is d. (*Beckmann, pp 157–158, 183–188. Cunningham, pp 712–715.*) Metritis, or infection of the uterus, is the most common infection that occurs after a cesarean section. A long labor and prolonged rupture of membranes are predisposing factors for metritis. In the presence of a pelvic abscess, usually signs of peritoneal irritation such as rebound tenderness, ileus, and decreased bowel sounds are present. Wound infections occur with an incidence of about 6% following cesarean deliveries. Fever usually begins on the fourth or fifth postoperative day, and erythema around the incision along with pus drainage is often present. In the case of a wound infection, first-line treatment involves draining the incision. Atelectasis can be a cause of postoperative fever, but the fever occurs generally in the first 24 h. In addition, on physical exam, atelectasis is generally accompanied by decreased breath sounds at the lung bases on auscultation. It more commonly occurs in women who have had general anesthesia, not an epidural like the patient described here. Septic pelvic thrombophlebitis occurs uncommonly as a sequela of pelvic infection. Venous stasis occurs in dilated pelvic veins; in the presence of bacteria, it can lead to septic thromboses. Diagnosis is usually made when persistent fever spikes occur after treatment for metritis. The patient usually has no uterine tenderness, and bowel function tends to be normal. Treatment is with intravenous heparin.

235. The answer is e. (*Beckmann, pp 185–186. Cunningham, pp 713–715.*) The etiology of metritis, like that of all pelvic infections, is polymicrobial. Therefore, the antibiotic coverage selected should treat aerobic and anaerobic organisms. Common aerobes associated with metritis are staphylococci, streptococci, enterococci, *Escherichia coli*, *Proteus*, and *Klebsiella*. The anaerobic organisms associated with pelvic infections are most commonly

Bacteroides, Peptococcus, Peptostreptococcus, and *Clostridium.* Generally, a broad-spectrum antibiotic, such as the cephalosporins cefotetan or cefoxitin, is administered intravenously. The antibiotic therapy is generally continued until the patient has been afebrile for at least 24 h. Bactrim is a sulfa drug that is commonly given orally to treat uncomplicated urinary tract infections. Dicloxacillin is commonly used orally to treat women with mastitis because it has good coverage against *Staphylococcus aureus,* which is the most common organism responsible for this infection. Ciprofloxacin, a quinolone, is useful in the treatment of complicated urinary tract infections. This medication is not recommended for pregnant or lactating women because animal studies show an association of fluoroquinolones with irreversible arthropathy.

236. The answer is a. *(Beckmann, pp 159–160. Cunningham, pp 1241–1245.)* This patient is exhibiting classic symptoms of postpartum depression. Postpartum depression develops in about 8 to 15% of women and generally is characterized by an onset about 2 weeks to 12 months postdelivery and an average duration of 3 to 14 months. Women with postpartum depression have the following symptoms: irritability, labile mood, difficulty sleeping, phobias, and anxiety. About 50% of women experience postpartum blues, or maternity blues, within 3 to 6 days after delivering. This mood disturbance is thought to be precipitated by progesterone withdrawal following delivery and usually resolves in 10 days. Maternity blues is characterized by mild insomnia, tearfulness, fatigue, irritability, poor concentration, and depressed affect. Postpartum psychosis usually has its onset within a few days of delivery and is characterized by confusion, disorientation, and loss of touch with reality. Postpartum psychosis is very rare and occurs in only 1 to 4 in 1000 births. Bipolar disorder or manic-depressive illness is a psychiatric disorder characterized by episodes of depression followed by mania.

237. The answer is a. *(Beckmann, pp 159–161. Cunningham, p 1243.)* Women experiencing postpartum blues usually do fine with reassurance alone, because this condition usually resolves spontaneously in a short period of time. Women with postpartum depression need referral to a psychiatrist who can administer psychotherapy and prescribe antidepressants. Haldol is an antipsychotic that might be administered in the treatment of postpartum psychosis. Sleep aids are not recommended. Electroconvulsive therapy would be used to treat depression only if a patient were unresponsive to pharmacologic therapy.

238. The answer is d. (*ACOG, Committee Opinion 260. Cunningham, 22/e, pp 643–644.*) The American Academy of Pediatrics and the American College of Obstetrics and Gynecology do not recommend that routine circumcision procedures be performed on newborn male infants. It is generally agreed that circumcision results in a decreased incidence of penile cancer, but there are no well-designed studies that indicate that circumcision results in a decreased incidence of urinary tract infections in babies or a decreased incidence of sexually transmitted diseases. When performed by an experienced person on a healthy, stable infant, circumcisions are generally safe procedures, although potential complications include infection and bleeding. Parents should discuss the risks and benefits of the procedure and obtain informed consent.

239. The answer is d. (*ACOG, Committee Opinion 260.*) Analgesia should always be provided to a newborn undergoing a circumcision procedure, because much evidence suggests that infants who undergo this procedure without pain medicine experience pain and stress. The administration of oral Tylenol or sucrose is not adequate for operative pain relief. Topical lidocaine cream, dorsal penile nerve block, and subcutaneous ring block are all effective and safe modalities to achieve analgesia in newborns undergoing a circumcision procedure.

240. The answer is c. (*Cunningham, p 642.*) An estimate of the gestational age of a newborn can be made rapidly by a physical exam immediately following delivery. Important physical characteristics that are evaluated are the sole creases, breast nodules, scalp hair, earlobes, and scrotum. In newborns who are 39 weeks gestational age or more, the soles of the feet will be covered with creases, the diameter of the breast nodules will be at least 7 mm, the scalp hair will be coarse and silky, the earlobes will be thickened with cartilage, and the scrotum will be full with extensive rugae. In infants that are 36 weeks or less, there will be an anterior transverse sole crease only, the breast nodule diameter will be 2 mm, the scalp hair will be fine and fuzzy, the earlobes will be pliable and lack cartilage, and the scrotum will be small with few rugae. In infants of gestational age between 37 and 38 weeks, the soles of the feet will have occasional creases on the anterior two-thirds of the feet, the breast nodule diameter will be 4 mm, the scalp hair will be fine and fuzzy, the earlobes will have a small amount of cartilage, and the scrotum will have some but not extensive rugae.

241. The answer is b. (*Cunningham, pp 637–638.*) The Apgar scoring system, applied at 1 min and again at 5 min, was developed as an aid to evaluate infants who require resuscitation. Heart rate, respiratory effort, muscle tone, reflex, irritability, and color are the five components of the Apgar score. A score of 0, 1, or 2 is given for each of the five components, and the total is added up to give one score. The table below demonstrates the scoring system.

Sign	0 Points	1 Point	2 Points
Heart rate	Absent	Below 100	Over 100
Respiratory effort	Absent	Slow, irregular	Good, crying
Muscle tone	Flaccid	Some extremity flexion	Active motion
Reflex irritability	No response	Grimace	Vigorous cry
Color	Blue, pale	Body pink, extremities blue	Completely pink

The baby described here receives an Apgar score of 9. One point is deducted for the baby not being completely pink and having blue extremities.

242. The answer is a. (*Cunningham, pp 638–639. Beckmann, p 147.*) The blood gas results described in this case are normal. Normal values for umbilical arterial samples are pH 7.25 to 7.3, P_{CO_2} 50 mmHg, P_{O_2} 20 mmHg, and bicarbonate 25 mEq. Acidemia is generally defined as a pH less than 7.20. Birth asphyxia generally refers to hypoxic injury so severe that the umbilical artery pH is less than 7.0, a persistent Apgar score is between 0 and 3 for more than 5 min, neonatal sequelae exist such as seizures or coma, and there is multiorgan dysfunction.

243. The answer is c. (*Cunningham, pp 641–642.*) The Centers for Disease Control recommends that all newborns receive routine immunization against hepatitis B prior to being discharged from the hospital. Only if the mother is positive for hepatitis B surface antigen should the neonate also be passively immunized with hepatitis B immune globulin. According to the Centers for Disease Control, all newborns should receive eye prophylaxis against chlamydia and gonorrhea with either silver nitrate, erythromycin ophthalmic ointment, or tetracycline ophthalmic ointment. Vitamin K is routinely administered to prevent hemorrhagic disease of the newborn;

breast milk contains only very small amounts of Vitamin K. Since the temperature of newborns drops very rapidly after birth, newly delivered infants must be monitored in a warm crib. All infants must be accurately identified via identification bands.

244. The answer is b. (*Cunningham, pp 699–704.*) According to the American Academy of Pediatrics, some of the benefits of nursing include a decrease in infant diarrhea, urinary tract infections, ear infections, and death from sudden infant death syndrome. Human milk is ideal food for neonates. It provides species- and age-specific nutrients for the baby. It has immunological factors and antibacterial properties and contains factors that act as biological signals to promote cellular growth. Breast-feeding can delay the resumption of ovulation and menses.

245. The answer is a. (*Cunningham, p 703.*) About 40% of women elect not to breast-feed. These women experience milk leakage, engorgement, and breast pain that begins 3 to 5 days postpartum. Ice packs applied to the breasts, a well-fitting bra or binder, and analgesics are all appropriate methods to manage engorged breasts. Bromocriptine, a drug used to lower prolactin levels and suppress lactation, is no longer recommended in postpartum women due to this medication being associated with an increased risk of stroke, myocardial infarctions, seizures, and psychiatric disturbances.

246. The answer is d. (*Beckmann, p 156.*) Use of an IUD, barrier methods, and hormonal contraceptive agents containing progestins are all appropriate methods of birth control for breast-feeding women. It is best for nursing mothers to avoid estrogen-containing contraceptives because estrogen preparations can inhibit lactation or decrease milk supply.

247. The answer is d. (*Beckmann, p 157. Droegemueller, p 902.*) Coitus can be painful in breast-feeding women because of an increase in vaginal dryness that is due to an associated hypoestrogenism. Water-soluble lubricants or estrogen cream applied topically to the vaginal mucosa can be helpful. In addition, the female superior position may be recommended during intercourse so that the woman can control the depth of penile penetration. Testosterone cream is sometimes used in postmenopausal women with vulvar atrophy, primarily in cases of lichen sclerosis. The side effects of local testosterone cream are clitoral hypertrophy and increased hair growth.

248. The answer is c. (*Cunningham, p 697. Beckmann, pp 409–410, 571.*) The uterus achieves its previous nonpregnant size by about 4 weeks postpartum. Subinvolution (cessation of the normal involution) of the uterus can occur in cases of retained placenta or uterine infection. In such cases, the uterus is larger and softer than it should be on bimanual exam. In addition, the patient usually experiences prolonged discharge and excessive uterine bleeding. With endometritis, the patient will also have a tender uterus on exam, and will complain of fever and chills. In adenomyosis, portions of the endometrial lining grow into the myometrium, causing menorrhagia and dysmenorrhea. On physical exam, the uterus is usually tender to palpation, boggy, and symmetrically enlarged. The patient described here has a physical exam most consistent with fibroids. Uterine leiomyomas would cause the uterus to be firm, irregular, and enlarged.

249–250. The answer is 249-c, 250-c. (*Cunningham, p 716. Beckmann, p 187.*) The incidence of incisional wound infection following cesarean delivery is approximately 6%. Risk factors that predispose to wound infections include obesity, diabetes, corticosteroid therapy, anemia, poor hemostasis, and immunosuppression. The use of preoperative prophylactic antibiotics decreases the incidence of wound infection to about 2%. Usually, incisional abscesses will cause a fever about postoperative day 4, and erythema, induration, and drainage from the incision are also frequently noted. Opening of the incision and surgical drainage are key to curing the infection. Broad-spectrum antimicrobial agents are also administered. In all cases of wound infection, the incision must be probed to rule out a wound dehiscence (separation of the wound involving the fascial layer). As long as the fascial layer is intact, the open wound is kept clean and allowed to heal by secondary intention.

Gynecology

Preventive Care and Health Maintenance

Questions

DIRECTIONS: Each of the items below contains a question followed by suggested responses. Select the **one best** response to each question.

251. A 75-year-old G2P2 presents to your GYN office for a routine exam. She tells you that she does not have an internist and does not remember the last time she had a physical exam. She says she is very healthy and denies taking any medication, including hormone replacement therapy. She is a nonsmoker and has an occasional cocktail with her dinner. She does not have any complaints. In addition, she denies any family history of cancer. The patient tells you that she is a widow and lives alone in an apartment in town. Her grown children have families of their own and live far away. She states that she is self-sufficient and spends her time visiting friends and volunteering at a local museum. Her blood pressure is 140/70. Her height is 5 ft 4 in. and she weighs 130 lb. Her physical exam is completely normal. Which of the following are the most appropriate screening tests to order for this patient?

a. Pap smear and mammogram
b. Pap smear, mammogram, and colonoscopy
c. Pap smear, mammogram, colonoscopy, and bone densitometry
d. Pap smear, mammogram, colonoscopy, bone densitometry, and TB skin test
e. Pap smear, mammogram, colonoscopy, bone densitometry, TB skin test, and auditory testing

252. A 72-year-old G5P5 presents to your office for well-woman exam. Her last exam was 7 years ago when she turned 65. She has routine checks and labs with her internist each year. Her last mammogram was 6 months ago and was normal. She takes a diuretic for hypertension. She is a retired school teacher. Her physical exam is normal. Which of the following is the best vaccination to recommend to this patient?

a. Diphtheria-pertussis
b. Hepatitis B vaccine
c. Influenza vaccine
d. Measles-mumps-rubella
e. Pneumocystis

253. A 65-year-old G3P3 presents to your office for annual checkup. She had her last well-woman exam 20 years before when she had a hysterectomy for fibroids. She denies any medical problems, except some occasional stiffness in her joints early in the morning. She takes a multivitamin daily. Her family history is significant for cardiac disease in both her parents and breast cancer in a maternal aunt at the age of 42 years of age. Her physical exam is normal. Which of the following is the most appropriate set of laboratory tests to order for this patient?

a. Lipid profile and fasting blood sugar
b. Lipid profile, fasting blood sugar, and TSH
c. Lipid profile, fasting blood sugar, TSH, and CA-125
d. Lipid profile, fasting blood sugar, TSH, and urinalysis
e. Lipid profile, fasting blood sugar, TSH, urinalysis, and CA-125

254. You are following up on the results of routine testing of a 68-year-old G4P3 for her well-woman examination. Her physical examination was normal for a postmenopausal woman. Her Pap smear revealed parabasal cells, her mammogram was normal, lipid profile was normal, and the urinalysis shows hematuria. Which of the following is the most appropriate next step in the management of this patient?

a. Colposcopy
b. Endometrial biopsy
c. Renal sonogram
d. Urine culture
e. No further treatment/evaluation is necessary if the patient is asymptomatic

255. A 74-year-old woman presents to your office for well-woman exam. Her last Pap smear and mammogram were 3 years ago. She has hypertension, high cholesterol, and osteoarthritis. She stopped smoking 15 years ago, and denies alcohol use. What is the leading cause of death in women of this patient's age?

a. Alzheimer's disease
b. Breast cancer
c. Cerebrovascular disease
d. Heart disease
e. Lung cancer
f. Trauma

256. A 16-year-old G0 female presents to your office for a routine annual gynecologic exam. She reports that she has previously been sexually active, but currently is not dating anyone. She has had three sexual partners in the past and says she diligently used condoms. She is a senior in high school and is doing well academically and has many friends. She lives at home with her parents and a younger sibling. She denies any family history of medical problems, but says her 80-year-old grandmother was recently diagnosed with breast cancer. She denies any other family history of cancer. She says she is healthy and has no history of medical problems or surgeries. She reports having had chickenpox. She smokes tobacco and drinks beer occasionally, but denies any illicit drug use. She had her first Pap smear and gynecologic exam last year with another doctor and reports that everything was normal. Her menses started at age 13 and are regular and light. She denies any dysmenorrhea. Her blood pressure is 90/60. Her height is 5 ft 6 in. and she weighs 130 lb. What is the leading cause of death in teenagers?

a. Suicide
b. Homicide
c. Motor vehicle accidents
d. Cancer
e. Heart disease

257. A 17-year-old G1P1 presents to your office for her yearly well-woman exam. She had an uncomplicated vaginal delivery last year. She has been sexually active for the past 4 years and has had 6 different sexual partners. Her menses occurs every 28 days and lasts for 4 days. She denies any intermenstrual spotting, postcoital bleeding, or vaginal discharge. She denies tobacco, alcohol, or illicit drug use. Which of the following are appropriate screening tests for this patient?

a. Pap test
b. Pap test and gonorrhea and chlamydia cervical cultures
c. Pap test and herpes simplex cultures
d. Pap test and hemoglobin level assessment
e. Pap test and hepatitis C antibody

258. A 15-year-old woman presents to your office for her first well-woman exam. She denies any medical problems or prior surgeries. She had chickenpox at age 4. Her menses started at the age of 12 and are regular. She has recently become sexually active with her 16-year-old boyfriend. She states that they use condoms for contraception. Her physical exam is normal. You obtain Pap smear and cervical cultures and order the appropriate laboratory testing. Which of the following vaccines is appropriate to administer to this patient?

a. Hepatitis A vaccine
b. Pneumococcal vaccine
c. Varicella vaccine
d. Hepatitis B vaccine
e. Influenza vaccine

259. A 16-year-old woman presents to your office for her well-woman exam. She denies any medical problems or prior surgeries. She states that her cycles are monthly. She is sexually active and uses oral contraceptive pills for birth control. Her physical exam is normal. As part of preventive health maintenance you recommend breast self-examination and instruct the patient how to do it. Which of the following is the best frequency and time to perform breast self-examinations?

a. Monthly, in the week prior to the start of the menstrual cycle
b. Monthly, in the week after cessation of menstrual cycle
c. Monthly, during the menstrual cycle
d. Every three months, in the week prior to the start of the menstrual cycle
e. Every six months, in the week prior to the start of the menstrual cycle

260. A 15-year-old woman presents to your office for her first well-woman exam. She has a history of asthma, for which she uses an inhaler as needed. She denies any prior surgeries. Her menses started at the age of 13 and are regular. She has recently become sexually active with her 17-year-old boyfriend. She states that they use condoms for contraception, but she is interested in something more effective. Which of the following is the most appropriate instrument to use when performing the Pap smear test in this patient?

a. Graves speculum
b. Pederson speculum
c. Pediatric speculum
d. Vaginoscope
e. Nasal speculum

261. A married 41-year-old G5P3114 presents to your office for a routine exam. This patient has been married for 20 years and is very happy being a stay-at-home mom. She is healthy and denies any medical problems except migraine headaches that are sometimes exacerbated by her menses. She reports that all her pregnancies were uncomplicated except for the development of gestational diabetes when she was pregnant with her last child. She drinks alcohol socially, and admits to smoking occasionally. She reports that her menses are regular and denies any dysmenorrhea or PMS. When questioned about her family history, she states that she thinks her grandmother was diagnosed with ovarian cancer when she was in her fifties. She denies a family history of any other cancers or medical diseases. She is tired of using condoms for contraception, and wants to discuss her options for birth control with you. She and her husband are sure that they do not want to have additional children in the future. Her BP is 140/90; height is 5 ft 5 in.; weight is 150 lb. Which of the following is the most common cause of death in women of this patient's age?

a. HIV
b. Cardiac disease
c. Accidents
d. Suicide
e. Cancer

262. A 44-year-old G6P3215 presents for her well-woman exam. She tells you that all of her deliveries were vaginal and that her largest child weighed 2900 g at birth. How many full-term pregnancies did this patient have?

a. 1
b. 2
c. 3
d. 5
e. 6

263. A 40-year-old G3P2012 presents for her well-woman exam. She has had two vaginal deliveries and her largest baby weighed 4000 g. She had a postpartum bilateral tubal ligation. Her menstrual cycles are regular every 28 days and last 5 days. She states that with cough she may occasionally lose some urine; otherwise she has no complaints. She denies any medical problems. On exam she weighs 56 kg and her blood pressure is 132/81. What type of speculum would be most appropriate to use when performing this patient's Pap test?

a. Graves speculum
b. Pederson speculum
c. Vaginoscope
d. Hysteroscope
e. Pediatric speculum

264. A 36-year-old G2P2 presents for her well-woman exam. She has had two spontaneous vaginal deliveries without complications; her largest child weighed 3500 g at birth. She uses oral contraceptive pills and denies any history of an abnormal Pap smear. She does not smoke, but drinks about four times per week. Her weight is 70 kg. Her vital signs are normal. After placement of the speculum, you note a clear cyst approximately 2.5 cm in size on the anterior lateral wall of the vagina on the right side. The cyst is nontender and does not cause the patient any dyspareunia or discomfort. Which of the following is the most likely diagnosis of this mass?

a. Bartholin's duct cyst
b. Gartner's duct cyst
c. Lipoma
d. Hematoma
e. Inclusion cyst

265. A 50-year-old G4P4 present for her well-woman exam. She had one cesarean delivery followed by three vaginal deliveries. Her menses stopped 1 year ago and she occassionally still has a hot flash. She tells you that about 10 years ago she was treated with a laser conization for carcinoma in situ of her cervix. Since that time, all of her Pap tests have been normal. What recommendation should you make regarding how frequently she should undergo Pap smear testing?

a. Every 3 months
b. Every 6 months
c. Every year
d. Every 2 years
e. Every 3 years

266. A 45-year-old G3P3 presents for her yearly examination. She last saw a doctor 7 years ago after she had her last child. She had three vaginal deliveries, the last of which was complicated by gestational diabetes and preeclampsia. She has not been sexually active in the past year. She once had an abnormal Pap smear for which she underwent cryotherapy. She denies any medical problems. Her family history is significant for coronary artery disease in her dad and a maternal aunt who developed ovarian cancer at the age of 67. Which of the following is best screening approach for this patient?

a. Pap smear and mammography
b. Pap smear, mammography, and cholesterol profile
c. Pap smear, mammography, cholesterol profile, and fasting blood sugar
d. Pap smear, mammography, cholesterol profile, fasting blood sugar, and serum CA-125

267. A 30-year-woman presents to your office with the fear of developing ovarian cancer. Her 70-year-old grandmother recently died from ovarian cancer. You discuss with her the risks factors and prevention for ovarian cancer. Which of the following can decrease a woman's risk of ovarian cancer?

a. Use of combination oral contraceptive therapy
b. Menopause after age 55
c. Nonsteroidal anti-imflammatory drugs
d. Nulliparity
e. Ovulation induction medications

268. A 42-year-old G4P3104 presents for her well-woman exam. She has had three vaginal deliveries and one cesarean delivery for breech. She states her cycles are regular and denies any sexually transmitted diseases. Currently she and her husband use condoms, but they hate the hassle of a coital-dependent method. She is interested in a more effective contraception because they do not want any more children. She reports occasional migraine headaches and had a serious allergic reaction to anesthesia as a child when she underwent a tonsillectomy. She drinks and smokes socially. She weighs 78 kg, and her blood pressure is 142/89. During her office visit, you counsel the patient at length regarding birth control methods. Which of the following is the most appropriate contraceptive method for this patient?

a. Intrauterine device
b. Bilateral tubal ligation
c. Combination oral contraceptives
d. Diaphragm
e. Transdermal patch

269. A 48-year-old G2P2 presents for her well-woman exam. She had two uneventful vaginal deliveries. She had a vaginal hysterectomy for fibroids and menorrhagia. She denies any medical problems, but has not seen a doctor in 6 years. Her family history is significant for stroke, diabetes, and high blood pressure. On exam she is a pleasant female, stands 5 feet 3 inches tall, and weighs 85 kg. Her blood pressure is 150/92, pulse 70, respiratory rate 14, and temperature 98.4. Her breast, lung, cardiac, abdomen, and pelvic exams are normal. The next appropriate step in the management of this patient's blood pressure is which of the following?

a. Beta-blocker
b. Calcium channel blocker
c. Diuretic
d. Diet, exercise, weight loss, and repeat blood pressure in 2 months

270. A 32-year-old female presents for her yearly exam. She has been smoking one package of cigarettes a day for the past 12 years. She wants to stop, and you make some recommendations to her. Which of the following is true regarding smoking cessation in women?

a. Ninety percent of those who stop smoking relapse within 3 months
b. Nicotine replacement in the form of chewing gum or transdermal patches has not been shown to be effective in smoking cessation programs
c. Smokers do not benefit from repeated warnings from their doctor to stop smoking
d. Stopping cold turkey is the only way to successfully achieve smoking cessation
e. No matter how long one has been smoking, smoking cessation appears to improve the health of the lungs

Preventive Care and Health Maintenance

Answers

251. The answer is c. (*Stenchever, pp 138–154. ACOG, Committee Opinion 292.*) In postmenopausal women, routine screening for colon cancer is recommended with a colonoscopy to be performed every 10 years. Alternatively, flexible sigmoidoscopy can be performed every 5 years along with a yearly fecal occult blood test. Mammography should be performed annually in all women over 50. Postmenopausal women who are not on hormone replacement therapy and all women 65 years or older should be screened for osteoporosis with a DEXA scan to determine bone mineral density. All women who have been sexually active should undergo yearly Pap test screening. After a woman has had three or more consecutive normal Pap smears, the Pap test may be performed less frequently in a low-risk woman. Tuberculosis skin testing need be performed only in individuals with HIV infection, those who have close contact with individuals suspected of having TB, those who are IV drug users, those who are residents of nursing homes or long-term-care facilities, or those who work in a profession that is health care–related. This patient does not have any risk factors that would necessitate TB testing.

252. The answer is c. (*Stenchever, pp 138–154. ACOG, Committee Opinion 292.*) Women over 65 should have all of the following immunizations: tetanus-diphtheria booster every 10 years, influenza virus vaccine annually, and a one-time pneumococcal vaccine. A hepatitis B vaccine would be indicated only in individuals at high risk (i.e., international travelers, intravenous drug users and their sexual contacts, those who have occupational exposure to blood or blood products, persons with chronic liver or renal disease, or residents of institutions for the developmentally disabled, and inmates of correctional institutions).

253. The answer is d. (*Stenchever, pp 138–154. ACOG, Committee Opinion 292.*) Women over 65 years old should undergo cholesterol testing every 3 to 5 years, fasting glucose testing every 3 years, screening for thyroid disease with a TSH every 3 to 5 years, and periodic urinalysis. CA-125 testing is not recommended for ovarian cancer screening in women who are at low risk for ovarian cancer.

254. The answer is d. (*Stenchever, pp 138–154. ACOG, Committee Opinion 292.*) A urinalysis that is positive for blood should be followed up with a urine culture to detect an asymptomatic urinary tract infection before further workup is done or referral to a urologist is made. Parabasal cells on a Pap smear indicate lack of estrogen and are a normal finding in postmenopausal women.

255. The answer is d. (*Stenchever, pp 138–154. ACOG, Committee Opinion 292.*) In order of decreasing incidence, the leading causes of death in women over 65 years old are the following: diseases of the heart, cancer, cerebrovascular diseases, chronic obstructive pulmonary diseases, pneumonia and influenza, diabetes mellitus, accidents, and Alzheimer's disease.

256. The answer is c. (*Stenchever, pp 138–154. ACOG, Committee Opinion 292.*) The leading causes of death in teenagers between the ages of 13 and 18 years old, in order of decreasing frequency, are as follows: motor vehicle accidents, homicide, suicide, cancer, all other accidents, diseases of the heart, congenital anomalies, and chronic obstructive pulmonary diseases.

257. The answer is b. (*Stenchever, pp 138–154. ACOG, Committee Opinion 292.*) All sexually active women at risk for STDs should undergo Pap smear and test screening for sexually transmitted diseases such as hepatitis B, gonorrhea, chlamydia, HIV, and syphilis. Hepatitis C virus testing is indicated only in persons with a history of injecting illegal drugs, those who have received blood transfusions before 1992, those with occupational exposure to blood products, or those undergoing chronic hemodialysis.

258. The answer is d. (*Stenchever, pp 138–154. ACOG, Committee Opinion 292.*) It would be appropriate for this patient to receive a hepatitis B vaccination, since it is recommended for all individuals with a history of multiple sexual partners. She is not a candidate for the varicella vaccine since she has had chickenpox. The hepatitis A vaccine is indicated for international travelers, illegal drug users, and health care workers. The pneumococcal vaccine is indicated in immunocompromised persons, those with chronic illnesses, and individuals over 65 years old. The influenza vaccine is especially indicated in pregnant women, individuals with chronic diseases, and those in long-term-care facilities.

259. The answer is b. (*Stenchever, pp 138–154. ACOG, Committee Opinion 292.*) When you teach a patient to perform a breast self-exam, you should recommend that it be performed monthly, a few days after the menses is over. It is best to perform the breast exam in both the erect and supine positions. Asymmetry of the breasts is common in most women, but any recent changes need to be reported. Any nipple discharge should be reported immediately to a physician, because it can be associated with an underlying tumor.

260. The answer is b. (*Stenchever, pp 138–154. ACOG, Committee Opinion 292.*) The two main types of specula commonly used to perform Pap smears are the Pederson and Graves specula. The Pederson speculum works best for nulliparous women and menopausal women with atrophic vaginas; the blades are flat and narrow and barely curve on the sides. The blades of the Graves speculum are wider, higher, and curved on the sides; they work better for parous women with looser vaginal walls. A child's vagina can best be examined using an instrument called a vaginoscope or some type of endoscope such as a hysteroscope. The Graves and Pederson speculums come in pediatric sizes to be used in virginal adults or young children. Nasal specula are too short to be used to examine the vagina in adults and children.

261. The answer is e. (*Stenchever, pp 138–154. ACOG, Committee Opinion 292.*) The leading causes of death in women ages 40 to 64 are, in order of decreasing incidence, are as follows: cancer, diseases of the heart, cerebrovascular diseases, accidents, chronic obstructive pulmonary disease, diabetes mellitus, chronic liver disease and cirrhosis, and pneumonia and influenza.

262. The answer is c. (*Stenchever, pp 138–154. ACOG, Committee Opinion 292.*) When taking an obstetric history on a patient, you must indicate the number of pregnancies (gravidity) and the outcome of each of these pregnancies (parity). More specifically, the parity is further subclassified into number of term deliveries, preterm deliveries, abortions (spontaneous or induced) or ectopics, and number of living children. Since this patient is a

G6P3215, she has been pregnant six times and has had three term deliveries, two preterm delivery, and one abortion and has five living children.

263. The answer is a. (*Stenchever, pp 138–154. ACOG, Committee Opinion 292.*) The Graves speculum is most appropriate for parous women because it has wide, curved blades that enhance visualization of the cervix in women with the relaxed perineum and loose vaginal walls that result from obesity and childbirth. Pederson specula have narrower blades and are most appropriate for nulliparous patients and postmenopausal patients with atrophic vaginas. Pediatric specula, vaginoscopes, and hysteroscopes are all used to examine infants or prepubertal children.

264. The answer is b. (*Stenchever, pp 138–154. ACOG, Committee Opinion 292.*) Gartner's duct cysts arise from embryonic remnants of the mesonephric duct that course along the outer anterior aspect of the vaginal canal. These are usually small and asymptomatic and are found incidentally during a pelvic exam. They can be followed conservatively unless the patient becomes symptomatic, at which time excision is recommended. Inclusion cysts are usually seen on the posterior lower vaginal surface. Inclusion cysts are the most common vaginal cysts and result from birth trauma or previous gynecologic surgery. Bartholin's duct cysts are the most common large cysts of the vulva. Bartholin's ducts open into a groove between the hymen and labia minora. Lipomas are benign, encapsulated tumors of fat cells; they are most commonly discovered in the labia major and are superficial in location. Hematomas of the vulva usually occur as a result of blunt trauma or straddle injury. Spontaneous hematomas can occur as a result of rupture of a varicose vein in pregnancy or the postpartum period.

265. The answer is c. (*Stenchever, pp 138–154. ACOG, Committee Opinion 292.*) The American College of Obstetricians and Gynecologists recommends that all women who have been sexually active or who have reached age 18 should undergo an annual Pap test. ACOG also states that, following three or more consecutive normal Pap tests, screening can be performed less frequently in low-risk women at the discretion of the physician. This patient is not considered to be a low-risk patient since she has a history of previous cervical pathology. Pap smear testing would be performed more frequently than annually in women who have recently been treated for cervical dysplasia or who are HIV-positive.

266. The answer is c. *(Stenchever, pp 138–154. ACOG, Committee Opinion 292.)* In women 40 to 64 years old, mammography should be performed every 1 to 2 years until age 50 and then annually. Cholesterol testing should be performed every 5 years. A fasting blood sugar should be performed periodically in women at high risk. This patient is at an increased risk of developing diabetes because she experienced gestational diabetes during pregnancy. Measuring CA-125 levels has not been shown to be effective in population-based screening for ovarian cancer. With her previous history of treatment for cervical dysplasia, yearly Pap smear is recommended.

267. The answer is a. *(Stenchever, p 957.)* Oral contraceptive use, multiparity, breast-feeding, and early menopause are all factors believed to decrease the risk of developing ovarian cancer because they reduce the number of years a woman spends ovulating. The use of combination oral contraceptives decreases the risk of developing ovarian cancer by about 40%. Nulliparity, increasing age, and fertility drugs all increase ovulatory cycles and therefore are risk factors for developing ovarian cancer. In the general population, the risk of developing ovarian cancer is about 1 to 1.5%. This risk increases to about 5% if a woman has one first-degree relative with ovarian cancer and to about 7% if she has two or more first-degree relatives with ovarian cancer.

268. The answer is a. *(Stenchever, pp 303–305, 312.)* An intrauterine device is a highly effective long-term method for which the patient has no contraindication. A bilateral tubal ligation would be another option; however, the patient had a serious allergic reaction to anesthesia as a child, and general anesthesia is required for female laparoscopic sterilization. The patient's smoking and age contraindicate the use of combination oral contraceptives. Migraine headaches accompanied by neurologic symptoms such as loss of vision, paresthesias, and numbness are generally considered to be a contraindication to combination oral contraceptive use. However, there are no studies that show a statistically significant increased risk of stroke in pill users who have migraine headaches. Use of a diaphragm is a coital-dependent action and the patient relates that that is not something she desires.

269. The answer is d. *(ACOG, Technical Bulletin 210.)* Hypertension is defined as a systolic blood pressure of 140 or greater and a diastolic blood pressure of 90 or greater. A single elevated diastolic blood pressure less than 100 mmHg should be treated but should be rechecked within 2 months. The first line of treatment for women with hypertension should be lifestyle changes: smoking cessation, weight loss, diet modification, stress management, and exercise. If after 3 months these measures have failed to lower blood pressure, then pharmacologic therapy should be instituted.

270. The answer is e. (*ACOG, Technical Bulletin 210.*) Cigarette smoking has been linked to many pathologic conditions, including coronary heart disease, obstructive pulmonary disease, and lung cancer. There are studies that demonstrate that smoking cessation is of benefit to pulmonary health regardless of how long one has smoked. Doctors should repeatedly counsel their patients to stop smoking, and follow-up visits to achieve these goals are effective. Nicotine replacement therapy and transdermal nicotine patches have increased the effectiveness of smoking cessation programs. Sixty-five percent of people who stop smoking will relapse within 3 months.

Benign and Malignant Disorders of the Breast and Pelvis

Questions

DIRECTIONS: Each item below contains a question followed by suggested responses. Select the **one best** response to each question.

271. A 50-year-old woman is diagnosed with cervical cancer. Which lymph node group would be the first involved in metastatic spread of this disease beyond the cervix and uterus?

a. Common iliac nodes
b. Parametrial nodes
c. External iliac nodes
d. Paracervical or ureteral nodes
e. Para-aortic nodes

272. A 21-year-old woman presents with left lower quadrant pain. An anterior 7-cm firm adnexal cyst is palpated. Ultrasound confirms a complex left adnexal mass with solid components that appear to contain bone and teeth. What percentage of these tumors are bilateral?

a. Less than 1%
b. 2 to 3%
c. 10 to 15%
d. 50%
e. Greater than 75%

273. A 54-year-old woman undergoes a laparotomy because of a pelvic mass. At exploratory laparotomy, a unilateral ovarian neoplasm is discovered that is accompanied by a large omental metastasis. Frozen section diagnosis confirms metastatic serous cystadenocarcinoma. Which of the following is the most appropriate intraoperative course of action?

a. Excision of the omental metastasis and ovarian cystectomy
b. Omentectomy and ovarian cystectomy
c. Excision of the omental metastasis and unilateral oophorectomy
d. Omentectomy and bilateral salpingo-oophorectomy
e. Omentectomy, total abdominal hysterectomy, and bilateral salpingo-oophorectomy

274. A 58-year-old woman is seen for evaluation of a swelling in her right vulva. She has also noted pain in this area when walking and during coitus. At the time of pelvic examination, a mildly tender, fluctuant mass is noted just outside the introitus in the right vulva in the region of the Bartholin's gland. Which of the following is the most appropriate treatment?

a. Marsupialization
b. Administration of antibiotics
c. Surgical excision
d. Incision and drainage
e. Observation

275. A 51-year-old woman is diagnosed with invasive cervical carcinoma by cone biopsy. Pelvic examination and rectal-vaginal examination reveal the parametrium to be free of disease, but the upper portion of the vagina is involved with tumor. Intravenous pyelography (IVP) and sigmoidoscopy are negative, but a computed tomography (CT) scan of the abdomen and pelvis shows grossly enlarged pelvic and periaortic nodes. This patient is classified at which of the following stages?

a. IIa
b. IIb
c. IIIa
d. IIIb
e. IV

Questions 276–277

A 35-year-old G3P3 with a Pap smear showing high-grade squamous intraepithelial lesion of the cervix (CIN III) has an inadequate colposcopy. Cone biopsy of the cervix shows squamous cell cancer that has invaded only 1 mm beyond the basement membrane. There are no confluent tongues of tumor, and there is no evidence of lymphatic or vascular invasion. The margins of the cone biopsy specimen are free of disease.

276. How should you classify or stage this patient's disease?
a. Carcinoma of low malignant potential
b. Microinvasive cancer, stage Ia1
c. Atypical squamous cells of undetermined significance
d. Carcinoma in situ
e. Invasive cancer, stage IIa

277. The patient now asks you for your advice on how to treat her cervical disease. Your best recommendation is for the patient to undergo which of the following?
a. Treatment with external beam radiation
b. Implantation of radioactive cesium into the cervical canal
c. Simple hysterectomy
d. Simple hysterectomy with pelvic lymphadenectomy
e. Radical hysterectomy

278. A woman is found to have a unilateral invasive vulvar carcinoma that is 2 cm in diameter but not associated with evidence of lymph node spread. Initial management should consist of which of the following?
a. Chemotherapy
b. Radiation therapy
c. Simple vulvectomy
d. Radical vulvectomy
e. Radical vulvectomy and bilateral inguinal lymphadenectomy

279. A patient is receiving external beam radiation for treatment of metastatic endometrial cancer. The treatment field includes the entire pelvis. Which of the following tissues within this radiation field is the most radiosensitive?

a. Vagina
b. Ovary
c. Rectovaginal septum
d. Bladder
e. Rectum

280. An intravenous pyelogram (IVP) shows hydronephrosis in the workup of a patient with cervical cancer otherwise confined to a cervix of normal size. This indicates which one of the following stages?

a. I
b. II
c. III
d. IV
e. V

281. A pregnant 35-year-old patient is at highest risk for the concurrent development of which of the following malignancies?

a. Cervix
b. Ovary
c. Breast
d. Vagina
e. Colon

282. Stage Ib cervical cancer is diagnosed in a young woman who wishes to retain her ability to have sexual intercourse. Your consultant has therefore recommended a radical hysterectomy. Assuming that the cancer is confined to the cervix and that intraoperative biopsies are negative, which of the following structures would not be removed during the radical hysterectomy?

a. Uterosacral and uterovesical ligaments
b. Pelvic nodes
c. The entire parametrium on both sides of the cervix
d. Both ovaries
e. The upper third of the vagina

283. A 24-year-old woman presents with new-onset right lower quadrant pain, and you palpate an enlarged, tender right adnexa. Which of the following sonographic characteristics of the cyst in this patient suggests the need for surgical exploration now instead of observation for one menstrual cycle?

a. Lack of ascites
b. Unilocularity
c. Papillary vegetation
d. Diameter of 5 cm
e. Demonstration of arterial and venous flow by Doppler imaging

284. A 70-year-old woman presents for evaluation of a pruritic lesion on the vulva. Examination shows a white, friable lesion on the right labia majora that is 3 cm in diameter. No other suspicious areas are noted. Biopsy of the lesion confirms squamous cell carcinoma. In this patient, lymphatic drainage characteristically would be first to which of the following nodes?

a. External iliac lymph nodes
b. Superficial inguinal lymph nodes
c. Deep femoral lymph nodes
d. Periaortic nodes
e. Internal iliac nodes

285. A 7-year-old girl is seen by her pediatrician for left lower quadrant pain. You are consulted because an ovarian neoplasm is identified by ultrasound. Which of the following is the most common ovarian tumor in this type of patient?

a. Germ cell
b. Papillary serous epithelial
c. Fibrosarcoma
d. Brenner tumor
e. Sarcoma botryoides

286. A 41-year-old woman undergoes exploratory laparotomy for a persistent adnexal mass. Frozen section diagnosis is serous carcinoma. Assuming that the other ovary is grossly normal, what is the likelihood that the contralateral ovary is involved in this malignancy?

a. 5%
b. 15%
c. 33%
d. 50%
e. 75%

287. A postmenopausal woman presents with pruritic white lesions on the vulva. Punch biopsy of a representative area is obtained. Which of the following histologic findings is consistent with the diagnosis of lichen sclerosus?

a. Blunting or loss of rete pegs
b. Presence of thickened keratin layer
c. Acute inflammatory infiltration
d. Increase in the number of cellular layers in the epidermis
e. Presence of mitotic figures

288. A 21-year-old woman returns to your office for evaluation of an abnormal Pap smear. The Pap smear showed a squamous abnormality suggestive of a high-grade squamous intraepithelial lesion (HGSIL). Colposcopy confirms the presence of a cervical lesion consistent with severe cervical dysplasia (CIN III). Which of the following human papilloma virus types is most often associated with this type of lesion?

a. HPV type 6
b. HPV type 11
c. HPV type 16
d. HPV type 42
e. HPV type 44

289. A 20-year-old woman presents complaining of bumps around her vaginal opening. The bumps have been there for several months and are getting bigger. Her boyfriend has the same type of bumps on his penis. On physical examination the patient has multiple 2- to 10-mm lesions around her introitus consistent with condyloma. Her cervix has no gross lesions. A Pap smear is done. One week later the Pap smear returns showing atypical squamous cells of undetermined significance (ASCUS). Reflex human papilloma virus (HPV) typing showed no high-risk HPV. Which of the following viral types is most likely responsible for the patient's condyloma?

a. HPV type 11
b. HPV type 16
c. HPV type 18
d. HPV type 45
e. HPV type 56

DIRECTIONS: Each group of questions below consists of lettered options followed by a set of numbered items. For each numbered item, select the **one** lettered option with which it is **most** closely associated. Each lettered option may be used once, more than once, or not at all.

Questions 290–295

Select the ovarian tumor from below that is most likely to be associated with the clinical picture.

a. Granulosa tumor
b. Sertoli-Leydig cell tumor
c. Immature teratoma
d. Gonadoblastoma
e. Krukenberg tumor

290. A 26-year-old G2P1 presents to the gynecologist complaining of increasing hair growth on her face, chest, and abomen, but the hair on her head is receding in the temporal regions. She also has had problems with acne. On physical examination the patient has significant amounts of coarse, dark hair on her face, chest, and abdomen. On pelvic examination she has an enlarged clitoris. She has a 7-cm left adnexal mass.

291. A 56-year-old postmenopausal female presents complaining of vaginal bleeding. Her uterus is slightly enlarged and she has a 6-cm right adnexal mass. Endometrial biopsy shows adenocarcinoma of the endometrium.

292. A 67-year-old woman is found to have bilateral adnexal masses while undergoing evaluation of her recently diagnosed colon cancer.

293. A 17-year-old woman is referred by her primary care physician for the evaluation of primary amenorrhea. On physical examination the patient has evidence of virilization. She also has a pelvic mass. During the workup of the patient she is found to have sex chromosome mosaicism (45X/46,XY).

294. A 19-year-old woman is undergoing exploratory laparotomy for a 9-cm right ovarian mass. The final pathology report shows shows evidence of glial tissue and immature cerebellar and cortical tissue.

295. A 51-year-old menopausal woman is undergoing exploratory laparotomy for bilateral adnexal masses. A frozen section is performed on the excised ovaries and shows significant numbers of signet cells.

Questions 296–301

Match the chemotherapeutic agents and common side effects.

a. Hemorrhagic cystitis
b. Renal failure
c. Tympanic membrane fibrosis
d. Necrotizing enterocolitis
e. Pulmonary fibrosis
f. Pancreatic failure
g. Ocular degeneration
h. Cardiac toxicity
i. Peripheral neuropathy
j. Bone marrow depression

296. Cyclophosphamide

297. Cisplatin

298. Taxol

299. Bleomycin

300. Doxorubicin

301. Vincristine

Questions 302–308

Match each figure with the correct description.

a. Well-differentiated adenocarcinoma of the endometrium (FIGO I/III)
b. Proliferative endometrium
c. Choriocarcinoma
d. Late secretory endometrium
e. Mixed Müllerian endometrial cancer
f. Mature cystic teratoma
g. Clear cell cancer of the endometrium

302.

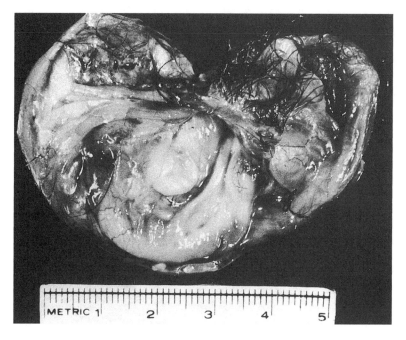

303.

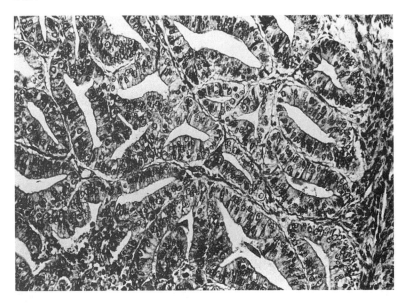

304.

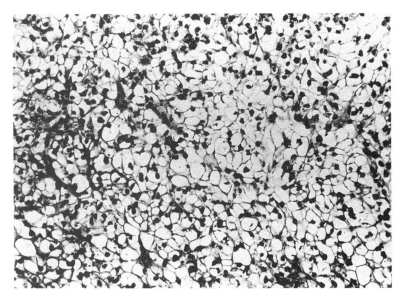

305.

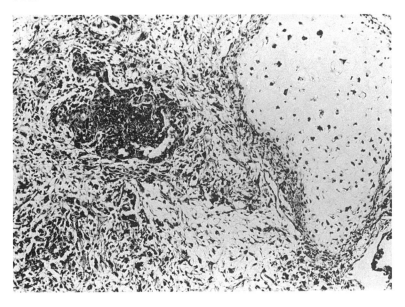

306.

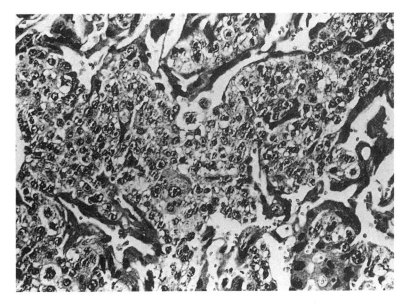

307.

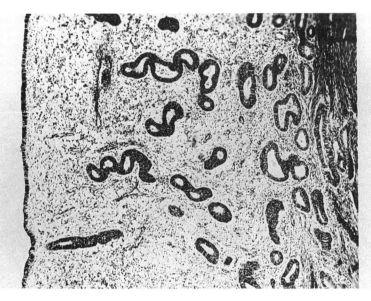

308.

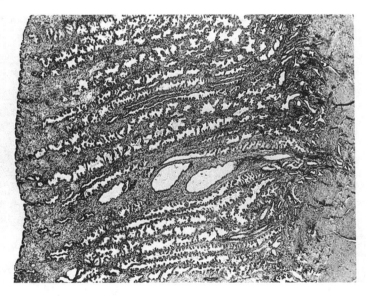

DIRECTIONS: Each item below contains a question followed by suggested responses. Select the **one best** response to each question.

309. A patient is diagnosed with carcinoma of the breast. Which of the following is the most important prognostic factor in the treatment of this disease?

a. Age at diagnosis
b. Size of tumor
c. Axillary metastases
d. Estrogen receptors on the tumor
e. Progesterone receptors on the tumor

310. A 25-year-old woman presents to you for routine well-woman examination. She has had two normal vaginal deliveries and is healthy. She smokes one pack of cigarettes per day. She has no gynecologic complaints. Her last menstrual period was 3 weeks ago. During the pelvic examination you notice that her left ovary is enlarged to 5 cm in diameter. Which of the following is the best recommendation to this patient?

a. Order CA-125 testing
b. Schedule outpatient diagnostic laparoscopy
c. Return to the office in 1 to 2 months to recheck the ovaries
d. Schedule a CT scan of the pelvis
e. Admit to the hospital for exploratory laparotomy

311. A 23-year-old woman presents to your office complaining of growths around her vaginal opening. Recently the growths have been itching and bleeding. On physical examination she has several broad-based lesions measuring 2 to 4 cm in diameter along the posterior fourchette. Although there is no active bleeding, the largest lesion appears to have been bleeding recently. Which of the following is the best way to treat this patient?

a. Weekly application of podophyllin in the office
b. Injection of 5-fluorouracil into the lesions
c. Self-application of imiquimod to the lesions by the patient
d. Weekly application of trichloroacetic acid in the office
e. Local excision

312. At the time of annual examination, a patient expresses concern over exposure to sexually transmitted diseases. During your pelvic examination, a single, indurated, nontender ulcer is noted on the vulva. Venereal Disease Research Laboratory (VDRL) and fluorescent treponemal antibody (FTA) tests are positive. Without treatment, the next stage of this disease is clinically characterized by which of the following?

a. Optic nerve atrophy and generalized paresis
b. Tabes dorsalis
c. Gummas
d. Macular rash over the hands and feet
e. Aortic aneurysm

313. A 24-year-old patient has returned from a yearlong stay in the tropics. Four weeks ago she noted a small vulvar ulceration that spontaneously healed. Now there is painful inguinal adenopathy with malaise and fever. You are considering the diagnosis of lymphogranuloma venereum (LGV). The diagnosis can be established by which of the following?

a. Staining for Donovan bodies
b. The presence of antibodies to *Chlamydia trachomatis*
c. Positive Frei skin test
d. Culturing *Haemophilus ducreyi*
e. Culturing *Calymmatobacterium granulomatis*

314. One day after a casual sexual encounter with a bisexual man recently diagnosed as antibody-positive for human immunodeficiency virus (HIV), a patient is concerned about whether she may have become infected. A negative antibody titer is obtained. To test for seroconversion, when is the earliest you should reschedule repeat antibody testing after the sexual encounter?

a. 1 to 2 weeks
b. 3 to 4 weeks
c. 6 to 12 weeks
d. 12 to 15 weeks
e. 26 to 52 weeks

315. A 20-year-old G3P0030 obese female comes to your office for a routine gynecologic exam. She is single, but is currently sexually active. She has a history of five sexual partners in the past, and became sexually active at age 15. She has had three first-trimester voluntary pregnancy terminations. She uses Depo-Provera for birth control, and reports occasionally using condoms as well. She has a history of genital warts, but denies any prior history of abnormal Pap smears. The patient denies use of any illicit drugs, but admits to smoking about one pack of cigarettes a day. Her physical exam is normal. However, 3 weeks later you receive the results of her Pap smear, which shows a high-grade squamous intraepithelial lesion (HGSIL). Which of the following factors in this patient's history does not increase her risk for cervical dysplasia?

a. Young age at initiation of sexual activity
b. Multiple sexual partners
c. History of genital warts
d. Use of Depo-Provera
e. Smoking

316. A 22-year-old woman presents for her first Pap smear. She has been sexually active with only one boyfriend since age 19. Her physical examination is completely normal. However, 2 weeks later her Pap smear results return showing high-grade squamous intraepithelial lesion (HGSIL). There were no endocervical cells seen on the smear. Which of the following is the most appropriate next step in the management of this patient?

a. Perform a cone biopsy of the cervix
b. Repeat the Pap smear to obtain endocervical cells
c. Order HPV typing on the initial Pap smear
d. Perform random cervical biopsies
e. Perform colposcopy and directed cervical biopsies

317. A 32-year-old woman consults with you for evaluation of an abnormal Pap smear done by a nurse practitioner at a family planning clinic. The Pap smear shows evidence of a high-grade squamous intraepithelial lesion (HGSIL). You perform a colposcopy in the office. Your colposcopic impression is mild cervical dysplasia (CIN I). Your biopsies show chronic cervicitis but no evidence of dysplasia. Which of the following is the most appropriate next step in the management of this patient?

a. Cryotherapy of the cervix
b. Laser ablation of the cervix
c. Conization of the cervix
d. Hysterectomy
e. Repeat the Pap smear in 3 to 6 months

318. A 55-year-old postmenopausal female presents to her gynecologist for a routine exam. She denies any use of hormone replacement therapy and does not report any menopausal symptoms. She denies the occurrence of any abnormal vaginal bleeding. She has no history of any abnormal Pap smears and has been married for 30 years to the same partner. She is currently sexually active with her husband on a regular basis. Two weeks after her exam, her Pap smear comes back as atypical glandular cells of undetermined significance (AGUS). Which of the following is the most appropriate next step in the management of this patient?

a. Re-Pap in 4 to 6 months
b. HPV testing
c. Hysterectomy
d. Cone biopsy
e. Colposcopy, endometrial biopsy, endocervical curettage

319. A 24-year-old G0 presents to your office complaining of vulvar discomfort. More specifically, she has been experiencing intense burning and pain with intercourse. The discomfort occurs at the vaginal introitus primarily with penile insertion into the vagina. The patient also experiences the same pain with tampon insertion and when the speculum is inserted during a gynecologic exam. The problem has become so bad that she can no longer have sex, which is causing problems in her marriage. She is otherwise healthy and denies any medical problems. She is experiencing regular menses and denies any dysmenorrhea. On physical exam, the region of the vulva around the vaginal vestibule has several punctate, erythematous areas of epithelium measuring 3 to 8 mm in diameter. Most of the lesions are located on the skin between the two Bartholin's glands. Each inflamed lesion is tender to touch with a cotton swab. Which of the following is the most likely diagnosis?

a. Vulvar vestibulitis
b. Atrophic vaginitis
c. Contact dermatitis
d. Lichen sclerosus
e. Vulvar intraepithelial neoplasia

320. You recently diagnosed a patient with vulvar vestibulitis and recommended that she wear loose clothing and cotton underwear and to stop using tampons. After 1 month she returns, reporting that her symptoms of intense burning and pain with intercourse have not improved. Which of the following treatment options is the best next step in treating this patient's problem?

a. Podophyllin
b. Surgical excision of the vestibular glands
c. Topical xylocaine
d. Topical trichloroacetic acid
e. Valtrex therapy

321. A 29-year-old G0 comes to your office complaining of a heavy vaginal discharge for the past 2 weeks. The patient describes the discharge as thin in consistency and of a grayish white color. She has also noticed a slight fishy vaginal odor that seems to have started with the appearance of the discharge. She denies any vaginal or vulvar prutitus or burning. She admits to being sexually active in the past, but has not had intercourse during the past year. She denies a history of any sexually transmitted diseases. She is currently on no medications with the exception of her birth control pills. Last month she took a course of amoxicillin for treatment of a sinusitis. On physical exam, the vulva appears normal and the cervix is not inflamed. There is a discharge present at the introitus. A copious, thin, whitish discharge is in the vaginal vault and adherent to the vaginal walls. The vaginal pH is 5.5 Wet smear of the discharge indicates the presence of clue cells. Which of the following is the most likely diagnosis?

a. Candidiasis
b. Bacterial vaginosis
c. Trichomoniasis
d. Physiologic discharge
e. Chlamydia

322. A 24-year-old G2P1 at 18 weeks gestation presents complaining of a foul-smelling vaginal discharge with irritation around the vaginal opening. Physical examination is consistent with bacterial vaginosis. Which of the following is the best treatment for this condition?

a. Reassurance
b. Oral Diflucan
c. Doxycycline 100 mg PO bid for 1 week
d. Metronidazole 500 mg PO bid for 1 week
e. Metronidazole 2 g PO single dose

323. A 20-year-old G2P0020 with an LMP 3 days ago presents to the emergency room complaining of a 24-hour history of increasing pelvic pain. This morning she experienced fever and chills, although she did not take her temperature. She reports no changes in her urine or bowel habits. She has had no nausea or vomiting. She denies any medical problems. Her only surgery was a laparoscopy performed last year for an ectopic pregnancy. She reports regular menses and denies dysmenorrhea. She is currently sexually active. She has a new sexual partner and had sexual intercourse with him just prior to her last menstrual period. She denies a history of any abnormal Pap smears or sexually transmitted diseases. Urine pregnancy test is negative. Urinalysis is completely normal. WBC is 18,000. Temperature is 102°F. On physical exam, her abdomen is diffusely tender with rebound. Bowel sounds are present but diminished. Which of the following diagnoses is most likely to cause this patient's symptoms?

a. Ovarian torsion
b. Endometriosis
c. Acute salpingitis
d. Kidney stone
e. Ruptured ovarian cyst

324. A 32-year-old women presents to the emergency room complaining of severe lower abdominal pain. She says she was diagnosed with pelvic inflammatory disease by her gynecologist last month but did not take the medicine that she was prescribed because it made her throw up. She has had fevers on and off for the past 2 weeks. In the emergency room the patient has a temperature of 101°F. Her abdomen is diffusely tender, but more so in the lower quadrants. She has diminished bowel sounds. On bimanual pelvic exam, bilateral adnexal masses are palpated. The patient is sent to the ultrasound department, and a transvaginal pelvic ultrasound demonstrates bilateral tuboovarian abscesses. Which of the following is the most appropriate next step in the management of this patient?

a. Admit the patient for emergent laparoscopic drainage of the abscesses
b. Call interventional radiology to perform CT-guided percutaneous drainage of the abscesses
c. Send the patient home and arrange for intravenous antibiotics to be administered by a home health agency
d. Admit the patient for intravenous antibiotic therapy
e. Admit the patient for exploratory laparotomy, TAH/BSO

325. A 36-year-old woman presents to the emergency room complaining of pelvic pain, fever, and vaginal discharge. She has had nausea and vomiting and cannot tolerate liquids at the time of her initial evaluation. The emergency room physician diagnoses her with pelvic inflammatory disease and asks you to admit her for treatment. Which of the following is the most appropriate antibiotic treatment regimen for this patient?

a. Doxycycline 100 mg PO twice daily for 14 days
b. Clindamycin 450 mg IV every 8 h plus gentamicin 1 mg/kg load followed by 1 mg/kg every 12 h
c. Cefoxitin 2 g IV q6h with doxycycline 100 mg IV twice daily
d. Ceftriaxone 250 mg IM plus doxycycline 100 mg PO twice daily for 14 days
e. Ofloxacin 400 mg PO twice daily for 14 days plus Flagyl 500 mg PO twice daily for 14 days

326. A 43-year-old G2P2 comes to your office complaining of an intermittent right nipple discharge that is bloody. She reports that the discharge is spontaneous and not associated with any nipple pruritus, burning, or discomfort. On physical exam, you do not detect any dominant breast masses or adenopathy. There are no skin changes noted. Which of the following conditions is the most likely cause of this patient's problem?

a. Breast cancer
b. Duct ectasia
c. Intraductal papilloma
d. Fibrocystic breast disease
e. Pituitary adenoma

327. A 28-year-old G0, LMP 1 week ago, presents to your gynecology clinic complaining of a mass in her left breast that she discovered on a routine breast self-exam in the shower. When you perform a breast exam on her, you palpate a 2-cm firm, nontender mass in the upper inner quadrant of the left breast that is well circumscribed and mobile. You do not detect any skin changes, nipple discharge, or lymphadenopathy. Which of the following is the most likely diagnosis?

a. Fibrocystic breast change
b. Fibroadenoma
c. Breast carcinoma
d. Fat necrosis
e. Cystosarcoma phyllodes

328. You have a patient who has undergone a routine screening ultrasound at 20 weeks gestation. The patient phones you immediately following the ultrasound because during the procedure the radiologist commented that she has several small fibroid tumors in her uterus. This is the patient's first pregnancy and she is most concerned regarding the possible sequelae these growths may have on the outcome of her pregnancy. As her obstetrician, which of the following should you tell her?

a. Fibroid necrosis and degeneration during pregnancy is common
b. Many women have fibroid tumors but most fibroids are asymptomatic during pregnancy
c. Progression to leiomyosarcoma is more common in pregnancy due to the hormonal effects of the pregnancy
d. Preterm labor occurs frequently, even in women with asymptomatic fibroid tumors
e. She will have to have a cesarean delivery because the fibroid tumors will obstruct the birth canal

329. A 55-year-old G3P3 with a history of fibroids comes to see you complaining of irregular vaginal bleeding. Last year she went 9 months without having a period and thought she was in menopause. But since then she has had irregular, spotty vaginal bleeding. The last time she bled was 5 weeks ago and was so heavy that she could not leave the house, fearing she would bleed through her clothes. She also complains of frequent hot flushes and emotional lability. She does not have any medical problems and is not taking any medications. She is a nonsmoker and denies any alcohol or drug use. Her gynecologic history is significant for cryotherapy of the cervix 10 years ago for moderate dysplasia. She has had three cesarean sections and a tubal ligation. On physical examination her uterus is 12 weeks in size and irregularly shaped. Her ovaries are not palpable. Which of the following is the most reasonable next step in the evaluation of this patient?

a. Schedule her for a hysterectomy
b. Insert a progesterone containing intrauterine device
c. Arrange for outpatient endometrial ablation
d. Perform an office endometrial biopsy
e. Arrange for outpatient conization of the cervix

330. A 57-year-old menopausal patient presents to your office for evaluation of postmenopausal bleeding. She is morbidly obese and has chronic hypertension and adult onset diabetes. An endometrial sampling done in the office shows complex endometrial hyperplasia with atypia, and a pelvic ultrasound done at the hospital demonstrates multiple, large uterine fibroids. Which of the following is the best treatment option for this patient?

a. Myomectomy
b. Total abdominal hysterectomy
c. Oral contraceptives
d. Uterine artery embolization
e. Oral progesterone

Benign and Malignant Disorders of the Breast and Pelvis

Answers

271. The answer is d. (*DiSaia, pp 55–62.*) The main routes of spread of cervical cancer include vaginal mucosa, myometrium, paracervical lymphatics, and direct extension into the parametrium. The prevalence of lymph node disease correlates with the stage of malignancy. Primary node groups involved in the spread of cervical cancer include the paracervical, parametrial, obturator, hypogastric, external iliac, and sacral nodes, essentially in that order. Less commonly, there is involvement in the common iliac, inguinal, and para-aortic nodes. In stage I, the pelvic nodes are positive in approximately 15% of cases and the para-aortic nodes in 6%. In stage II, pelvic nodes are positive in 28% of cases and para-aortic nodes in 16%. In stage III, pelvic nodes are positive in 47% of cases and para-aortic nodes in 28%.

272. The answer is c. (*Hoskins, p 987.*) Benign cystic teratomas (dermoids) are the most common germ cell tumors and account for about 20 to 25% of all ovarian neoplasms. They occur primarily during the reproductive years, but may also occur in postmenopausal women and in children. Dermoids are usually unilateral, but 10 to 15% are bilateral. Usually the tumors are asymptomatic, but they can cause severe pain if there is torsion or if the sebaceous material perforates, spills, and creates a reactive peritonitis.

273. The answer is e. (*Hoskins, pp 940–944.*) The survival of women who have ovarian carcinoma varies inversely with the amount of residual tumor left after the initial surgery. At the time of laparotomy, a maximum effort should be made to determine the sites of tumor spread and to excise all resectable tumor. Although the uterus and ovaries may appear grossly normal, there is a relatively high incidence of occult metastases to these organs; for this reason, they should be removed during the initial surgery.

Ovarian cancer metastasizes outside the peritoneum via the pelvic or para-aortic lymphatics, and from there into the thorax and the remainder of the body.

274. The answer is c. (*Hoskins, p 728.*) Although rare, adenocarcinoma of the Bartholin's gland must be excluded in women over 40 years of age who present with a cystic or solid mass in this area. The appropriate treatment in these cases is surgical excision of the Bartholin's gland to allow for a careful pathologic examination. In cases of abscess formation, both marsupialization of the sac and incision with drainage as well as appropriate antibiotics are accepted modes of therapy. In the case of the asymptomatic Bartholin's cyst, no treatment is necessary.

275. The answer is a. (*Hoskins, pp 827–828.*) Cervical cancer is still staged clinically. Physical examination, routine x-rays, barium enema, colposcopy, cystoscopy, proctosigmoidoscopy, and IVP are used to stage the disease. CT scan results, while clinically useful, are not used to stage the disease. Stage I disease is limited to the cervix. Stage Ia disease is preclinical (i.e., microscopic), while stage Ib denotes macroscopic disease. Stage II involves the vagina, but not the lower one-third, or infiltrates the parametrium, but not out to the pelvic side wall. IIa denotes vaginal but not parametrial extension, while IIb denotes parametrial extension. Stage III involves the lower one-third of the vagina or extends to the pelvic side wall; there is no cancer-free area between the tumor and the pelvic wall. Stage IIIa lesions have not extended to the pelvic wall, but involve the lower one-third of the vagina. Stage IIIb tumors have extension to the pelvic wall and/or are associated with hydronephrosis or a nonfunctioning kidney caused by tumor. Stage IV is outside the reproductive tract.

276–277. The answers are 276-b, 277-c. (*Hoskins, pp 793–794, 802–803.*) Microinvasive carcinoma of the cervix includes lesions within 3 mm of the base of the epithelium, with no confluent tongues or lymphatic or vascular invasion. The overall incidence of metastases in 751 reported cases is 1.2%. Simple hysterectomy is accepted therapy.

278. The answer is e. (*DiSaia, pp 153–160.*) Women who have invasive vulvar carcinoma usually are treated surgically. If the lesion is unilateral, is not associated with fixed or ulcerated inguinal lymph nodes, and does not involve the urethra, vagina, anus, or rectum, then treatment usually consists of radical vulvectomy and bilateral inguinal lymphadenectomy. If inguinal lymph nodes show evidence of metastatic disease, bilateral pelvic lymphadenectomy is usually performed. Radiation therapy, though not a routine part of the management of women who have early vulvar carcinoma, is employed (as an alternative to pelvic exenteration with radical vulvectomy) in the treatment of women who have local, advanced carcinoma.

279. The answer is b. (*DiSaia, pp 619–622.*) Different tissues tolerate different doses of radiation, but the ovaries are by far the most radiosensitive. They tolerate up to 2500 rads, while the other tissues listed tolerate between 5000 and 20,000 rads. Acute evidence of excessive radiation exposure includes tissue necrosis and inflammation, resulting in enteritis, cystitis, vulvitis, proctosigmoiditis, and possible bone marrow suppression. Chronic effects of excessive radiation exposure are manifest months to years after therapy and include vasculitis, fibrosis, and deficient cellular regrowth; these can result in proctitis, cystitis, fistulas, scarring, and stenosis.

Successful radiation depends on (1) the greater sensitivity of the cancer cell compared with normal tissue and (2) the greater ability of normal tissue to repair itself after irradiation. The maximal resistance to ionizing radiation depends on an intact circulation and adequate cellular oxygenation. Resistance also depends on total dose, number of portions, and time intervals. The relative resistance of normal tissue (cervix and vagina) in cervical cancer allows high surface doses approaching 15,000 to 20,000 rads to be delivered to the tumor with intracavitary devices, and, because of the inverse square law, significantly lower doses of radiation reach the bladder and rectum. The greater the fractionalization (number of portions the total dose is broken into), the better the normal tissue tolerance of that radiation dose; hence 5000 rads of pelvic radiation is usually given in daily fractions over 5 weeks, with approximately 200 rads being administered each day.

280. The answer is c. (*Hoskins, pp 790–791.*) By definition, a positive IVP would mean extension to the pelvic side wall and thus a stage III carcinoma, specifically stage IIIb. Such staging applies even if there is no palpable tumor beyond the cervix. In addition to examination, IVP, cystoscopy, and proctosigmoidoscopy are the diagnostic tests used to stage cervical cancer. However, it is important to understand that while the results of only certain tests are used to stage the cancer, this does not limit the physician from performing any other diagnostic tests (such as CT scans of the abdomen, pelvis, or chest) that in his or her judgment are required for appropriate medical care and decision making.

281. The answer is a. *(DiSaia, pp 1–16.)* Cervical cancer is a more common gynecologic malignancy in pregnancy than ovarian or breast cancer due to the fact that it is a disease of younger women. Management of cervical intraepithelial lesions is complicated in pregnancy because of increased vascularity of the cervix and because of the concern that manipulation of and trauma to the cervix can compromise continuation of the pregnancy. A traditional cone biopsy is indicated only in the presence of apparent microinvasive disease on a colposcopically directed cervical biopsy. Otherwise, more limited procedures such as shallow coin biopsies are more appropriate. If invasive cancer is diagnosed, the decision to treat immediately or wait until fetal viability depends in part on the gestational age at which the diagnosis is made and the severity of the disorder. Survival is decreased for malignancies discovered later in pregnancy. Radiation therapy almost always results in spontaneous abortion, in part because the fetus is particularly radiosensitive. Chemotherapy is associated with higher than expected rates of fetal malformations consistent with the antimetabolite effects of agents used. Specific malformations depend on the agent used and the time in pregnancy at which the exposure occurs.

282. The answer is d. *(DiSaia, pp 69–71.)* Radical hysterectomy was popularized by Meigs in the 1940s and has become a very safe procedure in skilled hands. It is most often used as primary treatment for early cervical cancer (stages Ib and IIa), and occasionally as primary treatment for uterine cancer. In either case, there must be no evidence of spread beyond the operative field, as suggested by negative intraoperative frozen section biopsies. The procedure involves excision of the uterus, the upper third of the vagina, the uterosacral and uterovesical ligaments, and all of the parametrium, and pelvic node dissection including the ureteral, obturator, hypogastric, and iliac nodes. Radical hysterectomy thus attempts to preserve the bladder, rectum, and ureters while excising as much as possible of the remaining tissue around the cervix that might be involved in microscopic spread of the disease. Ovarian metastases from cervical cancer are extremely rare. Preservation of the ovaries is generally acceptable, particularly in younger women, unless there is some other reason to consider oophorectomy.

283. The answer is c. (*DiSaia, pp 282–300.*) Approximately 20% of ovarian neoplasms are considered malignant on pathologic examination. However, all must be considered as placing the patient at risk. Given that most ovarian tumors are not found until significant spread has occurred, it is not unreasonable to attempt to operate on such patients as soon as there is a suspicion of tumor. Papillary vegetation, size greater than 10 cm, ascites, possible torsion, or solid lesions are automatic indications for exploratory laparotomy. In a younger woman, a cyst can be followed past one menstrual cycle to determine if it is a follicular cyst, since a follicular cyst should regress after onset of the next menstrual period. If regression does not occur, then surgery is appropriate. Doppler ultrasound imaging allows visualization of arterial and venous flow patterns superimposed on the image of the structure being examined; arterial and venous flow are expected in a normal ovary.

284. The answer is b. (*Hoskins, p 720.*) An important feature of the lymphatic drainage of the vulva is the existence of drainage across the midline. The vulva drains first into the superficial inguinal lymph nodes, then into the deep femoral nodes, and finally into the external iliac lymph nodes. The clinical significance of this sequence for patients with carcinoma of the vulva is that the iliac nodes are probably free of the disease if the deep femoral nodes are not involved. Unlike the lymphatic drainage from the rest of the vulva, the drainage from the clitoral region bypasses the superficial inguinal nodes and passes directly to the deep femoral nodes. Thus, while the superficial nodes usually also have metastases when the deep femoral nodes are implicated, it is possible for only the deep nodes to be involved if the carcinoma is in the midline near the clitoris.

285. The answer is a. (*DiSaia, p 285.*) The most common ovarian neoplasms in children are of germ cell origin, and about half of these tumors are malignant. Functioning ovarian tumors have been reported to produce precocious puberty in about 2% of affected patients. Epithelial tumors of the ovary, which are quite rare in prepubertal girls, are benign in approximately 90% of all cases; papillary serous cystadenocarcinoma is an example of such a malignant epithelial tumor. Stromal tumors (such as fibrosarcoma) and Brenner tumors are not seen in this age group. Sarcoma botryoides, a tumor seen in children, is a malignancy associated with Müllerian structures such as the vagina and uterus, including the uterine cervix.

286. The answer is c. (*Hoskins, pp 928–930.*) Serous carcinoma is the most common epithelial tumor of the ovary. On histologic examination, psammoma bodies can be seen in approximately 30% of these tumors. Bilateral involvement characterizes about one-third of all serous carcinomas. Although mesonephroid carcinomas tend to be associated with pelvic endometriosis, a similar association has not been demonstrated for serous carcinomas.

287. The answer is a. (*DiSaia, pp 41–42.*) Lichen sclerosus was formerly termed *lichen sclerosus et atrophicus,* but recent studies have concluded that atrophy does not exist. Patients with lichen sclerosus of the vulva tend to be older; they typically present with pruritus, and the lesions are usually white with crinkled skin and well-defined borders. The histologic appearance of lichen sclerosus includes loss of the rete pegs within the dermis, chronic inflammatory infiltrate below the dermis, the development of a homogenous subepithelial layer in the dermis, a decrease in the number of cellular layers, and a decrease in the number of melanocytes. Mechanical trauma produces bullous areas of lymphedema and lacunae, which are then filled with erythrocytes. Ulcerations and ecchymoses may be seen in these traumatized areas as well. Mitotic figures are rare in lichen sclerosus, and hyperkeratosis is not a feature. While a significant cause of symptoms, lichen sclerosus is not a premalignant lesion. Its importance lies in the fact that it must be distinguished from vulvar squamous cancer.

288–289. The answers are 288-c 289-a. (*Stenchever, pp 650–651, 864–868.*) The human papillomaviruses (HPV) are a group of double-stranded DNA viruses that infect epithelial cells. They do not cause systemic infection. There are numerous viruses within the group, and they are named by number according to the order of their discovery. Human papilloma viruses are sexually transmitted. HPV, in particular types 16, 18, and 31, have been linked to cervical neoplasia. HPV types 6 and 11 are associated with benign condyloma.

290–295. The answers are 290-b, 291-a, 292-e, 293-d, 294-c, 295-e. (*Griffiths, p 188.*) Sertoli-Leydig cell tumors, which represent less than 1% of ovarian tumors, may produce symptoms of virilization. Histologically, they resemble fetal testes; clinically, they must be distinguished from other functioning ovarian neoplasms as well as from tumors of the adrenal glands, since both adrenal tumors and Sertoli-Leydig tumors produce androgens. The androgen production can result in seborrhea, acne, menstrual irregularity, hirsutism, breast atrophy, alopecia, deepening of the voice, and clitoromegaly. Granulosa and theca cell tumors are often associated with excessive estrogen production, which may cause pseudoprecocious puberty, postmenopausal bleeding, or menorrhagia. These tumors are associated with endometrial carcinoma in 15% of patients. Because these tumors are quite friable, affected women frequently present with symptoms caused by tumor rupture and intraperitoneal bleeding. Gonadoblastomas frequently contain calcifications that can be detected by plain radiography of the pelvis. Women who have gonadoblastomas often have ambiguous genitalia. The tumors are usually small, and are bilateral in one-third of affected women. The malignant potential of immature teratomas correlates with the degree of immature or embryonic tissue present. The presence of choriocarcinoma can be determined histologically as well as by human chorionic gonadotropin (hCG) assays. The presence of choriocarcinoma in an immature teratoma worsens the prognosis. Krukenberg tumors are typically bilateral, solid masses of the ovary that nearly always represent metastases from another organ, usually the stomach or large intestine. They contain large numbers of signet ring adenocarcinoma cells within a cellular hyperplastic but nonneoplastic ovarian stroma.

296–301. **The answers are 296-a, 297-b, 298-j, 299-e, 300-h, 301-i.** (*Hoskins, pp 385–386, 393–394, 628–630.*) Cyclophosphamide is an alkylating agent that cross-links DNA and also inhibits DNA synthesis. Hemorrhagic cystitis and alopecia are common side effects. Cisplatin causes renal damage and neural toxicity. Patients must be well hydrated. Its mode of action does not fit a specific category. Taxol can produce allergic reactions and bone marrow depression. Bleomycin and doxorubicin are antibiotics whose side effects are pulmonary fibrosis and cardiac toxicity, respectively. Vincristine arrests cells in metaphase by binding microtubular proteins and preventing the formation of mitotic spindles. Peripheral neuropathy is a common side effect.

302–308. **The answers are 302-f, 303-a, 304-g, 305-e, 306-c, 307-b, 308-d.** (*Hoskins, pp 4–9, 607–610.*) The tumor in question 302 is an opened mature cystic teratoma (dermoid tumor) in which hair is visible.

The microscopic section in question 303 is a classical example of well-differentiated adenocarcinoma of the endometrium, showing cellular pleomorphism, nuclear atypia with mitoses, and back-to-back crowding of glands with obliteration of intervening stroma; the glandular architecture of the tissue is maintained, however. Endometrial cancer is categorized by both stage and grade. The differentiation of a carcinoma is expressed as its grade. Grade I lesions are well differentiated; grade II lesions are moderately well differentiated; grade III lesions are poorly differentiated. An increasing grade (i.e., a decreasing degree of differentiation) implies worsening prognosis. Tumors may be of a mixed cell type—for example, squamous and adenocarcinoma—or may be mucinous, serous, or clear.

Question 304 shows clear cell adenocarcinoma with large, pale staining cells. Clear cell carcinoma of the endometrium is similar to that arising in the cervix, vagina, and ovary, and the histologic appearance is similar in each of these organs. Diethylstilbestrol exposure has been associated with an increased incidence of vaginal and cervical clear cell carcinomas. The tumor's origins are suggested to be mesonephric duct remnants. The microscopic appearance of clear cell carcinoma is related to deposits of periodic acid–Schiff (PAS) stain–positive glycogen. These tumors characteristically occur in older women and are very aggressive.

The section in question 305 shows mixed Müllerian endometrial cancer. Mixed Müllerian tumors refer to the combination of heterologous elements—that is, tissue of different sources (cartilage in this picture).

Question 306 is an example of choriocarcinoma, showing sheets of malignant trophoblast. Malignant choriocarcinoma is a transformation of molar tissue or a de novo lesion arising from the placenta. There are significant degrees of cellular pleomorphism and anaplasia. Choriocarcinoma can be differentiated from invasive mole by the fact that the latter has chorionic villi and the former does not.

Question 307 and 308 show early- to midproliferative endometrium and late secretory endometrium, respectively. Proliferative and late secretory endometrium can be differentiated by the development of glandular tissue and secretory patterns. In question 307, the glands are just beginning to proliferate, and the section cuts through several coils as they course toward the surface epithelium on the left. In question 308, the glands are dilated and filled with amorphous (glycogen) material.

309. The answer is c. (*Hoskins, pp 1094–1095.*) Recognition of the high risk associated with axillary metastases for early death and poor 5-year survival has led to the use of postsurgical adjuvant chemotherapy in these patients. Patients who have estrogen- or progesterone-receptive tumors (i.e., receptor present or receptor-positive) are particular candidates for this adjuvant therapy, as 60% of estrogen-positive tumors will respond to hormonal therapy. Age and size of the tumor are certainly factors of importance, but they are secondary to the presence or absence of axillary metastases.

310. The answer is c. (*Stenchever, pp 506–507, 962.*) In young, menstruating women the most common reason for an enlargement of one ovary is the presence of a functional ovarian cyst. Functional cysts are physiologic, forming during the normal functioning of the ovaries. Follicular cysts are usually asymptomatic, unilateral, thin-walled, and filled with a watery, straw-colored fluid. Corpus luteum cysts are less common than follicular cysts. They are usually unilateral, but often appear complex, as they may be hemorrhagic. A patients with a corpus luteum cyst may complain of dull pain on the side of the affected ovary. Theca lutein cysts are the least common of the three types of functional ovarian cysts. They are almost always bilateral and are associated with pregnancy. Since the most common cause of a unilateral, asymptomatic ovarian cyst in a young, menstruating woman is a functional cyst, it is most reasonable to follow the patient conservatively and have her return after 1 to 2 months to recheck her ovary. More aggressive primary management with surgery is not indicated in a young, asymptomatic patient. CT scanning or pelvic ultrasonography may be indicated if the cyst is persistent. CA-125 is a cancer antigen expressed by approximately 80% of ovarian epithelial carcinomas. CA-125 testing is not very specific in women of childbearing age and is not useful for primary evaluation of an ovarian cyst in a young, asymptomatic patient.

311. The answer is e. (*Ransom 1997, p 53.*) The lesions are condyloma acuminatum, also known as venereal warts. This is a squamous lesion caused by a human papillomavirus (HPV). The lesion reveals a treelike growth microscopically with a mantle that shows marked acanthosis and parakeratosis. Treatment options include local excision, cryosurgery, application of podophyllin or trichloroacetic acid, and laser therapy, although podophyllum is not recommended for extensive disease because of toxicity (peripheral neuropathy). For intractable condyloma of the vagina, 5-fluorouracil can be employed. Medical treatment with podphyllum, imiquimod, trichloroacetic acid and 5-fluorouricil requires weeks or months of therapy to be effective. As this patient has large, bleeding lesions, local excision is the best treatment option.

312. The answer is d. (*Ransom 1997, p 52.*) Syphilis is a chronic disease produced by the spirochete *Treponema pallidum*. Because of the spirochete's extreme thinness, it is difficult to detect by light microscopy; therefore, spirochetes are diagnosed by use of a specially adapted technique known as dark-field microscopy. Clinically, syphilis is divided into primary, secondary, and tertiary (or late) stages. In primary syphilis a hard chancre develops. This is a painless ulcer with an indurated base that is usually found on the vulva, vagina, or cervix. Secondary syphilis is the result of hematogenous dissemination of the spirochetes and thus is a systemic disease. There are a number of systemic symptoms depending on the major organs involved. The classic rash of secondary syphilis is red macules and papules over the palms of the hands and the soles of the feet. The manifestations of late syphilis include optic atrophy, tabes dorsalis, generalized paresis, aortic aneurysm, and gummas of the skin and bones.

313. The answer is b. (*Ransom 1997, p 53.*) Lymphogranuloma venereum (LGV) is a chronic infection produced by *C. trachomatis*. The primary infection begins as a painless ulcer on the labia or vaginal vestibule; the patient usually consults the physician several weeks after the development of painful adenopathy in the inguinal and perirectal areas. Diagnosis can be established by culture or by demonstrating the presence of antibodies to *C. trachomatis*. The Frei skin test is no longer used because of its low sensitivity. The differential diagnosis includes syphilis, chancroid, granuloma inguinale, carcinoma, and herpes. Chancroid is a sexually transmitted disease caused by *H. ducreyi* that produces a painful, tender ulceration of the vulva. Donovan bodies are present in patients with granuloma inguinale, which is caused by *C. granulomatis*. Therapy for both granuloma inguinale and LGV is administration of tetracycline. Chancroid is successfully treated with either azithromycin or ceftriaxone.

314. The answer is c. (*Stenchever, pp 681–684.*) Persons at high risk for infection by human immunodeficiency virus (HIV) include homosexuals, bisexual males, women having sex with a bisexual or homosexual partner, intravenous drug users, and hemophiliacs. The virus can be transmitted through sexual contact, use of contaminated needles or blood products, and perinatal transmission from mother to child. The antibody titer usually becomes positive 6 to 12 weeks after exposure, and the presence of the antibody provides no protection against acquired immunodeficiency syndrome (AIDS). Because of occasional delayed appearance of the antibody after initial exposure, it is important to follow up patients for 1 year after exposure.

315. The answer is d. (*Droegemueller, pp 859–864.*) The occurrence of cervical squamous dysplasia/carcinoma is thought to be related to infection with the human papillomavirus (HPV), which is sexually transmitted. HPV causes genital warts. Women who begin sexual activity at a young age, have multiple sexual partners, do not use condoms, and have a history of sexually transmitted diseases are at an increased risk for cervical neoplasia. Alterations in immune function (such as in patients with HIV or on immunosuppressive therapy) place a patient at an increased risk of infection with HPV and therefore of cervical neoplasia. Women who smoke tobacco have an increased risk of developing cervical neoplasia. There is no known increased risk of cervical dysplasia due to use of DepoProvera. However, some studies support an association of increased risk of cervical adenocarcinoma with oral contraceptive use. The literature does not support an increased risk of squamous cell carcinoma of the cervix in women who smoke.

316. The answer is e. (*Stenchever, p 864.*) Any patient with a Pap smear result that comes back suggesting dysplasia of the cervix should undergo a colposcopy with subsequent directed biopsy of any abnormal-appearing areas and an endocervical curettage. High-grade results include possible moderate dysplasia, severe dysplasia, or carcinoma in situ. The colposcope is a type of microscope that allows the physician to examine the cervix at a magnification of 10 to 16×. Three percent acetic acid is applied to the cervix to help visualize any abnormal blood vessels or acetowhite areas that could represent areas of dysplasia. Abnormal areas are then biopsied for histologic analysis. In patients with an HGSIL Pap, there is no indication for repeating the smear or ordering HPV testing, because you need to immediately rule out a pathologic process. Repeating a Pap can produce a false-negative result, which can lead to a delay in treating the patient. Random cervical biopsies are not indicated because you can miss the abnormal areas. The indications for a cone biopsy would be (1) unsatisfactory colpo-scopic exam (i.e., the entire transformation zone cannot be seen); (2) a col-poscopically directed cervical biopsy that indicates the possibility of invasive disease; (3) neoplasm in the endocervix; or (4) cells seen on cervical biopsy that do not adequately explain the cells seen on cytologic exam-ination (i.e., the Pap).

317. The answer is c. *(Beckmann, pp 558–561.)* As discussed above in question 316, one of the indications for a cone biopsy is when the results of the cervical biopsy do not adequately explain the severity of the Pap smear. In about 10% of colposcopically directed cervical biopsies, there will be a substantial discrepancy between the Pap smear and the biopsy results (i.e., the biopsy is normal but the Pap indicates severely abnormal cells). A conization is required to rule out lesions higher in the endocervi-cal canal. Merely repeating the Pap smear is incorrect, because you may be delaying treatment of a serious problem. Once cervical dysplasia has been established, cryotherapy and laser ablation are viable treatment options. There is no indication for a hysterectomy in this patient.

318. The answer is e. *(Beckmann, pp 356–358.)* Approximately 0.5% of Pap smears come back with glandular cell abnormalities. These abnormali-ties can be associated with squamous lesions, adenocarcinoma in situ, or invasive adenocarcinoma. Therefore any patient with AGUS should undergo immediate colposcopy and ECC. In addition, postmenopausal women should have endometrial sampling. Hysterectomy or conization might be indicated based on results of the colposcopy; however, colposcopy must be performed initially.

319–320. The answers are 319-a, 320-c. *(Postgraduate Obstetrics and Gynecology. Stenchever, pp 487–488, 668, 1000–1002. Beckmann, p 538–539.)* Vulvar vestibulitis is a syndrome of unknown etiology. To make the diagnosis of this disorder, the following three findings must be present: (1) severe pain on vestibular touch or attempted vaginal entry, (2) tenderness to pressure localized within the vulvar vestibule, and (3) visible findings con-fined to vulvar erythema of various degrees. To treat vulvar vestibulitis, the first step is to avoid tight clothing, tampons, hot tubs, and soaps, which can all act as vulvar irritants. If this fails, topical treatments include lidocaine, estrogen, and steroids. Tricyclic antidepressants and intralesional interferon injections have also been used. For women refractory to medical therapy, surgical excision of the vestibular mucosa may be helpful. Valtrex (valacyclovir) is an antiviral medication used in the treatment of genital herpes and is not indicated for vulvar vestibulitis. Contact dermatitis is an inflammation and irritation of the vulvar skin due to a chemical irritant. The vulvar skin is usually red, swollen, and inflamed and may become weeping and eczemoid. Women with a contact dermatitis usually experience chronic vulvar tenderness, burning, and itching that can occur even when they are not engaging in intercourse. Atrophic vaginitis is a thinning and ulceration of the vaginal mucosa that occurs as a result of hypoestrogenism; thus this condition is usually seen in postmenopausal women not on any hormone replacement therapy. Lichen sclerosus is another atrophic condition of the vulva. It is characterized by diffuse, thin whitish epithelial areas on the labia majora, minora, clitoris, and perineum. In severe cases, it may be difficult to identify normal anatomic landmarks. The most common symptom of lichen sclerosus is chronic vulvar pruritus. Vulvar intraepithelial neoplasia (VIN) are precancerous lesions of the vulva that have a tendency to progress to frank cancer. Women with VIN complain of vulvar pruritus, chronic irritation, and raised lesions. These lesions are most commonly located along the posterior vulva and in the perineal body and have a whitish cast and rough texture.

321–322. The answers are 321-b, 322-d. (*Stenchever, pp 668–678. Beckmann, pp 370–371.*) Bacterial vaginosis is a condition is which there is an overgrowth of anaerobic bacteria in the vagina that replaces the normal lactobacillus. Women with this type of vaginitis complain of an unpleasant vaginal odor that is described as musty or fishy and a thin, gray-white vaginal discharge that is adherent to the vaginal walls. Vulvar irritation and pruritus are rarely present. To confirm the diagnosis of bacterial vaginosis, a wet smear is done. To perform a wet smear, saline is mixed with the vaginal discharge and clumps of bacteria and clue cells are identified. Clue cells are vaginal epithelial cells with clusters of bacteria adherent to their surfaces. In addition, a whiff test can be performed by mixing potassium hydroxide with the vaginal discharge. In cases of bacterial vaginosis, an amine-like odor will be detected. The treatment of choice for bacterial vaginosis is metronidazole (Flagyl) 500 mg given twice daily for 7 days. Pregnant women with symptomatic bacterial vaginosis (BV) should be treated the same way as nonpregnant women with BV. In cases of a normal or physiologic discharge, vaginal secretions are white, curdy, and odorless. In addition, normal vaginal secretions do not adhere to the vaginal side walls. In cases of candidiasis, patients commonly complain of vulvar burning, pain, pruritus, and erythema. The vaginal discharge tends to be white, highly viscous, granular, and adherent to the vaginal walls. A wet smear with potassium hydroxide can confirm the diagnosis by the identification of hyphae. Treatment of candidiasis can be achieved with the administration of topical imidazoles or triazoles or the oral medication Diflucan. *Trichomonas* vaginitis is the most common nonviral, nonchlamydial sexually transmitted disease of women. It is caused by the anaerobic, flagellated protozoan *T. vaginalis.* Women with *Trichomonas* vaginitis commonly complain of a copious vaginal discharge that may be white, yellow, green, or gray and that has an unpleasant odor. Some women complain of vulvar pruritus, which is primarily confined to the vestibule and labia minora. On physical exam, the vulva and vagina frequently appear red and swollen. Only a small percentage of women possess the classically described strawberry cervix. Diagnosis of trichomoniasis is confirmed with a wet saline smear. Under the microscope, the *Trichomonas* organisms can be visualized under high power; these organisms are unicellular protozoans that are spherical in shape with three to five flagella extending from one end. The recommended treatment for trichomoniasis is a one-time dose of 2 g metronidazole. *Chlamydia trachomatis* is an intracellular parasite that can cause an infection that may be manifested as cervicitis, urethritis, or salpingitis. Patients with mild cases may be asymptomatic. On physical exam, women with chlamydial infections may demonstrate a mucopurulent cervicitis. The diagnosis of chlamydia is suspected on clinical exam and confirmed with cervical cultures. Treatment for a chlamydial cervicitis is with oral azithromycin, 1 g, or doxycycline 100 mg twice daily for 7 days.

323–325. The answers are 323-c, 324-d, 325-c. (*Stenchever, pp 726–727.*) Ovarian torsion, appendicitis, acute salpingitis, and ruptured ovarian cyst are all commonly associated with fever, abdominal pain, and elevated white blood cell count. The timing of the symptoms of the patient in question 323 and her history of a new sexual partner point to the diagnosis of acute salpingitis. Ovarian torsion is associated with an adnexal mass. Pain from ruptured ovarian cysts usually occurs before menstruation. Although appendicitis is in the differential diagnosis, it is unlikely, as the patient in question 323 has no nausea or vomiting. In cases of kidney stone, urinalysis usually indicates the presence of blood. In addition, the pain is usually in the flank areas. Any patient with PID and a tuboovarian abscess should be hospitalized and given intravenous antibiotics. Any patient with TOAs who does not get better on broad-spectrum antibiotics should undergo surgical drainage of the abscesses via laparotomy, laparoscopy, or percutaneously under CT guidance.

The Centers for Disease Control's recommendation for inpatient management of PID includes the following:

1. Cefoxitin 2 g IV every 6 h or cefotetan 2 g IV every 12 h plus doxycycline 100 mg PO or IV twice daily
   or
2. Clindamycin 900 mg IV every 8 h plus gentamicin loading dose IV or IM (2 mg/kg) followed by maintenance dose (1.5 mg/kg) every 8 h

The Centers for Disease Control's recommendation for the outpatient management of PID includes the following:

1. Cefoxitin 2 g IM plus probenecid 1 g PO in a single dose concurrently or ceftriaxone 250 mg IM plus doxycycline 100 mg PO twice daily for 14 days
   or
2. Ofloxacin 400 mg PO two times a day for 14 days plus either clindamycin 450 mg PO four times a day or metronidazole 500 mg PO two times a day for 14 days.

326. The answer is c. (*Stenchever, pp 366–367.*) Nipple discharge can occur in women with either benign or malignant breast conditions. Approximately 10 to 15% of women with benign breast disease complain of nipple discharge. However, nipple discharge is present in only about 3% of women with breast malignancies. The most worrisome nipple discharges tend to be spontaneous, unilateral, and persistent. The color of nipple discharge does not differentiate benign from malignant breast conditions. The most common breast disorder associated with a bloody nipple discharge is an intraductal papilloma. However, breast carcinoma must always be ruled out in any patient complaining of a bloody nipple discharge. Sanguineous or serosanguineous nipple discharges can also be seen in women with duct ectasia and fibrocystic breast disease. Women with hyperprolactinemia due to a pituitary adenoma experience bilateral milky white nipple discharges.

327. The answer is b. (*Stenchever, pp 365–366. Beckmann, pp 420–421.*) This patient's breast mass is characteristic of a fibroadenoma. Fibroadenomas are the second most common benign breast disorder, after fibrocystic changes. They are characterized by being firm, solid, nontender, and freely mobile. Fibroadenomas have an average size diameter of 2.5 cm and are well circumscribed. These lesions most commonly occur in adolescents and women in their twenties. Fibrocystic changes occur in about one-third to one-half of reproductive-age women and represent an exaggerated response of the breast tissue to hormones. Patients with fibrocystic changes complain of bilateral mastalgia and breast engorgement preceding menses. On physical exam, diffuse bilateral nodularity is typically encountered. Cystosarcoma phyllodes are rare fibroepithelial tumors that constitute 1% of breast malignancies. These rapidly growing tumors are the most frequent breast sarcoma and occur most frequently in women in the fifth decade of life. Trauma to the breast can result in fat necrosis. Women with fat necrosis commonly present to the physician with a firm, tender mass that is surrounded by ecchymosis. Occasional skin retraction can occur, making this lesion difficult to differentiate from cancer. It is unlikely that this patient who presents in her twenties has breast cancer. Fine-needle aspiration or excisional biopsy must be performed to rule out the rare chance of malignancy, but breast cancer is not the most likely diagnosis based on the patient's age and lack of any other breast changes consistent with carcinoma (such as a fixed mass, skin retraction, or lymphadenopathy).

328. The answer is b. (*Beckmann, pp 571–574.*) Uterine fibroids or myomas are benign smooth-muscle tumors of the uterus. They are present in about 30% of American women. In pregnancy, most women with fibroids are asymptomatic and do not require therapy. Uterine myomas are hormonally responsive and grow in response to estrogen exposure. Uncommonly, during pregnancy a woman with fibroids may have an increase in size of these fibroids to the point where they outgrow their blood supply (carneous degeneration). Fibroid degeneration may lead to preterm labor. Uterine fibroids can also be associated with fetal malpresentation due to distortion of the endometrial cavity and postpartum atony due to inability of the uterine muscle to contract normally after delivery. Uterine leiomyosarcomas are smooth-muscle malignancies characterized by more than 5 mitoses per 10 hpf. These malignancies are not thought to arise from benign fibroids but occur de novo. Uterine leiomyosarcomas typically occur in postmenopausal women with a rapidly enlarging uterus.

329. The answer is d. (*Stenchever, pp 160, 232–233.*) Given this patient's age and symptoms, she is probably menopausal. Women with postmeno-pausal bleeding should be evaluated with an endometrial biopsy prior to any medical treatment or surgical intervention (such as hysterectomy or endometrial ablation). A pelvic ultrasound would also be helpful in the management of this patient and would offer information regarding the size and location of any uterine fibroids or polyps. There is no indication for conization of the cervix in this patient. Conization of the cervix is done for evaluation and treatment of cervical dysplasia.

330. The answer is b. (*Stenchever, pp 921–927.*) Postmenopausal patients with atypical complex hyperplasia of the endometrium have a 25 to 30% risk of having an associated endometrial carcinoma in the uterus. For this reason, hysterectomy is the recommended treatment for this patient. If hysterectomy is not medically advisable, progesterone treatment can be used. Myomectomy, or surgical removal of fibroid, is used in the treatment of premenopausal women with symptomatic uterine fibroids. The use of oral contraceptives is contraindicated in patients with atypical endometrial hyperplasia. There is no use for oral contraceptives in the treatment of postmenopausal bleeding.

Infertility, Endocrinology, and Menstrual Dysfunction

Questions

DIRECTIONS: Each item below contains a question followed by suggested responses. Select the **one best** response to each question.

331. You see five postmenopausal patients in the clinic. Each patient has one of the conditions listed, and each patient wishes to begin hormone replacement therapy today. Which one of the following patients would you start on therapy at the time of this visit?

a. Mild essential hypertension
b. Liver disease with abnormal liver function tests
c. Malignant melanoma
d. Undiagnosed genital tract bleeding
e. Treated stage III endometrial cancer

332. A mother brings her 12-year-old daughter in to your office for consultation. She is concerned because most of the other girls in her daughter's class have already started their period. She thinks her daughter hasn't shown any evidence of going into puberty yet. Knowing the usual first sign of the onset of puberty, you should ask the mother which of the following questions?

a. Has her daughter had any acne
b. Has her daughter started to develop breasts
c. Does her daughter have any axillary or pubic hair
d. Has her daughter started her growth spurt
e. Has her daughter had any vaginal spotting

333. A 9-year-old girl presents for evaluation of regular vaginal bleeding. History reveals thelarche at age 7 and adrenarche at age 8. Which of the following is the most common cause of this condition in girls?

a. Idiopathic
b. Gonadal tumors
c. McCune-Albright syndrome
d. Hypothyroidism
e. Tumors of the central nervous system

334. A 55-year-old woman presents to your office for consultation regarding her symptoms of menopause. She stopped having periods 8 months ago and is having severe hot flushes. The hot flushes are causing her considerable stress. What should you tell her regarding the psychological symptoms of the climacteric?

a. They are not related to her changing levels of estrogen and progesterone
b. They commonly include insomnia, irritability, frustration, and malaise
c. They are related to a drop in gonadotropin levels
d. They are not affected by environmental factors
e. They are primarily a reaction to the cessation of menstrual flow

335. A 58-year-old caucasian woman comes in to your office for advice regarding her risk factors for developing osteoporosis. She is 5 ft 1 in. tall and weighs 195 lb. She stopped having periods at age 49. She is healthy but she smokes one pack of cigarettes per day. She does not take any medications. She has never taken hormone replacement for menopause. Her mother died at age 71 after she suffered a spontaneous hip fracture. Which of the following will have the least effect on this patient's risk for developing osteoporosis?

a. Her family history
b. Her race
c. Her history of smoking cigarettes
d. Her menopause status
e. Her obesity

336. A mother brings her 14-year-old daughter in to the office for consultation. The mother says her daughter should have started her period by now. She is also concerned that she is shorter than her friends. On physical examination the girl is 4 ft 10 in. tall. She shows evidence of breast development at Tanner stage 2. She has no axillary or pubic hair. You reassure the mother that her daughter seems to be developing normally. Educating the mother and daughter, your best advice is to tell them which of the following?

a. The daughter will start her period when her breasts reach Tanner stage 5
b. The daughter will start her period then have her growth spurt
c. The daughter's period should start within 1 to 2 years since she has just started developing breast buds
d. The daughter will have her growth spurt, then pubic hair will develop, heralding the onset of menstruation
e. The daughter's period should start by age 18, but if she has not had her period by then, she should come back in for further evaluation

337. An 18-year-old consults you for evaluation of disabling pain with her menstrual periods. The pain has been present since menarche and is accompanied by nausea and headache. History is otherwise unremarkable, and pelvic examination is normal. You diagnose primary dysmenorrhea and recommend initial treatment with which of the following?

a. Ergot derivatives
b. Antiprostaglandins
c. Gonadotropin-releasing hormone (GnRH) analogues
d. Danazol
e. Codeine

338. An 18-year-old patient presents to you for evaluation because she has not yet started her period. On physical examination, she is 5 ft 7 in. tall. She has minimal breast development and no axillary or pubic hair. On pelvic examination she has a normally developed vagina. A cervix is visible. The uterus is palpable, as are normal ovaries. Which of the following is the best next step in the evaluation of this patient?

a. Draw her blood for a karyotype
b. Test her sense of smell
c. Draw her blood for TSH, FSH, and LH levels
d. Order an MRI of the brain to evaluate the pituitary gland
e. Prescribe a progesterone challenge to see if she will have a withdrawal bleed

339. A 7-year-old girl is brought in to see you by her mother because the girl has developed breasts and has a few pubic hairs starting to show up. Which of the following is the best treatment for the girl's condition?

a. Exogenous gonadotropins
b. Ethinyl estradiol
c. GnRH agonists
d. Clomiphene citrate
e. No treatment; reassure the mother that pubertal symptoms at age 7 are normal

340. A mother brings her daughter in to see you for consultation. The daughter is 17 years old and has not started her period. She is 4 ft 10 in. tall. She has no breast budding. On pelvic examination, she has no pubic hair. By digital examination the patient has a cervix and uterus. The ovaries are not palpable. As part of the workup, serum FSH and LH levels are drawn and both are high. Which of the following is the most likely reason for delayed puberty and sexual infantilism in this patient?

a. Adrenogenital syndrome (testicular feminization)
b. McCune-Albright syndrome
c. Kallman syndrome
d. Gonadal dysgenesis
e. Müllerian agenesis

341. While evaluating a 30-year-old woman for infertility, you diagnose a bicornuate uterus. You explain that additional testing is necessary because of the woman's increased risk of congenital anomalies in which organ system?

a. Skeletal
b. Hematopoietic
c. Urinary
d. Central nervous
e. Tracheoesophageal

342. A 39-year-old G3P3 complains of severe, progressive secondary dysmenorrhea and menorrhagia. Pelvic examination demonstrates a tender, diffusely enlarged uterus with no adnexal tenderness. Results of endometrial biopsy are normal. Which of the following is the most likely diagnosis?

a. Endometriosis
b. Endometritis
c. Adenomyosis
d. Uterine sarcoma
e. Leiomyoma

343. A 28-year-old G3P0 has a history of severe menstrual cramps, prolonged, heavy periods, chronic pelvic pain, and painful intercourse. All of her pregnancies were spontaneous abortions in the first trimester. A hysterosalpingogram she just had as part of the evaluation for recurrent abortion showed a large uterine septum. You have recommended surgical repair of the uterus. Of the patient's symptoms, which is most likely to be corrected by resection of the uterine septum?

a. Habitual abortion
b. Dysmenorrhea
c. Menometrorrhagia
d. Dyspareunia
e. Chronic pelvic pain

344. In an amenorrheic patient who has had pituitary ablation for a craniopharyngioma, which of the following regimens is most likely to result in an ovulatory cycle?

a. Clomiphene citrate
b. Pulsatile infusion of gonadotropin-releasing hormone (GnRH)
c. Continuous infusion of GnRH
d. Human menopausal or recombinant gonadotropin
e. Human menopausal or recombinant gonadotropin followed by human chorionic gonadotropin (hCG)

345. In the evaluation of a 26-year-old patient with 4 months of secondary amenorrhea, you order serum prolactin and β-hCG assays. The pregnancy test is positive, and the prolactin comes back at 100 ng/mL (normal <25 ng/mL in this assay). This patient requires which of the following?

a. Routine obstetric care
b. Computed tomography (CT) scan of her sella turcica to rule out pituitary adenoma
c. Repeat measurements of serum prolactin to ensure that values do not increase over 300 ng/mL
d. Bromocriptine to suppress prolactin
e. Evaluation for possible hypothyroidism

346. You have just performed diagnostic laparoscopy on a patient with chronic pelvic pain and dyspareunia. The patient had multiple implants of endometriosis on the uterosacral ligaments and ovaries and several on the rectosigmoid colon. At the time of the procedure you ablated all of the visible lesions on the peritoneal surfaces with the CO_2 laser. But because of the extent of the patient's disease you recommend postoperative medical treatment. Which of the following medications is the best option for the treatment of this patient's endometriosis?

a. Continuous unopposed oral estrogen
b. Dexamethasone
c. Danazol
d. Gonadotropins
e. Parlodel

347. A 28-year-old nulligravid patient complains of bleeding between her periods and increasingly heavy menses. Over the past 9 months she has had two dilation and curettages (D&Cs), which have failed to resolve her symptoms, and oral contraceptives and antiprostaglandins have not decreased the abnormal bleeding. Which of the following options is most appropriate at this time?

a. Perform a hysterectomy
b. Perform hysteroscopy
c. Perform endometrial ablation
d. Treat with a GnRH agonist
e. Start the patient on a high-dose progestational agent

348. You are treating a 31-year-old woman with danazol for endometriosis. You should warn the patient of potential side effects of prolonged treatment with the medication. When used in the treatment of endometriosis, which of the following changes should the patient expect?

a. Occasional pelvic pain, since danazol commonly causes ovarian enlargement
b. Lighter or absent menstruation, since danozol causes endometrial atrophy
c. Heavier or prolonged periods, since danozol causes endometrial hyperplasia
d. More frequent Pap smear screening, since danozol exposure is a risk factor for cervical dysplasia
e. Postcoital bleeding due to the inflammatory effect of danozol on the endocervical and endometrial glands

349. A patient presents to you for evaluation of infertility. She is 26 years old and has never been pregnant. She and her husband have been trying to get pregnant for 2 years. Her husband had a semen analysis and was told that everything was normal. The patient has a history of endometriosis diagnosed by laparoscopy at age 17. At the time she was having severe pelvic pain and dysmenorrhea. After the surgery the patient was told she had a few small implants of endometriosis on her ovaries and fallopian tubes and several others in the posterior cul-de-sac. She also had a left ovarian cyst, filmy adnexal adhesions and several subcentimeter serosal fibroids. You have recommended that she have a hysterosalpingogram as part of her evaluation for infertility. Which of the patient's following conditions can be diagnosed with a hysterosalpingogram?

a. Endometriosis
b. Hydrosalpinx
c. Subserous fibroids
d. Minimal pelvic adhesions
e. Ovarian cyst

350. During the evaluation of infertility in a 25-year-old female, a hysterosalpingogram showed evidence of Asherman syndrome. Which one of the following symptoms would you expect this patient to have?

a. Hypomenorrhea
b. Oligomenorrhea
c. Menorrhagia
d. Metrorrhagia
e. Dysmenorrhea

351. During the evaluation of secondary amenorrhea in a 24-year-old woman, hyperprolactinemia is diagnosed. Which of the following conditions could cause increased circulating prolactin concentration and amenorrhea in this patient?

a. Stress
b. Primary hyperthyroidism
c. Anorexia nervosa
d. Congenital adrenal hyperplasia
e. Polycystic ovarian disease

352. A 36-year-old morbidly obese woman presents to your office for evaluation of heavy menstruation with frequent bleeding between periods. An office endometrial biopsy shows complex hyperplasia of the endometrium without atypia. The hyperplasia is most likely related to the excess formation in the patient's adipose tissue of which of the following hormones?

a. Estriol
b. Estradiol
c. Estrone
d. Androstenedione
e. Dehydroepiandrosterone

353. A couple presents for evaluation of primary infertility. The evaluation of the woman is completely normal. The husband is found to have a left varicocele. If the husband's varicocele is the cause of the couple's infertility, what would you expect to see when evaluating the husband's semen analysis?

a. Decreased sperm count with an increase in the number of abnormal forms
b. Decreased sperm count with an increase in motility
c. Increased sperm count with an increase in the number of abnormal forms
d. Increased sperm count with absent motility
e. Azospermia

354. Your patient delivers a 7-lb 0-oz male infant at term. On physical examination the baby has normal-appearing male external genitalia. However, the scrotum is empty. No testes are palpable in the inguinal canals. At 6 months of age the boy's testes still have not descended. A pelvic ultrasound shows the testes in the pelvis, and there appears to be a uterus present as well. The presence of a uterus in an otherwise phenotypically normal male is due to which of the following?

a. Lack of Müllerian-inhibiting factor
b. Lack of testosterone
c. Increased levels of estrogens
d. 46,XX karyotype
e. Presence of ovarian tissue early in embryonic development

355. A 25-year-old woman presents to your office for evaluation of primary infertility. She has regular periods every 28 days. She has done testing at home with an ovulation kit, which suggests she is ovulating. A hysterosalpingogram demonstrates patency of both fallopian tubes. A progesterone level drawn in the midluteal phase is lower than expected. A luteal phase defect is suspected to be the cause of this patient's infertility. Which of the following studies performed in the second half of the menstrual cycle is helpful in making this diagnosis?

a. Serum estradiol levels
b. Urinary pregnanetriol levels
c. Endometrial biopsy
d. Serum follicle-stimulating hormone (FSH) levels
e. Serum luteinizing hormone (LH) levels

356. A 45-year-old woman who had two normal pregnancies 15 and 18 years ago presents with the complaint of amenorrhea for 7 months. She expresses the desire to become pregnant again. After exclusion of pregnancy, which of the following tests is next indicated in the evaluation of this patient's amenorrhea?

a. Hysterosalpingogram
b. Endometrial biopsy
c. Thyroid function tests
d. Testosterone and DHAS levels
e. LH and FSH levels

357. A 22-year-old woman consults you for treatment of hirsutism. She is obese and has facial acne and hirsutism on her face and periareolar regions and a male escutcheon. Serum LH level is 35 mIU/mL and FSH is 9 mIU/mL. Androstenedione and testosterone levels are mildly elevated, but serum DHAS is normal. The patient does not wish to conceive at this time. Which of the following single agents is the most appropriate treatment of her condition?

a. Oral contraceptives
b. Corticosteroids
c. GnRH
d. Parlodel
e. Wedge resection

358. An 18-year-old college student who has recently become sexually active is seen for severe primary dysmenorrhea. She does not want to get pregnant, and has failed to obtain resolution with heating pads and mild analgesics. Which of the following medications is most appropriate for this patient?

a. Prostaglandin inhibitors
b. Narcotic analgesics
c. Oxytocin
d. Oral contraceptives
e. Luteal progesterone

359. A 20-year-old female with Müllerian agenesis is undergoing laparoscopic appendectomy by a general surgeon. You are consulted intraoperatively because the surgeon sees several lesions in the pelvis suspicious for endometriosis. You should tell the surgeon which of the following?

a. Endometriosis cannot occur in patients with Müllerian agenesis since they do not have a uterus
b. Endometriosis is common in women with Müllerian agenesis since they have menstrual outflow obstruction
c. Endometriosis probably occurs in patients with Müllerian agenesis as a result of retrograde menstruation
d. Endometriosis may arise in patients with Müllerian agenesis as a result of coelomic metaplasia
e. Endometriosis cannot occur in patients with Müllerian agenesis because they have a 46,XY karyotype

360. A 19-year-old patient presents to your office with primary amenorrhea. She has normal breast and pubic hair development, but the uterus and vagina are absent. Diagnostic possibilities include which of the following?

a. XYY syndrome
b. Gonadal dysgenesis
c. Müllerian agenesis
d. Klinefelter syndrome
e. Turner syndrome

361. A 27-year-old woman presents to your office complaining of mood swings, depression, irritability, and breast pain each month in the week prior to her menstrual period. She often calls in sick at work because she cannot function when she has the symptoms. Which of the following medications is the best option for treating the patient's problem?

a. Progesterone
b. A short-acting benzodiazepine
c. A conjugated equine estrogen
d. A nonsteroidal anti-inflammatory drug (NSAID)
e. Selective serotonin reuptake inhibitors (SSRIs)

362. A 23-year-old woman presents for evaluation of a 7-month history of amenorrhea. Examination discloses bilateral galactorrhea and normal breast and pelvic examinations. Pregnancy test is negative. Which of the following classes of medication is a possible cause of her condition?

a. Antiestrogens
b. Gonadotropins
c. Phenothiazines
d. Prostaglandins
e. GnRH analogues

363. Which of the following pubertal events in girls is not estrogen-dependent?

a. Menses
b. Vaginal cornification
c. Hair growth
d. Reaching adult height
e. Production of cervical mucus

364. A 9-year-old girl has breast and pubic hair development. Evaluation demonstrates a pubertal response to a gonadotropin-releasing hormone (GnRH) stimulation test and a prominent increase in luteinizing hormone (LH) pulses during sleep. These findings are characteristic of patients with which of the following?

a.   Theca cell tumors
b.   Iatrogenic sexual precocity
c.   Premature thelarche
d.   Granulosa cell tumors
e.   Constitutional precocious puberty

365. An infertile couple presents to you for evaluation. A semen analysis from the husband is ordered. The sample of 2.5 cc contains 25 million sperm per milliliter; 65% of the sperm show normal morphology; 20% of the sperm show progressive forward mobility. You should tell the couple which of the following?

a.   The sample is normal but of no clinical value because of the low sample volume
b.   The sample is normal and should not be a factor in the couple's infertility
c.   The sample is abnormal because the percentage of sperm with normal morphology is too low
d.   The sample is abnormal due to an inadequate number of sperm per milliliter
e.   The sample is abnormal due to a low percentage of forwardly mobile sperm

366. You suspect that your infertility patient has an inadequate luteal phase. She should undergo an endometrial biopsy on which day of her menstrual cycle?

a.   Day 3
b.   Day 8
c.   Day 14
d.   Day 21
e.   Day 26

367. You have recommended a postcoital test for your patient as part of her evaluation for infertility. She and her spouse should have sexual intercourse on which day of her menstrual cycle as part of postcoital testing?

a.   Day 3
b.   Day 8
c.   Day 14
d.   Day 21
e.   Day 26

368. You ask a patient to call your office during her next menstrual cycle to schedule a hysterosalpingogram (HSG) as part of her infertility evaluation. Which day of the menstrual cycle is best for performing the HSG?

a. Day 3
b. Day 8
c. Day 14
d. Day 21
e. Day 26

369. You have recommended that your infertility patient return to your office during her next menstrual cycle to have her serum progesterone level checked. Which is the best day of the menstrual cycle to check her progesterone level if you are trying to confirm ovulation?

a. Day 3
b. Day 8
c. Day 14
d. Day 21
e. Day 26

370. Your patient is 43 years old and is concerned that she may be too close to menopause to get pregnant. You recommend that her gonadotropin levels be tested. Which is the best day of the menstrual cycle to check gonadotropin levels in this situation?

a. Day 3
b. Day 8
c. Day 14
d. Day 21
e. Day 26

371. A 22-year-old G0P0 comes to your office with a chief complaint of being too hairy. She reports that her menses started at age 13 and have always been very irregular. She also complains of acne and is currently seeing a dermatologist for the skin condition. She denies any medical problems, and her only surgery was an appendectomy at age 8. Height is 5 ft 5 in.; weight is 150 lb; BP is 100/60. On physical exam, there is sparse hair around the nipples, chin, and upper lip. No galactorrhea, thyromegaly, or temporal balding is noted. Pelvic exam is normal and there is no evidence of clitoromegaly. Which of the following is the most likely explanation for this patient's problem?

a. Idiopathic or constitutional hirsutism
b. Polycystic ovarian syndrome
c. Late-onset congenital adrenal hyperplasia
d. Sertoli-Leydig cell tumor of the ovary
e. Adrenal tumor

372. Your patient is a 23-year-old woman with primary infertility. She is 5 ft 4 in. tall and weighs 210 lb. She has had periods every 2 to 3 months since starting her period at age 12. She has a problem with acne and hair growth on her chin. Her mother had the same problem at her age and now has adult onset diabetes. On physical examination of the patient, you notice a few coarse, dark hairs on her chin and around her nipples. She has a normal-appearing clitoris. Her ovaries and uterus are normal to palpation. Which of the following blood tests has no role in the evaluation of this patient?

a. Total testosterone
b. 17 α-hydroxyprogesterone
c. DHEAS
d. Estrone
e. TSH

373. You have just diagnosed a 21-year-old infertile woman with polycystic ovarian syndrome. The remainder of the infertility evaluation, including the patient's hysterosalpingogram and her husband's semen analysis, were normal. Her periods are very unpredictable, usually coming every 3 to 6 months. She would like your advice on the best way to conceive now that you have made a diagnosis. Which of the following treatment options is the most appropriate first step in treating this patient?

a. Dexamethasone
b. Gonadotropins
c. Artificial insemination
d. Metformin
e. In vitro fertilization

374. A patient in your practice calls you in a panic because her 14-year-old daughter has been bleeding heavily for the past 2 weeks and now feels a bit dizzy and light-headed. The daughter experienced menarche about 6 months ago, and since that time her periods have been irregular and very heavy. You instruct the mother to bring her daughter to the emergency room. When you see the daughter in the emergency room, you note that she appears very pale and fatigued. Her blood pressure and pulse are 110/60 and 70, respectively. When you stand her up, her blood pressure remains stable, but her pulse increases to 100. While in the emergency room, you obtain a more detailed history. She denies any medical problems or prior surgeries and is not taking any medications. She reports that she has never been sexually active. On physical exam, her abdomen is benign. She will not let you perform a speculum exam, but the bimanual exam is normal. She is 5 ft 4 in. tall and weighs 95 lb. Which of the following blood tests is not indicated in the evaluation of this patient?

a. BHCG
b. Bleeding time
c. CBC
d. Type and screen
e. Estradiol level

375. A 32-year-old morbidly obese diabetic woman presents to your office complaining of prolonged vaginal bleeding. She has never been pregnant. Her periods were regular, monthly, and light until 2 years ago. At that time she started having periods every 3 to 6 months. Her last normal period was 5 months ago. She started having vaginal bleeding again 3 weeks ago, light at first. For the past week she has been bleeding heavily and passing large clots. On pelvic examination, the external genitalia is normal. The vagina is filled with large clots. A large clot is seen protruding through the cervix. The uterus is in the upper limit of normal in size. The ovaries are normal to palpation. Her urine pregnancy test is negative. Which of the following is the most likely diagnosis?

a. Uterine fibroids
b. Cervical polyp
c. Incomplete abortion
d. Chronic anovulation
e. Coagulation defect

376. One of your patients with polycystic ovarian syndrome presents to the emergency room complaining of prolonged, heavy vaginal bleeding. She is 26 years old and has never been pregnant. She was taking birth control pills to regulate her periods until 4 months ago. She stopped taking them because she and her spouse want to try to get pregnant. She thought she might be pregnant because she had not had a period since her last one on the birth control pills 4 months ago. She started having vaginal bleeding 8 days ago. She has been doubling up on superabsorbant sanitary napkins 5 to 6 times daily since the bleeding began. On arrival at the emergency room, the patient has a supine blood pressure of 102/64 with a pulse of 96. Upon standing, the patient feels light-headed. Her standing blood pressure is 108/66 with a pulse of 126. While you wait for lab work to come back, you order intravenous hydration. After 2 hours, the patient is no longer orthostatic. Her pregnancy test comes back negative, and her Hct is 31%. She continues to have heavy bleeding. Which of the following is the best next step in the management of this patient?

a. Perform a dilation and curettage
b. Administer a blood transfusion to treat her severe anemia
c. Send her home with a prescription for iron therapy
d. Administer high-dose estrogen therapy
e. Administer antiprostaglandins

377. A 29-year-old G0 who comes to your OB/GYN office complaining of PMS. On taking a more detailed history, you learn that the patient suffers from emotional lability and depression for about 10 days prior to her menses. She reports that once she begins to bleed she feels back to normal. The patient also reports a long history of premenstrual fatigue, breast tenderness, and bloating. Her previous health care provider placed her on oral contraceptives to treat her PMS 6 months ago. She reports that the pills have alleviated all her PMS symptoms except for the depression and emotional symptoms. Which of the following is the best next step in the treatment of this patient's problem?

a. Spironolactone
b. Evening primrose oil
c. Fluoxetine
d. Progesterone supplements
e. Vitamin B_6

378. A 51-year-old woman G3P3 presents to your office with a 6-month history of amenorrhea. She complains of debilitating hot flushes that awaken her at night; she wakes up the next day feeling exhausted and irritable. She tells you she has tried herbal supplements for her hot flushes, but nothing has worked. She is interested in beginning hormone replacement therapy (HRT), but is hesitant to do so because of its possible risks and side effects. The patient is very healthy. She denies any medical problems and is not taking any medication except calcium supplements. She has a family history of osteoporosis. Her height is 5 ft 5 in. and her weight is 115 lb. In counseling the patient regarding the risks and benefits of hormone replacement therapy, you should tell her that HRT (estrogen and progesterone) has been associated with which of the following?

a. An increased risk of colon cancer
b. An increased risk of uterine cancer
c. An increased risk of thromboembolic events
d. An increased risk of developing Alzheimer's disease
e. An increased risk of malignant melanoma

379. A 56-year-old woman presents to your office for her routine well-woman examination. She had a hysterectomy at age 44 for symptomatic uterine fibroids. She entered menopause at age 54 based on menopausal symptoms and an elevated FSH level. She started taking estrogen replacement therapy at that time for relief of her symptoms. She is fasting and would like to have her lipid panel checked while she is in the office today. You counsel the patient on the effects of estrogen therapy on her lipid panel. She should expect which of the following?

a.   An increase in her LDL
b.   An increase in her HDL
c.   An increase in her total cholesterol
d.   A decrease in her triglycerides
e.   A decrease in her HDL

380. A 48-year-old woman consults with you regarding menopausal symptoms. Her periods have become less regular over the past 6 months. Her last period was 1 month ago. She started having hot flushes last year. They have been getting progressively more frequent. She has several hot flushes during the day, and she wakes up twice at night with them as well. She has done quite a lot of reading about perimenopause, menopause, and hormone replacement therapy. She is concerned about the risks of taking female hormones. She wants to know what she should expect in regard to her hot flushes if she does not take hormone replacement. You should tell her which of the following?

a.   Hot flushes usually resolve spontaneously within 1 year of the last menstrual period
b.   Hot flushes are normal and rarely interfere with a woman's well-being
c.   Hot flushes usually resolve within 1 week after the initiation of HRT
d.   Hot flushes can begin several years before actual menopause
e.   Hot flushes are the final manifestation of ovarian failure and menopause

DIRECTIONS: Each group of questions below consists of lettered options followed by a set of numbered items. For each numbered item, select the **one** lettered option with which it is **most** closely associated. Each lettered option may be used once, more than once, or not at all.

Questions 381–385

For each description below, select the type of sexual precocity with which it is most likely to be associated.

a. True sexual precocity
b. Incomplete sexual precocity
c. Isosexual precocious pseudopuberty
d. Heterosexual precocious pseudopuberty
e. Precocity due to gonadotropin-producing tumors

381. Defined by the presence of virilizing signs in girls

382. Characterized by the presence of premature adrenarche, pubarche, or thelarche

383. Can arise from cranial tumors or hypothyroidism

384. Results from premature activation of the hypothalamic-pituitary system

385. Is frequently caused by ovarian tumors

Questions 386–390

Match each hysterosalpingogram with the correct description.

a. Bilateral hydrosalpinx
b. Unilateral hydrosalpinx with intrauterine adhesions
c. Unilateral hydrosalpinx with a normal uterine cavity
d. Bilateral proximal occlusion
e. Salpingitis isthmica nodosa
f. Bilateral normal spillage

386.

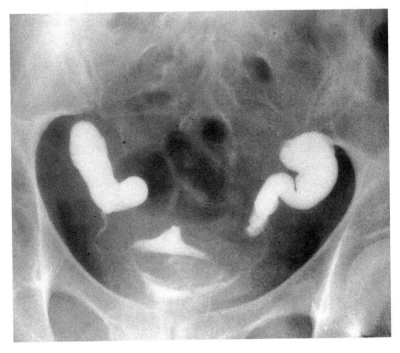

387.

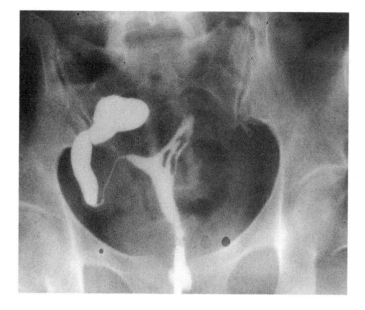

388.

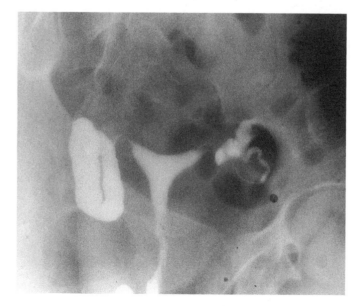

389.

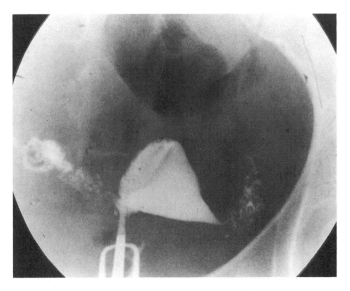

390.

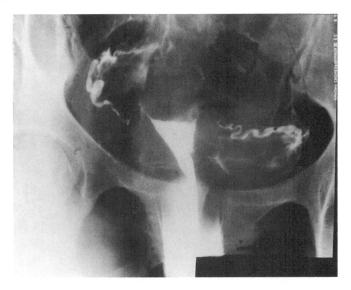

Infertility, Endocrinology, and Menstrual Dysfunction

Answers

331. The answer is a. *(Speroff, pp 718–755.)* Absolute contraindications to postmenopausal hormone replacement therapy include the presence of estrogen-dependent tumors (breast or uterus), active thromboembolic disease, undiagnosed genital tract bleeding, active severe liver disease, or malignant melanoma. Past or current history of hypertension, diabetes, or biliary stones does not automatically disqualify a patient for hormone replacement therapy.

332. The answer is b. *(Stenchever, pp 280–288, Speroff, pp 386–391.)* In the United States, the appearance of breast buds (thelarche) is usually the first sign of puberty, generally occurring between the ages of 9 and 11 years. This is subsequently followed by the appearance of pubic and axillary hair (adrenarche or pubarche), the adolescent growth spurt, and finally menarche. On average, the sequence of developmental changes requires a period of 4.5 years to complete, with a range of 1.5 to 6 years. The average ages of adrenarche/pubarche and menarche are 11.0 and 12.8 years, respectively. These events are considered to be delayed if thelarche has not occurred by the age of 13, adrenarche by the age of 14, or menarche by the age of 16. Girls with delayed sexual development should be fully evaluated for delayed puberty, including central, ovarian, systemic, or constitutional causes.

333. The answer is a. *(Stenchever, pp 280–288, Speroff, pp 392–403.)* In North America, pubertal changes before the age of 8 years in girls and 9 years in boys are regarded as precocious. Although the most common type of precocious puberty in girls is idiopathic, it is essential to ensure close long-term follow-up of these patients to ascertain that there is no serious underlying pathology, such as tumors of the central nervous system or ovary. Only 1 to 2% of patients with precocious puberty have an estrogen-producing ovarian tumor as the causative factor. McCune-Albright syndrome (polyostotic fibrous dysplasia) is also relatively rare and consists of fibrous dysplasia and cystic degeneration of the long bones, sexual precocity, and café au lait spots on the skin. Hypothyroidism is a cause of precocious puberty in some children, making thyroid function tests mandatory in these cases. Tumors of the central nervous system as a cause of precocious puberty occur more commonly in boys than in girls; they are seen in about 11% of girls with precocious puberty.

334. The answer is b. (*Ransom, 2000, pp 593–598.*) Psychological symptoms during the climacteric occur at a time when much is changing in a woman's life. Steroid hormone levels are dropping, and the menses is stopping. However, studies show these two factors to be unrelated to emotional symptoms in most women. Many factors, such as hormonal, environmental, and intrapsychic elements, combine to cause the symptoms of the climacteric such as insomnia; vasomotor instability (hot flushes, hot flashes); emotional lability; and genital tract atrophy with vulvar, vaginal, and urinary symptoms.

335. The answer is e. (*Speroff, pp 652–672.*) A major menopausal health issue is osteoporosis, which can result in fractures of the vertebral bodies, humerus, upper femur, forearm, or ribs. Patients with vertebral fractures experience back pain, gastrointestinal motility disorders, restrictive pulmonary symptoms, and loss of mobility. There may be a gradual decrease in height as well. Although all races experience osteoporosis, white and Asian women lose bone earlier and at a more rapid rate than black women. Thin women and those who smoke are at increased risk for developing osteoporosis. Physical activity increases the mineral content of bone in postmenopausal women.

336. The answer is c. (*Stenchever, pp 280–288. Speroff, pp 365–387.*) Significant emotional concerns develop when puberty is delayed. By definition, if breast development has not begun by age 13, delayed puberty should be suspected. Menarche usually follows about 1 to 2 years after the beginning of breast development; if menarche is delayed beyond age 16, delayed puberty should be investigated. Appropriate laboratory tests include circulating pituitary and steroid hormone levels, karyotypic analysis, and central nervous system (CNS) imaging when indicated. An FSH value greater than 40 mIU/mL defines hypergonadotropic hypogonadism as a cause of delayed pubertal maturation. Hypergonadotropic hypogonadism is seen in girls with gonadal dysgenesis, such as occurs with Turner syndrome. Since gonadal dysgenesis is such a common cause of absent pubertal development, hypergonadotropic hypogonadism is frequently—but not invariably—found in these patients.

337. The answer is b. *(Scott, p 613.)* Dysmenorrhea is considered secondary if associated with pelvic disease such as endometriosis, uterine myomas, or pelvic inflammatory disease. Primary dysmenorrhea is associated with a normal pelvic examination and with ovulatory cycles. The pain of dysmenorrhea is usually accompanied by other symptoms (nausea, fatigue, diarrhea, and headache) which may be related to excess of prostaglandin $F_{2\alpha}$. The two major drug therapies effective in dysmenorrhea are oral contraceptives and antiprostaglandins. GnRH analogues are used in several gynecologic conditions, but would not be first-line therapy for primary dysmenorrhea. Danazol is used for the treatment of endometriosis and ergot derivatives for hyperprolactinemia. Analgesics such as codeine or narcotics would generally be employed only in very severe cases when no other treatment provides adequate relief. Treatment will reduce the number of women incapacitated by menstrual symptoms to about 10% of those treated. Contrary to past beliefs, psychological factors play only a minor role in dysmenorrhea.

338. The answer is b. *(Scott, pp 603–604. Speroff, pp 450–451.)* Testicular feminization is a syndrome of androgen insensitivity in genetic males, characterized by a normal 46,X genotype, normal female phenotype during childhood, tall stature, and "normal" breast development with absence of axillary and pubic hair. Breast development (gynecomastia) occurs in these males because high levels of circulating testosterone (which cannot act at its receptor) are aromatized to estrogen, which then acts on the breast. The external genitalia develop as those of a female because testosterone cannot masculinize them, while the Müllerian structures are absent because of testicular secretion of Müllerian-inhibiting factor in utero. Gonadal dysgenesis (e.g., 45,X Turner syndrome) is characterized by short stature and absence of pubertal development; in these girls the ovaries are either absent or streak gonads that are nonfunctional. In either case, estrogen production is possible, and therefore isosexual pubertal development does not occur. Kallmann's syndrome (hypogonadotropic hypogonadism), the most likely diagnosis in this patient, should be suspected in an amenorrheic patient of normal stature with delayed or absent pubertal development, especially when associated with the classic finding of anosmia. Testing the sense of smell with coffee or perfume is a simple way to screen for this disorder. These individuals have a structural defect of the CNS involving the hypothalamus and the olfactory bulbs (located in close proximity to the hypothalamus) such that the hypothalamus does not secrete GnRH in normal pulsatile fashion, if at all. Other causes of minimal or absent pubertal development with normal stature include malnutrition; anorexia nervosa; severe systemic disease; and intensive athletic training, particularly ballet and running.

339. The answer is c. (*Speroff, pp 372–384.*) Precocious puberty is diagnosed if a young girl develops pubertal changes before age 8 or menarche before age 10. Precocious puberty can be treated by agents that reduce gonadotropin levels by exerting negative feedback in the hypothalamic-pituitary axis or that directly inhibit gonadotropin secretion from the pituitary gland. Until about 10 years ago, the greatest experience in the treatment of idiopathic central precocious puberty was with medroxyprogesterone acetate (MPA). MPA was usually administered intramuscularly in a dose of 100 to 200 mg/wk, or orally at 20 to 40 mg/d. Currently, the most effective treatment for central precocious puberty is the use of a long-acting GnRH agonist, such as leurolide (Lupron) and others. These drugs act by downregulating pituitary gonadotropes, eventually decreasing the secretion of FSH and LH, which are inappropriately stimulating the ovaries of these patients. As a result of this induced hypogonadotropic state, ovarian steroids (estrogens, progestins, and androgens) are suppressed back to prepubertal levels and precocious pubertal development stops or regresses. During the first 1 or 2 weeks of therapy there is a flare-up effect of increased gonadotropins and sex steroids, a predicted side effect of these medications. At the time of expected puberty, the GnRH analogue is discontinued and the pubertal sequence resumes.

340. The answer is d. (*Speroff, pp 345–350. Adashi, pp 1008–1015.*) Delayed puberty is a rare condition, usually differentiated into hypergonadotropic (high FSH and LH levels) hypogonadism or hypogonadotropic (low FSH and LH) hypogonadism. The most common cause of hypergonadotropic hypogonadism is gonadal dysgenesis (i.e., the 45,X

Turner syndrome). Hypogonadotropic hypogonadism can be seen in patients with hypothalamic-pituitary or constitutional delays in development. Kallmann syndrome presents with amenorrhea, infantile sexual development, low gonadotropins, normal female karyotype, and anosmia (the inability to perceive odors). In addition to these conditions, many other types of medical and nutritional problems can lead to this type of delayed development (e.g., malabsorption, diabetes, regional ileitis, and other chronic illness). Congenital adrenal hyperplasia leads to early pubertal development, although in girls the development is not isosexual (not of the expected sex) and would therefore include hirsutism, clitoromegaly, and other signs of virilization. Complete Müllerian agenesis is a condition in which the Müllerian ducts either fail to develop or regress early in fetal life. These patients have a blind vaginal pouch and no upper vagina, cervix, or uterus, and they present with primary amenorrhea. However, because ovarian development is not affected, secondary sexual characteristics develop normally despite the absence of menarche, and gonadotropin levels are normal. The McCune-Albright syndrome involves the constellation of precocious puberty, café au lait spots, and polyostotic fibrous dysplasia.

341. The answer is c. *(Speroff, p 1079.)* Failed fusion of the Müllerian ducts can give rise to several types of uterine anomalies, of which bicornuate uterus is a representative type. This condition is associated with a higher risk of obstetric complications, such as an increase in the rate of second-trimester abortion and premature labor. If these pregnancies go to term, malpresentations such as breech and transverse lie are more frequent. Also, prolonged labor (probably due to inadequate muscle development in the uterus), increased bleeding, and a higher incidence of fetal anomalies caused by defective implantation of the placenta all occur more commonly than in normal pregnancies. An intravenous pyelogram or urinary tract ultrasound is mandatory in patients with Müllerian anomalies since approximately 30% of patients with Müllerian anomalies have coexisting congenital urinary tract anomalies. In bicornuate uterus (termed *uterus bicornis unicollis*), there is a double uterine cavity (bicornis) and a single cervix (unicollis) with a normal vagina.

342. The answer is c. *(Stenchever, pp 554–557.)* Adenomyosis is a condition in which normal endometrial glands grow into the myometrium. Symptomatic disease primarily occurs in multiparous women over the age of 35 years, compared to endometriosis, in which onset is considerably younger. Patients with adenomyosis complain of dysmenorrhea and menorrhagia, and the classical examination findings include a tender, symmetrically enlarged uterus without adnexal tenderness. Although patients with endometriosis can have similar complaints, the physical examination of these patients more commonly reveals a fixed, retroverted uterus, adnexal tenderness and scarring, and tenderness along the uterosacral ligaments. Leiomyoma is the most common pelvic tumor, but the majority are asymptomatic and the uterus is irregular in shape. Patients with endometritis can present with abnormal bleeding, but endometrial biopsies show an inflammatory pattern. Uterine sarcoma is rare, and presents in older women with postmenopausal bleeding and nontender uterine enlargement.

343. The answer is a. *(Speroff, pp 1079–1080.)* Habitual abortion is the most important indication for surgical treatment of women who have a double uterus. The abortion rate in women who have a double uterus is two to three times greater than that of the general population. Therefore, women who present with habitual abortion should be evaluated to detect a possible double uterus. Hysterosalpingography, hysteroscopy, ultrasound, CT, and magnetic resonance imaging (MRI) are all potentially useful imaging modalities in this investigation. Dysmenorrhea, premature delivery, dyspareunia, and menometrorrhagia are other, less important indicators for surgical intervention.

344. The answer is e. *(Stenchever, pp 1182–1187.)* This patient would be unable to produce endogenous gonadotropin, since her pituitary has been ablated. The patient will therefore need to be given exogenous gonadotropin in the form of human menopausal gonadotropin (hMG), which contains an extract of urine from postmenopausal women with follicle-stimulating hormone (FSH) and luteinizing hormone (LH) in various ratios. Recombinant human FSH (rhFSH) is now also available. Carefully timed administration of hCG, which takes the place of an endogenous LH surge, will be needed to complete oocyte maturation and induce ovulation. Clomiphene citrate acts by competing with endogenous circulating estrogens for estrogen-binding sites in the hypothalamus. Therefore, it blocks the normal negative feedback of the endogenous estrogens and stimulates release of endogenous GnRH. However, the pituitary will not respond in this patient. Endogenous or exogenous GnRH cannot stimulate the release of FSH or LH in this woman because the pituitary gland is nonfunctional.

345. The answer is a. *(Stenchever, pp 1126–1127.)* There is a marked increase in levels of serum prolactin during gestation to over 10 times those values found in nonpregnant women. If this woman were not pregnant, the prolactin value could easily explain the amenorrhea and further evaluation of hyperprolactinemia would be necessary. The physiologic significance of increasing prolactin in pregnancy appears to involve preparation of the breasts for lactation.

346. The answer is c. *(Speroff, pp 1114–1120.)* Medical treatment of endometriosis currently involves a selection of four medications—oral contraceptive pills (OCPs), continuous progestins, danazol, and GnRH analogues. Surgery, both via a laparoscopic approach and laparotomy, is also used to treat endometriosis. One of the first medical treatments for endometriosis was the uninterrupted (acyclic) administration of high-dose birth-control pills for prolonged periods of time. Today this regimen is not used as often as it once was. Progestin therapy can lead to subjective and objective improvement in patients with endometriosis. Problems with continuous progestin therapy include breakthrough bleeding and depression. Overall, however, the side effects of progestin therapy are less than those seen with other treatments in most patients. Progestin therapy is generally reserved for patients who do not desire fertility. Danazol is an isoxazol derivative of 17α-ethinyl testosterone; it has been characterized as a pseudomenopausal treatment for endometriosis. Side effects include weight gain, edema, decreased breast size, acne, and other menopausal symptoms. GnRH agonists are the most recent addition to our armamentarium against endometriosis. These agents produce a medical oophorectomy. Collaborative studies have confirmed that fertility rates and symptom relief are similar between GnRH analogues and other medications. At the present time, conservative surgery compares favorably with administration of danazol in the management of mild to moderate endometriosis. Surgery is definitely indicated in patients with severe disease, those who fail hormonal therapy, or in the older infertile patient. Dexamethasone is not a treatment for endometriosis, and unopposed estrogen therapy would probably exacerbate the disease. Gonadotropins are used for ovulation induction, and Parlodel is a dopamine agonist used in the treatment of hyperprolactinemia.

347. The answer is b. *(Stenchever, pp 1085–1093.)* In patients with abnormal bleeding who are not responding to standard therapy, hysteroscopy should be performed. Hysteroscopy can rule out endometrial polyps or small fibroids, which, if present, can be resected. In patients with heavy abnormal bleeding who no longer desire fertility, an endometrial ablation can be performed. If a patient has completed childbearing and is having significant abnormal bleeding, a hysteroscopy, rather than a hysterectomy, would still be the procedure of choice to rule out easily treatable disease. Treatment with a GnRH agonist would only temporarily relieve symptoms.

348. The answer is b. (*Speroff, p 1115.*) Danazol is a progestational compound derived from testosterone that is used to treat endometriosis. It induces a pseudomenopause but does not alter basal gonadotropin levels. It appears to act as an antiestrogen and causes endometrial atrophy. Cyclic menses return almost immediately on withdrawal of danazol. It is felt that the endometrium is poorly developed with danazol use and that three menstrual cycles should be allowed to pass before conception so as to avoid a higher risk of spontaneous abortion, which could result from implantation in this poorly developed endometrium.

349. The answer is b. (*Speroff, pp 1040.*) A hysterosalpingogram is a procedure in which 3 to 6 mL of either an oil- or water-soluble contrast medium is injected through the cervix in a retrograde fashion to outline the uterine cavity and fallopian tubes. Spill of contrast medium into the peritoneal cavity proves patency of the fallopian tubes. By outlining the uterine cavity, abnormalities such as bicornuate or septate uterus, uterine polyps, or submucous myomas can be diagnosed, while tubal opacification allows identification of such conditions as salpingitis isthmica nodosum and hydrosalpinx. However, pelvic abnormalities outside the uterine cavity and fallopian tube (such as subserous fibroids, ovarian tumors, endometriosis, or minimal pelvic adhesions) are possibly not visible with this study, and hence a false-negative report could be generated. Some studies have shown a therapeutic effect resulting in an increased rate of pregnancy in the months immediately following the hysterosalpingogram.

350. The answer is a. (*Speroff, p 419.*) Because of the decreased amount of functional endometrium, progressive hypomenorrhea (lighter menstrual flow) or amenorrhea is common. Oligomenorrhea is defined as infrequent, irregular uterine bleeding greater than 35 days apart, often due to anovulation. Ovulation is not affected in Asherman's syndrome; therefore, ovulatory patients with Asherman's syndrome may continue to have regular periods. The best diagnostic study is the hysterosalpingogram under fluoroscopy. Hysteroscopy with lysis of adhesions is the treatment of choice. Prophylactic antibiotics may improve success rates.

351. The answer is a. *(Speroff, pp 427–447.)* In anorexia nervosa, prolactin, thyroid-stimulating hormone (TSH), and thyroxine levels are normal, FSH and LH levels are low, and cortisol levels are elevated. Prolactin is under the control of prolactin-inhibiting factor (PIF), which is produced in the hypothalamus. Many drugs (e.g., the phenothiazines), stress, hypothalamic lesions, stalk lesions, and stalk compression decrease PIF. In hypothyroidism, elevated TRH acts as a prolactin-releasing hormone to cause release of prolactin from the pituitary; hyperthyroidism is not associated with hyperprolactinemia. There are many other conditions, such as acromegaly and pregnancy, that are associated with elevated prolactin levels. Hyperandrogenic conditions such as congenital adrenal hyperplasia or polycystic ovarian disease are not typically associated with hyperprolactinemia.

352. The answer is c. *(Stenchever, pp 921–927, 1220–1221.)* In premenopausal adult women, most of the estrogen in the body is derived from ovarian secretion of estradiol, but a significant portion comes also from the extraglandular conversion of androstenedione to estrone. To a lesser extent, testosterone conversion to estradiol also contributes to the estrogen milieu. Muscle and adipose tissue are the major sites of aromatization. When there is an increase in fat cells, as in obese persons, estrogen levels will be higher, because adipose tissue exhibits a greater aromatization of androstenedione to estrone than does muscle.

353. The answer is a. *(Keye, pp 559–561, 629–637.)* The incidence of varicoceles in the general population is about 15%, but 40% of males with infertility are found to have varicoceles. Because of the anatomy and physiology, varicoceles are more likely to occur on the left side. There is no correlation between the size of the varix and prognosis for fertility. The characteristic stress pattern seen with varicoceles is decreased number of sperm, decreased motility, and increased abnormal forms. How the varicocele causes abnormal semen quality, and the relationship between varicocele, semen abnormalities, and male infertility (especially when semen quality appears normal) is unclear.

354. The answer is a. (*Speroff, pp 325–327.*) Remember that the Müllerian structures appear during embryonic development in both males and females. Female gonads do not secrete Müllerian-inhibiting factor (MIF), and the Müllerian structures persist. Male testes secrete MIF, which causes regression of Müllerian structures. Anything that prevents MIF secretion in genetic males will result in persistence of Müllerian structures into the postnatal period. Persons who appear to be normal males but who possess a uterus and fallopian tubes have such a failure of Müllerian-inhibiting factor. Their karyotype is 46,XY, testes are present, and testosterone production is normal. When the testes are located intraabdominally, orchidectomy is required to prevent malignant degeneration in these ectopic gonads.

355. The answer is c. (*Speroff, pp 1031–1036, 1179.*) An abnormal luteal phase is defined as ovulation with a poor progestational effect in the second half of the cycle. Luteal function is usually evaluated at the endometrium, which is inadequately prepared for embryo implantation. Endometrial biopsy is crucial to the diagnosis of this defect because the endometrium will be out of phase with the time of cycle in these patients. For example, a biopsy taken on day 26 of the cycle will resemble endometrium of day 22 because of decreased progesterone stimulation. Progesterone levels in the midluteal phase less than 7 ng/mL are suggestive of a luteal phase defect but not diagnostic. Pregnanetriol is a breakdown product of 17-hydroxyprogesterone, and levels are not helpful in diagnosing this condition. Determination of the level of pregnanediol, which is a metabolic product of progesterone excreted in the urine, is helpful. Serum luteinizing hormone levels have no correlation with the presence of luteal phase defect.

356. The answer is e. (*Ransom, 1997, p 136. Speroff, pp 634–635.*) This patient has secondary amenorrhea, which rules out abnormalities associated with primary amenorrhea such as chromosomal abnormalities and congenital Müllerian abnormalities. The most common reason for amenorrhea in a woman of reproductive age is pregnancy, which should be evaluated first. Other possibilities include chronic endometritis or scarring of the endometrium (Asherman syndrome), hypothyroidism, and ovarian failure. The latter is the most likely diagnosis in a woman at this age. In addition, emotional stress, extreme weight loss, and adrenal cortisol insufficiency can bring about secondary amenorrhea. A hysterosalpingogram is part of an infertility workup that may demonstrate Asherman syndrome, but it is not indicated until premature ovarian failure has been excluded. Persistently elevated gonadotropin levels (especially when accompanied by low serum estradiol levels) are diagnostic of ovarian failure.

357. The answer is a. (*Speroff, p 916–917.*) This patient has polycystic ovarian syndrome (PCOS), diagnosed by the clinical picture, abnormally high LH-to-FSH ratio (which should normally be approximately 1:1), and elevated androgens but normal DHAS. DHAS is a marker of adrenal androgen production; when normal, it essentially excludes adrenal sources of hyperandrogenism. Several medications have been used to treat hirsutism associated with PCOS. For many years contraceptives were the most frequently used agents; they can suppress hair growth in up to two-thirds of treated patients. They act by directly suppressing ovarian steroid production and increasing hepatic-binding globulin production, which binds circulating hormone and lowers the concentration of metabolically active (free unbound) androgen. However, clinical improvement can take as long as 6 months to manifest. Other medications that have shown promise include medroxyprogesterone acetate, spironolactone, cimetidine, and GnRH agonists, which suppress ovarian steroid production. However, GnRH analogues are expensive and have been associated with significant bone demineralization after only 6 months of therapy in some patients. Surgical wedge resection is no longer considered an appropriate therapy for PCOS given the success of pharmacologic agents and the ovarian adhesions that were frequently associated with this surgery.

358. The answer is d. (*Stenchever, pp 1065–1066.*) Conservative measures for treating dysmenorrhea include heating pads, mild analgesics, sedatives or antispasmodic drugs, and outdoor exercise. In patients with dysmenorrhea there is a significantly higher than normal concentration of prostaglandins in the endometrium and menstrual fluid. Prostaglandin synthase inhibitors such as indomethacin, naproxen, ibuprofen, and mefenamic acid are very effective in these patients. However, for patients with dysmenorrhea who are sexually active, oral contraceptives will provide needed protection from unwanted pregnancy and generally alleviate the dysmenorrhea. The OCPs minimize endometrial prostaglandin production during the concurrent administration of estrogen and progestin.

359. The answer is d. (*Stenchever, pp 532–534. Speroff, pp 1103–1108.*) Retrograde menstruation is currently believed to be the major cause of endometriosis. Supporting this belief are the following findings: inversion of the uterine cervix into the peritoneal cavity can cause monkeys to develop endometriosis; endometrial tissue is viable outside the uterus; and blood can issue from the ends of the fallopian tubes of some women during menstruation. The fact that endometrial implants can occur in the lung implies that lymphatic or vascular routes of spread of the disease also are possible. Another theory of the etiology of endometriosis entails the conversion of celomic epithelium into glands resembling those of the endometrium. Endometriosis in men, or in women without Müllerian structures, is an example of this causative mechanism.

360. The answer is c. (*Speroff, pp 420–421.*) Since this patient has other signs of pubertal development that are sex steroid–dependent, we can conclude some ovarian function is present. This excludes such conditions as gonadal dysgenesis and hypothalamic-pituitary failure as possible causes of her primary amenorrhea. Müllerian defects are the only plausible cause, and the diagnostic evaluation in this patient would be directed toward both confirmation of this diagnosis and establishment of the exact nature of the Müllerian defect. Müllerian agenesis, also known as Mayer-Rokitansky-Küster-Hauser syndrome, presents as amenorrhea with absence of a vagina. The incidence is approximately 1 in 10,000 female births. The karyotype is 46,XX. There is normal development of breasts, sexual hair, ovaries, tubes, and external genitalia. There are associated skeletal (12%) and urinary tract (33%) anomalies. Treatment generally consists of progressive vaginal dilation or creation of an artificial vagina with split-thickness skin grafts (McIndoe procedure). Testicular feminization, or congenital androgen insensitivity syndrome, is an X-linked recessive disorder with a karyotype of 46,XY. These genetic males have a defective androgen receptor and/or downstream signal transduction mechanism (in the genome) such that the androgenic signal does not have its normal tissue-specific effects. This accounts for 10% of all cases of primary amenorrhea. The patient presents with an absent uterus and blind vaginal canal. However, in these patients the amount of sexual hair is significantly decreased. Although there is a 25% incidence of malignant tumors in these patients, gonadectomy should be deferred until after full development is obtained. In other patients with a Y chromosome, gonadectomy should be performed as early as possible to prevent masculinization. Patients with gonadal dysgenesis present with lack of secondary sexual characteristics. Patients with Klinefelter syndrome typically have a karyotype of 47,XXY and a male phenotype. Causes of primary amenorrhea, in descending order of frequency, are gonadal dysgenesis, Müllerian agenesis, and testicular feminization. XYY syndrome and Turner syndrome often present with menstrual difficulties, but these patients have a uterus.

361. The answer is e. *(Speroff, pp 535–539.)* Premenstrual syndrome is a constellation of symptoms that occur in a cyclic pattern, always in the same phase of the menstrual cycle. These symptoms usually occur 7 to 10 days before the onset of menses. Examples of symptoms reported include edema, mood swings, depression, irritability, breast tenderness, increased appetite, and cravings for sweets. The etiology is unclear. Therapy has included oral contraceptives, danazol, bromocriptine, evening primrose oil, and aerobic exercise. Controlled studies have been performed with most of the different treatment regimens with variable, unreproducible, and generally disappointing results that are probably the result of patient heterogeneity because of difficulty in diagnosing this condition. Of all the medications studied, SSRIs have shown the greatest efficacy in PMS treatment.

362. The answer is c. *(Speroff, pp 583–585.)* Amenorrhea and galactorrhea may be seen when something causes an increase in prolactin secretion or action. The differential diagnosis involves several possible causes. Excessive estrogens, such as with birth control pills, can reduce prolactin-inhibiting factor, thus raising serum prolactin level. Similarly, intensive suckling (during lactation and associated with sexual foreplay) can activate the reflex arc that results in hyperprolactinemia. Many antipsychotic medications, especially the phenothiazines, are also known to have mammotropic properties. Hypothyroidism appears to cause galactorrhea secondary to thyrotropin-releasing hormone (TRH) stimulation of prolactin release. When prolactin levels are persistently elevated without obvious cause (e.g., in breast-feeding), evaluation for pituitary adenoma becomes necessary.

363. The answer is c. *(Scott, pp 615–618. Ransom, 1997, pp 570–580.)* The presence of estrogen in a pubertal girl stimulates the formation of secondary sex characteristics, including development of breasts, production of cervical mucus, and vaginal cornification. As estrogen levels increase, menses begins and ovulation is maintained for several decades. Ovarian estrogen production late in puberty is at least in part responsible for termination of the pubertal growth spurt, thereby determining adult height.

Decreasing levels of estrogen are associated with lower frequency of ovulation, eventually leading to menopause. Hair growth during puberty is caused by androgens from the adrenal gland and, later, the ovary.

364. The answer is e. (*Speroff, pp 372–374.*) These GnRH results and LH pulses are seen in normal puberty. Normal signs of puberty involve breast budding (thelarche, 9.8 years), pubic hair (pubarche, 10.5 years), and menarche (12.8 years). Besides an increase in androgens and a moderate rise in FSH and LH levels, one of the first indications of puberty is an increase in the amplitude and frequency of nocturnal LH pulses. In patients with idiopathic true precocious puberty, the pituitary response to GnRH is identical to that in girls undergoing normal puberty. Iatrogenic sexual precocity (i.e., the accidental ingestion of estrogens), premature thelarche, and ovarian tumors are examples of sexual precocity independent of GnRH, FSH, and LH function.

365. The answer is e. (*Speroff, pp 1143–1150.*) Because of the variability in semen specimens from the same person, preferably three specimens should be evaluated over the course of an investigation for infertility. A normal semen analysis will demonstrate at least 20 million sperm per milliliter, over 60% of the sperm with a normal shape, a volume of between 2 and 6 mL, and at least 50% of the sperm with progressive forward motility.

366–370. The answers are 366-e, 367-c, 368-b, 369-d, 370-a. (*Adashi, pp 1898–1913. Speroff, pp 1026–1029, 1033–1035.*) The diagnostic evaluation of an infertile couple should be thorough and completed as rapidly as possible. The primary diagnostic steps in the workup of the infertile couple include (1) documentation of ovulation by measurement of basal body temperature (BBT) or mid–luteal phase serum progesterone; (2) semen analysis; (3) postcoital test; (4) hysterosalpingogram; and (5) endometrial biopsy. Women should record their BBT for evidence of ovulation. In addition, serial serum progesterone levels may be helpful to confirm ovulation. Serum progesterone values should be obtained 7 days after ovulation and may also be helpful in evaluating inadequate luteal phase. An endometrial biopsy may also provide valuable information regarding the status of the luteal phase. The biopsy is obtained 12 days after the thermogenic shift, or 2 to 3 days before the expected onset of menses, on about day 26 of a 28-day cycle. A postcoital test is an in vivo test that evaluates the interaction of sperm and cervical mucus. It is performed during the periovulatory period up to 12 h after coitus. The cervical mucus is obtained, and its quantity and quality as well as its interaction with the sperm are evaluated. The hysterosalpingogram is performed in the midfollicular phase in order to evaluate the fallopian tubes and the contour of the uterine cavity; it should not be done while the patient is menstruating or after ovulation has occurred. Although gonadotropin levels are not routinely evaluated, they should be obtained in the early follicular phase when testing is indicated (e.g., in cases where there is a history of oligoovulation).

371. The answer is b. *(Beckmann, pp 472–480.)* Sertoli-Leydig cell tumors, also known as adroblastomas or arrhenoblastomas, are testosterone-secreting ovarian neoplasms. These tumors usually occur in women between the ages of 20 and 40 and tend to be unilateral and reach a size of 7 to 10 cm. Women with a Sertoli-Leydig cell tumor tend to have very high levels of testosterone (>200 ng/dL) and rapidly develop virilizing characteristics such as temporal balding, clitoral hypertrophy, voice deepening, breast atrophy, and terminal hair between the breasts and on the back. Women with constitutional or idiopathic hirsutism have greater activity of 5α-reductase than do unaffected women. They have hirsutism with a diagnostic evaluation that gives no explanation for the excess hair. Women with attenuated congenital adrenal hyperplasia are hirsute due to an increase in adrenal androgen production caused by a deficiency in 21-hydroxylase. Polycystic ovarian syndrome is the most common cause of androgen excess and hirsutism. Selective insulin resistance is thought to be central to the etiology of this syndrome.

372. The answer is d. *(ACOG, Practice Bulletin 41.)* Thyroid dysfunction and hyperprolactinemia can both be associated with hirsutism, and therefore it is important to check levels of TSH and prolactin. In order to rule out congenital adrenal hyperplasia due to a deficiency in 21-hydroxylase, a 17α-hydroxyprogesterone level should be drawn. Very high levels of total testosterone would indicate the presence of an androgen-secreting ovarian tumor. Elevated levels of dehydroepiandrostenedione would be consistent with PCOS. There is no role for ordering an isolated estrone level in the workup and evaluation of hirsutism.

373. The answer is d. *(Speroff, pp 1186–1187. ACOG, Practice Bulletin 41. Beckmann, p 479.)* Oral contraceptives have long been used in the management of PCOS because they suppress pituitary luteinizing hormone secretion, suppress ovarian androgen secretion, and increase circulating SHBG. Medications such as metformin that improve insulin sensitivity have been used to treat PCOS. Spironolactone, which is a diuretic and aldosterone agonist, has been used to treat PCOS because it binds to the androgen receptor as an antagonist. Weight loss is recommended as part of the treatment for women with PCOS because it reduces hyperinsulinemia. Metformin use is a simple step in the attempt to induce ovulation in patients with PCOS. Insulin is thought to act on the ovary to stimulate androgen secretion. In addition, hyperinsulinemia decreases SHBG. There is no role for the use of dexamethasone to treat PCOS. Glucocorticoid therapy is indicated in cases of congenital adrenal hyperplasia.

374. The answer is e. (*Beckmann, pp 468–470. Speroff, pp 553–560, 566–567.*) The case presented is a typical representation of a patient with dysfunctional uterine bleeding due to anovulation. The onset of menarche in young women is typically followed by approximately 5 years of irregular cycles that result from anovulation secondary to immaturity of the hypothalamic-pituitary axis. Uterine cancer, cervical polyps, or cervical pathology would be rare in a girl this age. These other causes of abnormal bleeding would be more common in older women. Of course pregnancy should always be considered as a possible cause in all women of reproductive age. Appropriate lab tests to order in the emergency room would be a BHCG (to rule out pregnancy), a bleeding time (20% of adolescents with dysfunctional uterine bleeding have a coagulation defect), and type and screen (since she is orthostatic she may require a blood transfusion). A CBC will show the degree of blood loss this patient has suffered. Measuring an estradiol level would serve no purpose in the workup of this patient.

375. The answer is d. (*Beckmann, pp 468–470. Speroff, pp 553–560, 566–567.*) This patient presents an example of chronic anovulation in an older woman. She gives a classic history of changing from regular, monthly periods to irregular, infrequent episodes of vaginal bleeding. Patients with chronic anovulation often have underlying medical problems such as diabetes, thyroid problems, or polycystic ovarian syndrome. A patient with uterine fibroids may have heavy periods, but the regularity of the periods is not affected unless the patient has underlying ovulatory dysfunction. A cervical polyp would clearly be seen on physical examination and, like uterine fibroids, would not affect the timing of menstruation. Patients with cervical polyps often complain of bleeding between periods, usually provoked by sexual intercourse. Since the patient's pregnancy test is negative, she cannot have an incomplete abortion. Patients with coagulation defects have problems with heavy periods from the time of menarche.

376. The answer is d. (*Beckmann, pp 468–470. Speroff, pp 553–560, 566–567.*) The administration of high-dose estrogen therapy is the preferred way to manage this patient. In women who have suffered heavy and acute bleeding due to anovulation, 25 mg of conjugated estrogen can be administered every 4 h until the bleeding abates. The estrogen will help stop the bleeding by building up the endometrium and stimulating clotting at the capillary level. Since the bleeding is heavy and acute, a D&C will not help stop the bleeding, because the lining is already thinned and atrophic. In older women, a D&C might be helpful in obtaining tissue for pathology to rule out endometrial cancer. In this young patient who is resuscitated and stabilized with intravenous fluids, there is no indication for a blood transfusion as long as the bleeding abates. Iron therapy alone would not be adequate for this patient; the bleeding must be stopped first. Antiprostaglandins have no role in curtailing hemorrhage in a woman suffering from anovulation. They have been used with some success in ovulatory women who have heavy cycles or in women with menorrhagia caused by use of the intrauterine device. It is thought that prostaglandin synthetase inhibitors reduce the amount of bleeding by promoting vasoconstriction and platelet aggregation.

377. The answer is c. (*Speroff, pp 535–539.*) The only medications that have been shown in randomized, double-blind, placebo-controlled trials to be consistently effective in treating the emotional symptoms of PMS are the selective serotonin reuptake inhibitors. Such antidepressants include fluoxetine, sertraline, and paroxetine. Some women can be effectively treated by limiting use of the medication to the luteal phase.

378. The answer is c. (*Beckmann, pp 484–490. Speroff, pp 689–754.*) It is well established that the use of ERT/HRT increases the user's risk of a thromboembolic event two- to threefold. The use of combined HRT does not increase the risk of uterine cancer, colon cancer, or Alzheimer's disease.

There is much literature to support the idea that HRT use decreases the risk of colon cancer and possibly Alzheimer's disease. There is no scientific evidence that HRT use affects the incidence of malignant melanoma.

379. The answer is b. *(Beckmann, pp 484–490. Speroff, pp 689–754.)* Estrogen use decreases total cholesterol and LDL and increases HDL and triglycerides.

380. The answer is d. *(Beckmann, pp 484–490. Speroff, pp 689–754.)* The hot flush is the first physical symptom of declining ovarian function. More than 95% of perimenopausal/menopausal women experience these vasomotor symptoms. Hot flushes may begin several years before the cessation of menstruation. When a woman experiences a hot flush, she typically feels a sudden sensation of heat over the chest and face that lasts between 1 and 2 min. This feeling of heat is followed by a sensation of cooling or a cold sweat. The entire hot flush lasts about 3 min total. Estrogen therapy will usually cause resolution of the hot flush within 3 to 6 weeks. Without estrogen therapy, hot flushes on average resolve spontaneously within 2 to 3 years after cessation of menstruation. Although hot flushes are normal, they may interfere with a woman's sleep, causing significant interference with her sense of well-being.

381–385. The answers are 381-d, 382-b, 383-a, 384-a, 385-c. *(Ransom, 1997, pp 271–275.)* True sexual precocity in girls is characterized by normal gonadotropin levels (as opposed to expected low prepubertal gonadotropin levels) and a normal ovulatory pattern. It represents premature activation of a normally operating hypothalamic-pituitary axis. Although it is usually idiopathic, true sexual precocity can arise from cerebral causes such as tumors or a history of encephalitis or meningitis, as well as from hypothyroidism, polyostotic fibrous dysplasia, neurofibromatosis, and other disorders. In girls who have precocious pseudopuberty, the endocrine glands, usually under neoplastic influences, produce elevated amounts of estrogens (isosexual precocious pseudopuberty) or androgens (heterosexual precocious pseudopuberty). Ovarian tumors appear to be the most common cause of isosexual precocious pseudopuberty; some ovarian tumors, including dysgerminomas and choriocarcinomas, can produce so much gonadotropin that pregnancy tests are positive. Incomplete sexual precocity, which is usually idiopathic, is characterized by only partial sexual maturity, such as premature thelarche or premature adrenarche (pubarche). Incomplete sexual precocity can be accompanied by abnormal function of the central nervous system (e.g., mental deficiency). Gonadotropin levels are frequently normal in these patients. In gonadotropin-producing tumors, high levels of gonadotropins such as FSH are produced with subsequent production of estrogen. Examples of these rare tumors are hepatoma, chorioepithelioma, and presacral tumors.

386–390. The answers are 386-a, 387-b, 388-c, 389-e, 390-f. *(Rock, pp 550–555. Speroff, p 1040. Stenchever, pp 233–236.)* Hysterosalpingography is an important tool in the evaluation of infertility. It provides information regarding the shape of the uterine cavity and the patency of the tubes. Tubal factors, many of which follow from sexually transmitted diseases, are an important cause of infertility. The figure in question 386 displays bilateral hydrosalpinx and clubbing of the tubes with no evidence of any spillage into the peritoneal cavity. The uterine cavity in this HSG is normal. In the figure in question 387, there is unilateral hydrosalpinx and evidence of adhesions within the uterine cavity consistent with Asherman syndrome. There is no filling of the other tube. In the figure in question 388, one tube fills and has unilateral hydrosalpinx; the other shows loculation and minimal fluid accumulation. The uterine cavity here is normal, in contrast to the cavity shown in question 387. The figure in question 389 shows salpingitis isthmica nodosa, in which there is a characteristic "salt-and-pepper" pattern of tubal filling and evidence of a diverticulum of the tube on one side. The figure in question 390 shows normal filling and spillage of contrast media. This is a normal hysterosalpingogram. None of the figures show bilateral proximal occlusion.

Pelvic Relaxation and Urology

Questions

DIRECTIONS: Each item below contains a question followed by suggested responses. Select the **one best** response to each question.

391. A 50-year-old woman complains of leakage of urine. After genuine stress urinary incontinence, which of the following is the most common cause of urinary leakage?

a. Detrusor dyssynergia
b. Unstable bladder
c. Unstable urethra
d. Urethral diverticulum
e. Overflow incontinence

392. A 65-year-old woman complains of leakage of urine. Which of the following is the most common cause of this condition in such patients?

a. Anatomic stress urinary incontinence
b. Urethral diverticula
c. Overflow incontinence
d. Unstable bladder
e. Fistula

393. A 59-year-old woman undergoes vaginal hysterectomy and anteroposterior repair for uterine prolapse. Which of the following is a complication of this procedure that often develops within 2 weeks of surgery?

a. Dyspareunia
b. Stress urinary incontinence
c. Nonfistulous fecal incontinence
d. Enterocele
e. Vaginal vault prolapse

394. A 53-year-old postmenopausal woman, gravida 3, para 3, presents for evaluation of troublesome urinary leakage 6 weeks in duration. Which of the following is the most appropriate first step in this patient's evaluation?

a. Urinalysis and culture
b. Urethral pressure profiles
c. Intravenous pyelogram
d. Cystourethrogram
e. Urethrocystoscopy

395. A postmenopausal woman is undergoing evaluation for fecal incontinence. She has no other diagnosed medical problems. She lives by herself and is self-sufficient, oriented, and an excellent historian. Physical examination is completely normal. Which of the following is the most likely cause of this patient's condition?

a. Rectal prolapse
b. Diabetes
c. Obstetric trauma
d. Senility
e. Excessive caffeine intake

396. You are discussing surgical options with a patient with symptomatic pelvic relaxation. Partial colpocleisis (Le Fort procedure) may be more appropriate than vaginal hysterectomy and anterior and posterior (A&P) repair for patients in which of the following circumstances?

a. Do not desire retained sexual function
b. Need periodic endometrial sampling
c. Have had endometrial dysplasia
d. Have cervical dysplasia that requires colposcopic evaluation
e. Have a history of urinary incontinence

397. A 65-year-old woman presents to your office for evaluation of genital prolapse. She has a history of chronic hypertension, well controlled with a calcium channel blocker. She has had three full-term spontaneous vaginal deliveries. The last one was 9 lb and required forceps to deliver the head. She says she had a large tear in the vagina involving the rectum during the last delivery. She has a history of chronic constipation and often uses a laxative to help her have a bowel movement. She has smoked for more than 30 years and has a smoker's cough. She entered menopause at age 52 but has never taken hormone replacement therapy. Which of the following factors is least important in the subsequent development of genital prolapse in this patient?

a. Chronic cough
b. Chronic constipation
c. Chronic hypertension
d. Childbirth trauma
e. Menopause

398. A 63-year-old woman is undergoing a total abdominal hysterectomy (TAH) for atypical edometrial hyperplasia. She mentioned to her doctor two weeks prior to the surgery that she has had problems with leakage of urine with straining and occasional episodes of urinary urgency. A urine culture at that visit is negative. She has had preoperative cystometrics done in the doctor's office showing loss of urine during valsalva maneuvers along with evidence of detrusor instability. The doctor has elected to do a retropubic bladder neck suspension following the TAH. A Marshall-Marchetti-Krantz procedure (MMK) is done to attach the bladder neck to the pubic symphysis. The patient does well after her surgery and is released from the hospital on postoperative day 3. Which of the following should her doctor advise her prior to her discharge?

a. Urinary retention is very common after an MMK procedure and often requires long-term self-catheterization
b. She has a 5% risk of enterocele formation
c. The MMK procedure is highly effective, with greater than 90% long-term cure rate
d. Osteitis pubis occurs in approximately 10% of patients after an MMK but is easily treated with oral antibiotics
e. She will not need any additional treatment for her bladder dysfunction

399. A 30-year-old G3P3 is being evaluated for urinary urgency, urinary frequency, and dysuria. She also complains of pain with insertion when attempting intercourse. She frequently dribbles a few drops of urine after she finishes voiding. She has had three full-term spontaneous vaginal deliveries. Her last baby weighed more than 9 lb. She had multiple sutures placed in the vaginal area after delivery of that child. She also has a history of mutiple urinary tract infections since she was a teenager. On pelvic examination she has a 1-cm tender suburethral mass. With palpation of the mass, a small amount of blood-tinged pus is expressed from the urethra. Which of the following is the most likely cause of this patient's problem?

a. Urethral polyp
b. Urethral fistula
c. Urethral stricture
d. Urethral eversion
e. Urethral diverticulum

400. A patient is seen on the second postoperative day after a difficult abdominal hysterectomy complicated by hemorrhage from the left uterine artery pedicle. Multiple sutures were placed into this area to control bleeding. The patient now has fever, left back pain, left costovertebral angle tenderness, and hematuria. An ultrasound examination shows that fluid has accumulated in the left flank. A ureteral injury is diagnosed. If the injury had been recognized at the time of surgery, which of the following procedures could have been recommended?

a. Percutaneous nephrostomy
b. Placement of a ureteral stent without anastomosis
c. Intraperitoneal drainage without anastomosis
d. Ureteroureteral anastomosis
e. Ureteral reimplantation into the bladder

401. A 44-year-old woman complains of urinary incontinence. She loses urine when she laughs, coughs, and plays tennis. Urodynamic studies are performed in the office with a mutiple-channel machine. If this patient has genuine stress urinary incontinence, which of the following do you expect to see on the cystometric study?

a. An abnormally short urethra
b. Multiple unihibited detrusor contractions
c. Total bladder capacity of 1000 cc
d. Normal urethral pressure profile
e. First urge to void at 50 cc

402. A 59-year-old G4P4 presents to your office complaining of losing urine when she coughs, sneezes, or engages in certain types of strenuous physical activity. The problem has gotten increasingly worse over the past few years, to the point where the patient finds her activities of daily living compromised secondary to fear of embarrassment. She denies any other urinary symptoms such as urgency, frequency, or hematuria. In addition, she denies any problems with her bowel movements. Her prior surgeries include tonsillectomy and appendectomy. She has adult-onset diabetes and her blood sugars are well controlled with oral glucophage. The patient has no history of any gynecologic problems in the past. She has four children who were all delivered vaginally. Their weights ranged from 8 to 9 lb. Her last delivery was forceps-assisted. She had a third-degree laceration with that birth. She is currently sexually active with her partner of 25 years. She has been menopausal for 4 years and has never taken any hormone replacement therapy. Her height is 5 ft 6 in., and she weighs 190 lb. Her blood pressure is 130/80. Based on the patient's history, which of the following is the most likely diagnosis?

a. Overflow incontinence
b. Stress incontinence
c. Urinary tract infection
d. Detrusor instability
e. Vesicovaginal fistula

403. A 49-year-old G4P4 presents to your office complaining of a 2-month history of leakage of urine every time she exercises. She has had to limit her physical activities due to the loss of urine. She has had burning with urination and some blood in her urine for the past few days. Which of the following is the best next step in the evaluation and management of this patient?

a. Physical exam
b. Placement of a pessary
c. Urinalysis with urine culture
d. Cystoscopy
e. Office cystometrics

404. A 46-year-old woman presents to your office complaining of something bulging from her vagina for the past year. It has been getting progressively more prominent. She has started to notice that she leaks urine with laughing and sneezing. She still has periods regularly every 26 days. She is married. Her husband had a vasectomy for contraception. After appropriate evaluation, you diagnose a second-degree cystocele. She has no uterine prolapse or rectocele. Which of the following is the best treatment plan to offer this patient?

a. Anticholinergic medications
b. Surgical correction with a bladder neck suspension procedure
c. Placement of a pessary
d. Antibiotic therapy with Bactrim
e. Le Fort colpocleisis

405. An obese 46-year-old G6P1051 with type 1 diabetes since age 12 presents to your office complaining of urinary incontinence. She has been menopausal since age 44. Her diabetes has been poorly controlled for years due to her noncompliance with insulin therapy. She often cannot tell when her bladder is full, and she will urinate on herself without warning. Which of the following factors in this patient's history has contributed the most to the development of her urinary incontinence?

a. Menopause
b. Obesity
c. Obstetric history
d. Age
e. Diabetic status

406. A 76-year-old woman presents for evaluation of urinary incontinence. She had a hysterectomy for fibroid tumors of the uterus at age 48. After complete evaluation, you determine that the patient has genuine stress urinary incontinence. On physical examination she has a hypermobile urethra, but there is no cystocele or rectocele. There is no vaginal vault prolapse. Office cystometrics confirms genuine stress urinary incontinence. Which of the following surgical procedures should you recommend to this patient?

a. Kelly plication
b. Anterior and posterior colporrhaphy
c. Burch procedure
d. Abdominal sacral colpopexy
e. Lefort colpocleisis

407. A patient presents to your office approximately 2 weeks after having a total vaginal hysterectomy with anterior colporrhaphy and Burch procedure for uterine prolapse and stress urinary incontinence. She complains of a constant loss of urine throughout the day. She denies any urgency or dysuria. Which of the following is the most likely explanation for this complaint?

a. Failure of the procedure
b. Urinary tract infection
c. Vesicovaginal fistula
d. Detrusor instability
e. Diabetic neuropathy

408. A 90-year-old G5P5 with multiple medical problems is brought into your gynecology clinic accompanied by her granddaughter. The patient has hypertension, chronic anemia, coronary artery disease, and osteoporosis. She is mentally alert and oriented and lives in an assisted living facility. She takes numerous medications, but is very functional at the current time. She is a widow and not sexually active. Her chief complaint is a sensation of heaviness and pressure in the vagina. She denies any significant urinary or bowel problems. On performance of a physical exam, you note that the cervix is just inside the level of the introitus. Based on the physical exam, which of the following is the most likely diagnosis?

a. Normal exam
b. First-degree uterine prolapse
c. Second-degree uterine prolapse
d. Third-degree uterine prolapse
e. Complete procidentia

409. An 86-year-old woman presents to your office for her well-woman examination. She has no complaints. On pelvic examination performed in the supine and upright positions, the patient has second-degree prolapse of the uterus. Which of the following is the best next step in the management of this patient?

a. Reassurance
b. Placement of a pessary
c. Vaginal hysterectomy
d. Le Fort procedure
e. Anterior colporrhaphy

410. An 81-year-old woman presents to your office complaining that her uterus fell out 2 months ago. She has multiple medical problems, including chronic hypertension, congestive heart failure, and osteoporosis. She is limited to sitting in a wheelchair due to her health problems. Her fallen uterus causes significant pain. On physical examination, the patient is frail and requires assistance with getting on the examination table. She has complete procidentia of the uterus. Which of the following is the most appropriate next step in the management of this patient?

a. Reassurance
b. Placement of a pessary
c. Vaginal hysterectomy
d. Le Fort procedure
e. Anterior colporrhaphy

411. A 78-year-old woman with chronic obstructive pulmonary disease, chronic hypertension, and history of myocardial infarction requiring angioplasty presents to your office for evaluation of something hanging out of her vagina. She had a hysterectomy for benign indications at age 48. For the past few months she has been experiencing the sensation of pelvic pressure. Last month she felt a bulge at the vaginal opening. Two weeks ago something fell out of the vagina. On pelvic examination the patient has total eversion of the vagina. There is a superficial ulceration at the vaginal apex. Which of the following is the best next step in the management of this patient?

a. Biopsy the vaginal ulceration
b. Schedule abdominal sacral colpopexy
c. Place a pessary
d. Prescribe oral estrogen
e. Prescribe topical vaginal estrogen cream

412. A 40-year-old G3P3 comes to your office for a routine annual GYN exam. She tells you that she gets up several times during the night to void. On further questioning, she admits to you that during the day she sometimes gets the urge to void, but sometimes cannot quite make it to the bathroom. She attributes this to getting older and is not extremely concerned, although she often wears a pad when she goes out in case she loses some urine. This patient is very healthy otherwise and does not take any medication on a regular basis. She still has regular, monthly menstrual periods. She has had three normal spontaneous vaginal deliveries of infants weighing between 7 and 8 lb. An office dipstick of her urine does not indicate any blood, bacteria, WBCs, or protein. Her urine culture is negative. Based on her office presentation and history, which of the following is the most likely diagnosis?

a. Urinary stress incontinence
b. Urinary tract infection
c. Overflow incontinence
d. Bladder dyssynergia
e. Vesicovaginal fistula

413. A 38-year-old woman presents to your office complaining of urinary incontinence. Her symptoms are suggestive of urge incontinence. She admits to drinking several large glasses of iced tea and water on a daily basis because her mother always told her to drink lots of liquids to lower her risk of bladder infections. Urinalysis and urine culture are negative. After confirming the diagnosis with physical examination and office cystometrics, which of the following treatments should you recommend to the patient as the next step in the management of her problem?

a. Instruct her to start performing Kegel exercises
b. Tell her to hold her urine for 6 hours at a time to enlarge her bladder capacity
c. Instruct her to eliminate excess water and caffeine from her daily fluid intake
d. Prescribe an anticholinergic
e. Schedule cystoscopy

414. A 45-year-old woman with previously documented urge incontinence continues to be symptomatic after following your advice for conservative self-treatment. Which of the following is the best next step in management?

a. Prescribe Ditropan (oxybutynin chloride)
b. Prescribe Estrogen therapy
c. Schedule a retropubic suspension of the bladder neck
d. Refer her to a urologist for urethral dilation
e. Schedule a voiding cystourethrogram

415. An 18-year-old G0 comes to see you complaining of a 3-day history of urinary frequency, urgency, and dysuria. She panicked this morning when she noticed the presence of bright red blood in her urine. She also reports some midline lower abdominal discomfort. She had intercourse for the first time 5 days ago and reports that she used condoms. On physical exam, there are no lacerations of the external genitalia, there is no discharge from the cervix or in the vagina, and the cervix appears normal. Bimanual exam is normal except for mild suprapubic tenderness. There is no flank tenderness, and the patient's temperature is normal. Which of the following is the most likely diagnosis?

a. *Chlamydia* cervicitis
b. Pyelonephritis
c. Acute cystitis
d. Acute appendicitis
e. Monilial vaginitis

416. A 28-year-old woman presents to your office with symptoms of a urinary tract infection. This is her second infection in 2 months. You treated the last infection with Bactrim DS for three days. Her symptoms never really improved. Now she has worsening lower abdominal discomfort, dysuria, and frequency. She has had no fever or flank pain. Physical examination shows only mild suprapubic tenderness. Which of the following is the best next step in the evaluation of this patient?

a. Urine culture
b. Intravenous pyelogram
c. Cystoscopy
d. Wet smear
e. CT scan of the abdomen with contrast

417. You have diagnosed a healthy, sexually active 24-year-old female patient with an uncomplicated acute urinary tract infection. Which of the following is the likely organism responsible for this patient's infection?

a. *Chlamydia*
b. *Pseudomonas*
c. *Klebsiella*
d. *E. coli*
e. *Candida albicans*

418. A 32-year-old woman presents to your office with dysuria, urinary frequency, and urinary urgency for 24 hours. She is healthy but is allergic to sulfa drugs. Urinalysis shows large blood, leukocytes, and nitrites in her urine. Which of the following medications is the best to treat this patient's condition?

a. Dicloxacillin
b. Bactrim
c. Nitrofurantoin
d. Azithromycin
e. Flagyl

419. You are seeing a patient in the emergency room who complains of fever, chills, flank pain, and blood in her urine. She has had severe nausea and started vomiting after the fever developed. She was diagnosed with a urinary tract infection 3 days ago by her primary care physician. The patient never took the antibiotics that she was prescribed because her symptoms improved after she started drinking cranberry juice. The patient has a temperature of 102°F. She has severe right-sided CVA tenderness. She has severe suprapubic tenderness. Her clean-catch urinalysis shows a large amount of ketones, RBCs, WBCs, bacteria, and squamous cells. Which of the following is the most appropriate next step in the management of this patient?

a. Tell her to take the oral antibiotics that she was prescribed and give her a prescription of Phenergan rectal suppositories
b. Admit the patient for IV fluids and IV antibiotics
c. Admit the patient for diagnostic laparoscopy
d. Admit the patient for an intravenous pyelogram and consultation with a urologist
e. Arrange for a home health agency to go to the patient's home to administer IV fluids and oral antibiotics

420. A 22-year-old woman has been seeing you for treatment of recurrent urinary tract infections over the past 6 months. She married 6 months ago and became sexually active at that time. She seems to become symptomatic shortly after having sexual intercourse. Which of the following is the most appropriate recomendation for this patient to help her with her problem?

a. Refer her to a urologist
b. Schedule an IVP
c. Prescribe prophylactic urinary antispasmodic
d. Prescribe suppression with an antibiotic
e. Recommend use of condoms to prevent recurrence of the UTIs

Pelvic Relaxation and Urology

Answers

391. The answer is b. (*Scott, pp 768–770.*) Stress incontinence is the involuntary loss of urine when intravesical pressure exceeds the maximum urethral pressure in the absence of detrusor activity. The most common cause of urinary incontinence is incompetence of the urethral sphincter, termed *genuine stress incontinence.* The other major cause of incontinence is unstable bladder. An unstable bladder is the occurrence of involuntary, uninhibited detrusor contractions of greater than 15 cmH$_2$O with simultaneous urethral relaxation. Up to approximately 60% of patients presenting with incontinence may have unstable bladder. Other causes of urinary incontinence are less common and include overflow secondary to urinary retention, congenital abnormalities, infections, fistulas, detrusor dyssynergia, and urethral diverticula. Detrusor dyssynergia implies that when the patient has an uninhibited detrusor contraction, there is simultaneous contraction of the urethral or periurethral striated muscle (normally there is urethral relaxation with a detrusor contraction). This is generally seen in patients with neurologic lesions. Urethral diverticula classically present with dribbling incontinence after voiding.

392. The answer is d. (*Scott, pp 767–768.*) As patients age, the incidence of vesicle instability or unstable bladder increases dramatically. Although estrogen has been reported to decrease urgency, frequency, and nocturia in menopausal women, its effect on correction of stress urinary incontinence or vesicle instability is unclear. In the elderly population there are also many transient causes of incontinence that the physician should consider. These include dementia, medications (especially α-adrenergic blockers), decreased patient mobility, endocrine abnormalities (hypercalcemia, hypothyroidism), stool impaction, and urinary tract infections.

393. The answer is b. (*Stenchever, pp 791–794.*) Many patients who have uterine prolapse or a large protuberant cystocele will be continent because of urethral obstruction caused by the cystocele or prolapse. In fact, at times these patients may need to reduce the prolapse in order to void. Following surgical repair, if the urethrovesical junction is not properly elevated, urinary incontinence may result. This incontinence may present within the first few days following surgery. Dyspareunia can be caused by shortening of the vagina or constriction at the introitus after healing is complete. If the vaginal vault is not properly suspended and the uterosacral ligaments plicated, vaginal vault prolapse or enterocele may occur at a later date. Fecal incontinence is not a complication of vaginal hysterectomy with repair. It may occur, however, if a fistula is formed through unrecognized damage to the rectal mucosa.

394. The answer is a. (*Scott, p 753. Rock, pp 1088–1089.*) When patients present with urinary incontinence, a urinalysis and culture should be performed. In patients diagnosed with a urinary tract infection, treatment should be initiated and then the patient should be reevaluated. It is not uncommon for symptoms of urinary leakage to resolve after appropriate therapy. After obtaining the history and physical examination and evaluating a urinalysis (including urine culture), initial evaluation of the incontinent patient includes a cystometrogram, check for residual urine volume, stress test, and urinary diary. A cystometrogram is a test that determines urethral and bladder pressures as a function of bladder volume; also noted are the volumes and pressures when the patient first has the sensation of need to void, when maximal bladder capacity is reached, and so on. Residual urine volume is determined by bladder catheterization after the patient has voided; when urine remains after voiding, infection and incontinence may result.

395. The answer is c. (*Rock, pp 1211–1213.*) The most common cause of fecal incontinence is obstetric trauma with inadequate repair. The rectal sphincter can be completely lacerated, but as long as the patient retains a functional puborectalis sling, a high degree of continence will be maintained. Generally the patient is continent of formed stool but not of flatus. Other causes of fecal incontinence include senility, central nervous system (CNS) disease, rectal prolapse, diabetes, chronic diarrhea, and inflammatory bowel disease. While rectal prolapse, CNS disease, and senility are thus potential causes of this condition, they can be excluded by the history of the patient in the question. Approximately 20% of all diabetics complain of fecal incontinence. Therapy for fecal incontinence includes bulk-forming and antispasmodic agents, especially in those patients presenting with diarrhea. All caffeinated beverages should be stopped. Biofeedback and electrical stimulation of the rectal sphincter are other possible conservative treatments. Surgical repair of a defect is indicated when conservative measures fail, when the defect is large, or when symptoms warrant a more aggressive treatment approach.

396. The answer is a. *(Rock, pp 375–378.)* Partial colpocleisis by the Le Fort procedure is reasonable for elderly patients who are not good candidates for vaginal hysterectomy and anterior and posterior (A&P) repair as treatment for vaginal and uterine prolapse. The technique involves partial denudation of opposing surfaces of the vaginal mucosa followed by surgical apposition, thereby resulting in partial obliteration of the vagina. Patients who are candidates for this procedure must have no evidence of cervical dysplasia or endometrial hyperplasia, have an atrophic endometrium, and no longer desire sexual function since the vagina is essentially obliterated and there is no longer access to the cervix or uterus via the vagina. Urinary incontinence can be a side effect of this procedure, so care must be exercised in the denudation of vaginal mucosa near the bladder. In a patient who already has urinary incontinence, the Le Fort operation would be relatively contraindicated. An A&P repair essentially involves excision of redundant mucosa along the anterior and posterior walls of the vagina, at the same time strengthening the vaginal walls by suturing the lateral paravaginal fascia together in the midline.

397. The answer is c. *(Rock, pp 951–962.)* All the factors mentioned in the question are commonly seen in patients with genital relaxation (with formation of an enterocele, rectocele, cystocele, or urethrocele, alone or in combination) and uterine prolapse. Undoubtedly, the most important factor is the actual quality of the tissue itself. There is a much lower incidence of uterine prolapse and enterocele formation in black and Asian patients in comparison with whites. Any factors that increase abdominal pressure can aggravate or further deteriorate the prolapse. Although the actual number of deliveries is probably not important, traumatic deliveries, especially those in which the rectal sphincter is lacerated or improperly repaired, have been associated with pelvic relaxation. Chronic hypertension is not a risk factor for genital prolapse.

398. The answer is b. *(Stenchever, pp 625–627.)* There are many procedures that will provide successful correction of stress urinary incontinence.

One of the abdominal procedures that successfully cures stress incontinence is the Marshall-Marchetti-Krantz (MMK) procedure, which involves the attachment of the periurethral tissue to the symphysis pubis. The long-term cure rate for an MMK procedure is around 80%. In approximately 1 to 2% of patients undergoing the procedure, the painfully debilitating condition of osteitis pubis will develop. Treatment of this aseptic inflammation of the symphysis is suboptimal, and the course is usually chronic. Urinary retention after an MMK procedure occasionally occurs, but the problem usually resolves within 1 week. Short-term intermittent or indwelling catheterization is the treatment for urinary retention. Enteroceles may occur in approximately 5% of women who have undergone the MMK procedure. In addition to the surgery, the patient in question will require medical treatment for her incontinence as her preoperative cystometrics showed evidence of detrusor instability.

399. The answer is e. (*Stenchever, pp 618–620.*) Urethral diverticula occur in 3 to 4% of all women. The typical symptoms include urinary frequency, urgency, dysuria, hematuria, and dyspareunia. Frequently, patients will have a history of frequent UTIs, dribbling, or incontinence. A urethral diverticulum is often palpable as a mass on the anterior vaginal wall under the urethra. Although urethral polyps, eversion, fistula, and stricture may present with similar symptoms, there is no suburethral mass present.

400. The answer is e. (*Rock, pp 1156–1157.*) Implanting a severed ureter into the bladder is the procedure of choice, especially when the ureteral transection is near the bladder, as would be expected in this case. Following an injury to the ureter during surgery, a drain should be placed extraperitoneally, not intraperitoneally. If a polyethylene catheter is inserted, it should be placed above the site of injury so that urine is drained before arrival at the site of injury. Ureteroureteral anastomosis should be done only if reimplantation into the bladder is not feasible.

401. The answer is d. (*Stenchever, pp 614–616.*) As a catheter is introduced for performing a cystometrogram, measurement of residual urine is obtained. During the cystometrogram, a normal first sensation is of fullness felt at 100 mL. Urge is felt at approximately 350 mL, with maximum capacity at 450 mL. The primary reason to perform a cystometrogram is to rule out uninhibited detrusor contractions. The urethral pressure profile is normal in women with genuine stress urinary incontinence.

402. The answer is b. *(Beckmann, pp 385–386, 393. Stenchever, pp 621–622.)* This patient's history is most consistent with a diagnosis of urinary stress incontinence. Genuine stress incontinence is a condition of immediate involuntary loss of urine when intravesical pressure exceeds the maximum urethral pressure in the absence of detrusor activity. Patients with this condition complain of bursts of urine loss with physical activity or a cough, laugh, or sneeze. The cause of stress incontinence is structural, due to a cystocele or urethrocele. In cases of overflow incontinence, patients experience a continuous loss of a small amount of urine and associated symptoms of fullness and pressure. Overflow incontinence is usually due to obstruction or loss of neurologic control. Women with detrusor instability/dyssynergia have a loss of bladder inhibition and complain of urgency, frequency, and nocturia. Vesicovaginal fistulas are uncommon and usually occur as a complication of benign gynecologic procedures. Women with this complication usually present with a painless and continuous loss of urine from the vagina. Sometimes the uncontrolled loss of urine is not continuous but related to a change in position or posture. In the case of urinary tract infections, women usually present with symptoms of frequency, urgency, nocturia, dysuria, and hematuria.

403. The answer is a. *(Beckmann, pp 388–390.)* In this patient with presumed urinary stress incontinence by history, the next step in the evaluation of this patient would be the performance of a physical exam to document a cystocele, urethrocele, or other evidence of pelvic relaxation. A urine culture, cystoscopy, and cystometrics may also be part of the workup for this patient's chief complaint, but the physical exam should be the very next step. Placement of a pessary is one of the treatments for a cystocele, once the diagnosis has been made.

404. The answer is b. *(Beckmann, pp 389–394.)* Surgical therapy for stress urinary incontinence due to cystocele and loss of urethral support involves suspension of the bladder neck via Kelly plication, retropubic suspension (Marshall-Marchetti-Krantz and Burch procedures), or sling procedures (Pereyra and Stamey procedures). Placement of a pessary is an option to relieve a cystocele, but is not ideal in this patient, who is sexually active. Antibiotics such as Bactrim would be used to treat a urinary tract infection, but would not affect stress incontinence. A Le Fort procedure is performed in patients with vaginal vault prolapse and pelvic relaxation who are poor surgical candidates and not sexually active. The procedure involves obliterating the vaginal canal to provide support to the pelvic structures. Anticholinergic drugs such as Ditropan (oxybutynin chloride) are used to relax the bladder in the treatment of bladder dyssynergia.

405. The answer is e. *(Beckmann, pp 385–387.)* In pelvic relaxation, there is a loss of connective tissue support adjacent to the reproductive tract organs and in the perineum. Natural aging of the tissue, intrinsic weaknesses due to genetics, birth trauma, hypoestrogenism, and chronic elevation of intraabdominal pressure due to obesity, cough, or heavy lifting are all factors that contribute to pelvic relaxation. Diabetes can result in neuropathy, which can affect the neurologic control of the bladder, but this medical condition is not a cause of pelvic relaxation.

406. The answer is c. *(Beckmann, pp 391–392.)* The Burch procedure is the most appropriate surgical treatment for stress urinary incontinence in this patient. Kelly plication is an older procedure used to suspend the urethra and has a lower cure rate for stress incontinence than the Burch procedure. The Burch procedure suspends the bladder neck to Cooper's ligament of the pubic bone using an abdominal approach. Anterior and posterior colporrhaphy are procedures used to correct cystoceles and rectoceles and are not indicated in this patient. Sacral colpopexy is a procedure to repair prolapse of the vagina by suspending the vaginal vault from the sacrum. Le Fort colpocleisis is used in patients with uterine or vaginal prolapse.

407. The answer is c. *(Stenchever, pp 793–794. Beckmann, pp 392–393.)* Both vesicovaginal and ureterovaginal fistulas are complications that occur rarely after benign gynecologic procedures. Seventy-five percent of fistulas occur after abdominal hysterectomies and 25% occur as a result of vaginal operations. Classically, urinary tract fistulas present with painless and continuous loss of urine 8 to 12 days after surgery. Urinary tract infections and bladder dyssynergia present with dysuria, urgency, and frequency. Since this patient has no symptoms of stress incontinence, failure of the procedure would not be the correct answer.

408. The answer is c. *(Beckmann, pp 387–388.)* The degree or severity of pelvic relaxation is rated on a scale of 1 to 3, based on the descent of the organ or structure involved. First-degree prolapse involves descent limited to the upper two-thirds of the vagina. Second-degree prolapse is present when the structure is at the vaginal introitus. In cases of third-degree pro-lapse, the structure is outside the vagina. Total procidentia of the uterus is the same as a third-degree prolapse, which means that the uterus would be located outside the body.

409–410. The answers are 409-a, 410-b. *(Stenchever, pp 577–583, 585–586. Beckmann, pp 389–391.)* Uterine prolapse that does not bother the patient or cause her any great discomfort does not require treatment. This especially applies to our patient, who is elderly and a poor surgical candi-date. Placement of a pessary provides mechanical support to pelvic tissue, while hysterectomy and the Le Fort procedure are surgical treatments for prolapse. An anterior colporrhaphy is a surgical method to reduce a cysto-cele. Pessaries provide mechanical support for the pelvic organs. These devices come in a variety of sizes and shapes and are placed in the vagina to provide support. Pessaries are ideal for patients who are not good surgical candidates. Their complications include vaginal trauma, necrosis, discharge from inflammation, and urinary stress incontinence.

411. The answer is e. *(Stenchever, pp 583–585.)* Vaginal vault prolapse occurs in up to 18% of patients who have undergone hysterectomy. Symp-toms include pelvic pressure, backache, and a mass protruding from the vagina. Depending upon the duration of the prolapse the patient may also have vaginal ulcerations from the rubbing of the prolapsed vagina against the undergarments. This patient is a poor surgical candidate given her mul-tiple medical problems; therefore abdominal sacral colpopexy is contra-indicated. For the same reasons she should not be given oral estrogen treatment. The preferred treatment is to have her apply a topical estrogen cream to the lesion and the prolapsed vagina to help with healing of the ulcer. If the ulcer does not resolve, biopsy is indicated. A pessary may be tried, but only after the ulcer has healed.

412–414. The answers are 412-d, 413-c, 414-a. *(Stenchever, pp 629–630. Beckmann, p 389.)* The presentation of the patient in question 412 is most consistent with bladder dyssynergia (urge incontinence). Urge incontinence is the involuntary loss of urine associated with a strong desire to void. Most urge incontinence is caused by detrusor or bladder dys-synergia in which there is an involuntary contraction of the bladder dur-ing distension with urine. The management of urge incontinence includes bladder training, elimination of excess caffeine and fluid intake, biofeed-back, or medical therapy. If conservative measures fail, treatment with anti-cholinergic drugs (oxybutynin chloride), β-sympathomimetic agonists (metaproterenol sulfate), Valium, antidepressants (imipramine hydrochloride), and dopamine agonists (Parlodel) have been successful. These pharmacologic agents will relax the detrusor muscle. In postmenopausal women who are not on estrogen replacement therapy, estrogen therapy may improve urinary control. Kegel exercises may strengthen the pelvic musculature and improve bladder control in women with stress urinary incontinence.

415–420. The answers are 415-c, 416-a, 417-d, 418-c, 419-b, 420-d.
(*Stenchever, pp 616–621. Beckmann, pp 393–394.*) Approximately 15 to 20% of women develop urinary tract infections (cystitis) at some point during their lives. Cystitis is diagnosed when a clean-catch urine sample has a concentration of at least 100,000 bacteria per milliliter of urine and when the patient suffers the symptoms of dysuria, frequency, urgency, and pain. The most common etiology of urinary tract infections is *E. coli*. Treatment of a urinary tract infection involves obtaining a culture and starting a patient on an antibiotic regimen of sulfa or nitrofurantoin, which have good coverage against *E. coli* and are relatively inexpensive. Patients treated for a urinary tract infection should have a follow-up culture done 10 to 14 days after the initial diagnosis to document a cure. Patients treated for a UTI who have persistent symptoms after treatment should have a urine culture performed to evaluate for the presence of resistant organisms. Patients with acute pyelonephritis may be treated on an outpatient basis unless they cannot tolerate oral antibiotic therapy or show evidence of sepsis. Women who experience recurrent urinary tract infections with intercourse benefit from voiding immediately after intercourse. If this treatment method fails, then prophylactic treatment with an antibiotic effective against *E. coli* may help prevent recurrent UTIs. Urinary antispasmodics do not prevent infection.

Human Sexuality and Contraception

Questions

DIRECTIONS: Each item below contains a question followed by suggested responses. Select the **one best** response to each question.

421. A 20-year-old gravida 0 and her partner, a 20-year-old man, present for counseling for sexual dysfunction. Prior to their relationship, neither had been sexually active. Both deny any medical problems. In medical experience, which type of male or female sexual dysfunction has the lowest cure rate?

a. Premature ejaculation
b. Vaginismus
c. Primary impotence
d. Secondary impotence
e. Female orgasmic dysfunction

422. A 28-year-old G3P3 presents to your office for contraceptive counseling. She denies any medical problems or sexually transmitted diseases. You counsel her on the risks and benefits of all contraceptive methods. Which of the following is the most common form of contraception used by reproductive-age women in the United States?

a. Pills
b. Condom
c. Diaphragm
d. Intrauterine device (IUD)
e. Permanent sterilization

423. A 20-year-old woman presents to your office for her well-woman exam. She has recently become sexually active and desires an effective contraceptive method. She has no medical problems, but family history is significant for breast cancer in a maternal aunt at the age of 42. She is worried about getting cancer from taking birth control pills. You discuss with her the risks and benefits of contraceptive pills. You tell her that which of the following neoplasms has been associated with the use of oral contraceptives?

a. Breast cancer
b. Ovarian cancer
c. Endometrial cancer
d. Hepatic cancer
e. Hepatic adenoma

424. A 39-year-old G3P3 presents for her postpartum exam and desires a long-term contraceptive method but is unsure if she wants sterilization. She has been happily married for 15 years and denies any sexually transmitted diseases. Her past medical history is significant for mild hypertension, for which she takes a low-dose diuretic. She is considering an intrauterine device and wants to know how it works. Which of the following is the best explanation for the mechanism of the action of the intrauterine device (IUD)?

a. Hyperperistalsis of the fallopian tubes accelerates oocyte transport and prevents fertilization
b. A subacute or chronic bacterial endometritis interferes with implantation
c. Premature endometrial sloughing associated with menorrhagia causes early abortion
d. A sterile inflammatory response of the endometrium prevents implantation
e. Cervical mucus is rendered impenetrable to migrating sperm

425. A 21-year-old G0 presents to your office because her menses is 2 weeks late. She states that she is taking her birth control pills correctly; she may have missed a day at the beginning of the pack, but took it as soon at she remembered. She denies any medical problems, but 3 or 4 weeks ago she had a "viral stomach flu" and missed 2 days of work for nausea, vomiting, and diarrhea. Her cycles are usually regular even without contraceptive pills. She has been on the pill for 5 years and recently developed some midcycle bleeding, which usually lasts about 2 days. She has been sexually active with the same partner for the past 3 months and has a history of chlamydia 3 years ago. She has had a total of 10 sexual partners. A urine pregnancy test is positive. Which of the following is the major cause of unplanned pregnancies in women using oral contraceptives?

a. Breakthrough ovulation at midcycle
b. High frequency of intercourse
c. Incorrect use of oral contraceptives
d. Gastrointestinal malabsorption
e. Development of antibodies

426. An intrauterine pregnancy of approximately 10 weeks gestation is confirmed in a 30-year-old G5P4 woman with an IUD in place. The patient expresses a strong desire for the pregnancy to be continued. On examination, the string of the IUD is noted to be protruding from the cervical os. Which of the following is the most appropriate course of action?

a. Leave the IUD in place without any other treatment
b. Leave the IUD in place and continue prophylactic antibiotics throughout pregnancy
c. Remove the IUD immediately
d. Terminate the pregnancy because of the high risk of infection
e. Perform a laparoscopy to rule out a heterotopic ectopic pregnancy

427. A 34-year-old G1P1 with a history of pulmonary embolism presents to your office to discuss contraception. Her cycles are regular. She has a history of pelvic inflammatory disease last year, for which she was hospitalized. She has currently been sexually active with the same partner for the past year. She wants to use condoms and a spermicide. You counsel her on the risks and benefits. Which of the following statements is true regarding spermicides found in vaginal foams, creams, and suppositories?

a. The active agent in these spermicides is nonoxynol-9
b. The active agent in these spermicides is levonorgestrel
c. Effectiveness is higher in younger users
d. Effectiveness is higher than that of the diaphragm
e. These agents are associated with an increased incidence of congenital malformations

428. A 32-year-old woman presents to your office for her well-woman exam. She is also worried because she has not been able to achieve orgasm with her new partner, with whom she has had a relationship for the past 3 months. She had three prior sexual partners and achieved orgasm with them. She is taking a combined oral contraceptive pill for birth control and an antihypertensive medication for chronic hypertension. She has also been on fluoxetine for depression for the past 2 years. She smokes one pack per day and drinks one drink per week. She had a cervical cone biopsy for severe cervical dysplasia 6 months ago. Which of the following is the most likely cause of her sexual dysfunction?

a. Clonidine
b. Contraceptive pill
c. Disruption of cervical nerve pathways
d. Fluoxetine
e. Nicotine

429. A 20-year-old woman presents to your office for a well-woman exam. She has been sexually active with one male partner for the past year. She has not achieved orgasm with her partner. On further questioning, she has never achieved orgasm with other partners or with masturbation or the use of a vibrator. Which of the following statements is true regarding her condition?

a. It is unrelated to partner behavior
b. The influence of orthodox religious beliefs is still of major etiologic significance
c. It is unrelated to partner sexual performance
d. It is not associated with a history of rape
e. It always has an underlying physical etiology

430. A 23-year-old woman presents to your office with the complaint of a red splotchy rash on her chest that occurs during intercourse. It is nonpuritic and painless. She states that it usually resolves within a few minutes to a few hours after intercourse. Which of the following is the most likely cause of the rash?

a. Allergic reaction to her partner's phermones
b. Decreased systolic blood pressure during the plateau phase
c. Increased estrogen during the excitement phase
d. Vasocongestion during the excitement phase
e. Vasocongestion during the orgasmic phase

431. A 19-year-old woman presents for voluntary termination of pregnancy 6 weeks after her expected (missed) menses. She previously had regular menses every 28 days. Pregnancy is confirmed by β-human chorionic gonadotropin (β-hCG), and ultrasound confirms expected gestational age. Which of the following techniques for termination of pregnancy would be safe and effective in this patient at this time?

a. Dilation and evacuation (D&E)
b. Hypertonic saline infusion
c. Suction dilation and curettage (D&C)
d. 15-methyl α-prostaglandin injection
e. Hysterotomy

432. A 48-year-old woman presents to your office with the complaint of vaginal dryness during intercourse. She denies any medical problems or prior surgeries and does not take any medications. She still has regular menstrual cycles every 28 days. She denies any sexually transmitted diseases. She describes her sexual relationship with her husband as satisfying. Her physical exam is normal. Components of the natural lubrication produced by the female during sexual arousal and intercourse include which of the following?

a. Fluid from Skene's glands
b. Mucus produced by endocervical glands
c. Viscous fluid from Bartholin's glands
d. Transudate-like material from the vaginal walls
e. Uterotubal fluid

433. A 62-year-old woman presents for annual examination. Her last spontaneous menstrual period was 9 years ago, and she has been reluctant to use postmenopausal hormone replacement because of a strong family history of breast cancer. She now complains of diminished interest in sexual activity. Which of the following is the most likely cause of her complaint?

a. Decreased vaginal length
b. Decreased ovarian function
c. Alienation from her partner
d. Untreatable sexual dysfunction
e. Physiologic anorgasmia

434. A 22-year-old nulliparous woman has recently become sexually active. She consults you because of painful coitus, with the pain located at the vaginal introitus. It is accompanied by painful involuntary contraction of the pelvic muscles. Other than confirmation of these findings, the pelvic examination is normal. Which of the following is the most common cause of this condition?

a. Endometriosis
b. Psychogenic causes
c. Bartholin's gland abscess
d. Vulvar atrophy
e. Ovarian cyst

435. A 39-year-old patient is contemplating discontinuing birth control pills in order to conceive. She is concerned about her fertility at this age, and inquires about when she can anticipate resumption of normal menses. You counsel her that by 3 months after discontinuation of birth control pills, what proportion of patients will resume normal menses?

a. 99%
b. 95%
c. 80%
d. 50%
e. 5%

436. A 36-year-old woman presents to your office for contraception. She has had three vaginal deliveries without complications. Her medical history is significant for hypertension, controlled with a lose dose diuretic, and a seizure disorder. Her last seizure was 12 years ago. Currently she does not take any antiepileptic medications. She also complains of stress-related headaches that are relieved with an over-the-counter pain medication. She denies any history of surgeries. She is divorced, smokes one pack of cigarettes per day and has three to four alcoholic drinks per week. On exam her vital signs include weight 90 kg, blood pressure 126/80, pulse 68, respiratory rate 16, and temperature 97.6. Her exam is normal except for some lower-extremity nontender varicosities. She has taken birth control pills in the past and wants to restart them because they help with her cramps. Which of the following would contradict the use of combination oral contraceptive pills in this patient?

a. Varicose veins
b. Tension headache
c. Seizure disorders
d. Smoking in a woman over 35 years of age
e. Mild essential hypertension

437. A 30-year-old woman presents for a physical examination for work. She denies any medical problems or surgeries in the past. She has had no pregnancies. She is sexually active and has been using oral contraceptive pills for the past 6 years. She denies any allergies to medications. On exam her weight is 62 kg, blood pressure 120/78, pulse 76, respiratory rate 15, temperature 98.4°F. Her physical exam is normal. Laboratory evaluation is also done. Which direct effect of birth control pills could be noted in the laboratory results?

a. Decreased glucose tolerance
b. Decreased binding globulins
c. Decreased high-density lipoprotein (HDL) cholesterol
d. Decreased triglycerides
e. Decreased hemoglobin concentration

438. A 32-year-old woman presents to your office to discuss contraception. She has recently stopped breast-feeding her 8-month-old son and wants to stop her progestin-only pill because her cycles are irregular on it. You recommend a combination pill to help regulate her cycle. You also mention that with estrogen added the contraceptive efficacy is also higher. In combination birth control pills, which of the following is the primary contraceptive effect of the estrogenic component?

a. Conversion of ethinyl estradiol to mestranol
b. Atrophy of the endometrium
c. Suppression of cervical mucus secretion
d. Suppression of luteinizing hormone (LH) secretion
e. Suppression of follicle-stimulating hormone (FSH) secretion

439. A 22-year-old woman presents to your office for her well-woman exam and contraception. She has no medical problems or prior surgeries. She does not smoke or drink. Her vital signs and physical exam are normal. You explain the risks and benefits of combination oral contraceptive pills to the patient. She wants to know how they will keep her from getting pregnant. Which of the following mechanisms best explains the contraceptive effect of birth control pills that contain both synthetic estrogen and progestin?

a. Direct inhibition of oocyte maturation
b. Inhibition of ovulation
c. Production of uterine secretions that are toxic to developing embryos
d. Impairment of implantation hyperplastic changes of the endometrium
e. Impairment of sperm transport due to uterotubal obstruction

440. Five patients present for contraceptive counseling, each requesting that an IUD be inserted. Which of the following is a recognized contraindication to the insertion of an IUD?

a. Pelvic inflammatory disease
b. Previous pregnancy with an IUD
c. Dysfunctional uterine bleeding
d. Cervical conization
e. Chorioamnionitis in previous pregnancy

441. A 30-year-old woman presents to your office for her well-woman exam and contraception. She has two prior vaginal deliveries without any complications. Her medical and surgical histories are negative. Her family history is significant for coronary heart disease in her father and breast cancer in her mother diagnosed at the age of 62 years. In addition to effective contraception, health benefits for women taking oral combination contraceptives include which of the following?

a. Decreased risk of lung cancer
b. Decreased incidence of benign breast disease
c. Decreased diastolic hypertension
d. Decreased risk of cervical cancer
e. Decreased incidence of thromboembolism

442. A couple presents to your office to discuss permanent sterilization. They have three children and are sure they do not want any more. You discuss the risk and benefits of surgical sterilization. Which of the following statements is true regarding surgical sterilizations?

a. They cannot be performed immediately postpartum
b. They have become the second most common method of contraception for white couples between 20 and 40 years of age in the United States
c. They can be considered effective immediately in females (bilateral tubal ligation)
d. They can be considered effective immediately in males (vasectomy)
e. Tubal ligation should be performed in the secretory phase of the menstrual cycle

443. A couple presents to your office to discuss sterilization. They are very happy with their four children and do not want any more. You discuss with them the pros and cons of both female and male sterilization. The 34-year-old male undergoes a vasectomy. Which of the following is the most frequent immediate complication of this procedure?

a. Infection
b. Impotence
c. Hematoma
d. Spontaneous reanastomosis
e. Sperm granulomas

DIRECTIONS: Each group of questions below consists of lettered options followed by a set of numbered items. For each numbered item, select the **one** lettered option with which it is **most** closely associated. Each lettered option may be used once, more than once, or not at all.

Questions 444–448

For each female patient seeking contraception, select the method that is medically contraindicated for that patient.

a. Oral contraceptives
b. IUD
c. Condoms
d. Laparoscopic tubal ligation
e. Diaphragm

444. A woman with multiple sexual partners

445. A woman with a history of deep vein thrombosis

446. A woman with moderate cystocele

447. A woman with severely reduced functional capacity as a result of chronic obstructive lung disease

448. A woman with a known latex allergy

Questions 449–455

For the following methods of contraception, select the most appropriate rate of use effectiveness (percentage of pregnancies per year of actual patient use).

a. 80%
b. 40%
c. 15 to 25%
d. 5 to 15%
e. 3 to 10%

449. Rhythm method

450. IUD

451. Diaphragm

452. Postcoital douche

453. Oral contraceptive

454. Condom and spermicidal agent

455. Condom alone

Questions 456–460

For each situation involving oral contraceptives, select the most appropriate response.

a. Stop pills and resume after 7 days
b. Continue pills as usual
c. Continue pills and use an additional form of contraception
d. Take an additional pill
e. Stop pills and seek a medical examination

456. Nausea during first cycle of pills

457. No menses during 7 days following 21-day cycle of correct use

458. Pill forgotten for 1 day

459. Pill forgotten for 3 continuous days

460. Light bleeding at midcycle during first month on pill

Human Sexuality and Contraception

Answers

421. The answer is c. (*Stenchever, pp 185–190.*) In a 5-year follow-up study of couples treated by Masters and Johnson, the cure rates for vaginismus and premature ejaculation approached 100%. Orgasmic dysfunction was corrected in 80% of women, and secondary impotence (impotence despite a history of previous coital success) resolved in 70% of men. Primary impotence (chronic and complete inability to maintain an erection sufficient for coitus) had the worst prognosis, with cure reported in only approximately 50% of cases. Other therapists report very similar statistics.

422. The answer is e. (*Stenchever, pp 296–297.*) In studies of contraceptive methods used by reproductive-age women in the United States, 34.1% used permanent sterilization (tubal ligation by any method for themselves or vasectomy for their partners). Oral contraception was used by 28%, and barrier methods of contraception were used by 17.5% of women surveyed.

423. The answer is e. (*Stenchever, pp 316–320.*) Beginning with high-dose combination contraceptive pills used more than 20 years ago, pills have been studied extensively for a possible association with neoplasia. There is only scant evidence from this experience that use of oral contraceptives increases the risk of any type of cancer. Actually, the progestational component of combination pills (or progestin-only minipills) may confer a protective effect against carcinoma of the breast and endometrium, and avoiding ovulation may decrease the risk of developing ovarian carcinoma. A slightly higher risk of cervical carcinoma was observed in some studies of users of oral contraceptives. These studies were not controlled, however, for confounding variables such as multiple partners or age at onset of sexual intercourse, and it is generally believed now that any increased risk in contraceptive pill users would be attributable to these other factors and not to the steroids themselves. Although the risk of developing benign liver adenomas is increased somewhat in users of oral contraceptives, the risk of hepatic carcinoma is not increased.

424. The answer is d. *(Speroff, p 980.)* It is currently believed that alteration in the cellular and biochemical components of the endometrium occurs with the IUD, culminating in the development of a sterile inflammatory reaction. Polymorphonuclear leukocytes, giant cells, plasma cells, and macrophages are seen in the endometrium after placement. Biochemical changes in the endometrium include changing levels of lysosomal hydrolases, glycogen deposition, oxygen composition, total proteins, acid and alkaline phosphatases, urea phospholipids, and RNA/DNA ratios. IUDs treated with copper and progesterone exert additional effects. In sum, these cellular and biochemical effects result in an endometrium that is not conducive to implantation. No effects on the fallopian tubes or systemic hormone levels have been identified, nor is a bacterial endometritis produced.

425. The answer is c. *(Speroff, pp 873–874.)* The pregnancy rate with birth control pills, based on theoretical effectiveness, is 0.1%. However, the pregnancy rate in actual use is 0.7%. This increase is due to incorrect use of the pills. Breakthrough ovulation on combination birth control pills, when the pills are taken correctly, is thought to be a very rare occurrence. Unintended pregnancy in women correctly using oral contraceptive pills is not related to sexual frequency, gastrointestinal disturbances, or the development of antibodies.

426. The answer is c. *(Stenchever, pp 341–343.)* Although there is an increased risk of spontaneous abortion, and a small risk of infection, an intrauterine pregnancy can occur and continue successfully to term with an IUD in place. However, if the patient wishes to keep the pregnancy and if the string is visible, the IUD should be removed in an attempt to reduce the risk of infection, abortion, or both. Although the incidence of ectopic pregnancies with an IUD was at one time thought to be increased, it is now recognized that in fact the overall incidence is unchanged. The apparent increase is the result of the dramatic decrease in intrauterine implantation without affecting ectopic implantation. Thus, while the overall probability of pregnancy is dramatically decreased, when a pregnancy does occur with an IUD in place, there is a higher probability that it will be an ectopic one. With this in mind, in the absence of signs and symptoms suggestive of an ectopic pregnancy, especially after ultrasound documentation of an intrauterine pregnancy, laparoscopy is not indicated. The incidence of heterotopic pregnancy, in which intrauterine and extrauterine implantation occur, is no higher than approximately 1 in 2500 pregnancies.

427. The answer is a. (*Stenchever, pp 299–300. Ransom, 1997, p 95. Ransom, 2000, p 12.*) All spermicides contain an ingredient, usually nonoxynol-9, that immobilizes or kills sperm on contact. Spermicides provide a mechanical barrier and need to be placed into the vagina before each coital act. Their effectiveness increases with increasing age of the women who use them, probably due to increased motivation. The effectiveness of spermicides is similar to that of the diaphragm, and increases with the concomitant use of condoms. Although it has been reported that contraceptive failures with spermicides may be associated with an increased incidence of congenital malformations, this finding has not been confirmed in several large studies and is not believed to be valid. Levonorgestrel is a synthetic progestational agent found in several combination oral contraceptive pills.

428. The answer is a. (*Stenchever, pp 185–190.*) Clonidine, an antihypertensive agent, can cause inhibition of orgasm in women. Selective serotonin reuptake inhibitors usually decrease libido. In women sensitive to hormonal changes, combination contraceptive pills can decrease free testosterone and decrease libido. Masters and Johnson identified the clitoris as the center of sexual satisfaction in women. Orgasm and sexual gratification has been associated with nerve endings in the clitoris, mons pubis, labia, and pressure receptors in the pelvis. Even though the cervix has a rich nerve supply, there is no scientific evidence that it plays a role in the sexual response.

429. The answer is b. (*Stenchever, p 190.*) Many factors can contribute to the development of primary orgasmic dysfunction in women. By definition, these women will not have been able to achieve orgasm through any means at any time in their lives; reasons for their dysfunction can include the influence of orthodox religious or rigid familial beliefs, dissatisfaction with their partners' behavioral or social traits, or past trauma such as rape. Sexual dysfunction, particularly premature ejaculation in a male partner, can reinforce a woman's orgasmic dysfunction.

430. The answer is d. (*Stenchever, pp 185–186.*) The response of women to sexual stimulation is generalized and affects many different organ systems. During the excitement or seduction phase vasocongestion leads to breast engorgment and the development of a rash on the breasts, chest, and epigastric area, which is called the "sex flush." Heart rate and blood pressure also increase during this phase. Vasocongestion also occurs in the clitoris, labia, and vagina, and a transudative lubricant develops in the vagina. The plateau phase is marked by greater vasocongestion throughout the body and retraction of the clitorus. During the orgasmic phase, the sexual tension is released via muscular contractions throughout the body, but notably in the vagina, anus, and uterus. Changes in hormones such as estrogen are not part of the sexual response.

431. The answer is c. (*Rock, pp 485–497.*) Surgical abortion is among the safest procedures in medicine, with a serious complication rate in the first trimester of less than 1% and a mortality of only 1/20 that of term delivery. In the first trimester, suction dilation and curettage is the method of choice. The oral agent RU-486 followed by injection of prostaglandin has been shown to be highly effective and safe in European trials. It is effective up to about 9 weeks of gestation. 15-methyl α-prostaglandin can be used as an intramuscular abortifacient, as can prostaglandin E_2 suppositories or intra-amniotic prostaglandin $F2_\alpha$ for second-trimester induction of preterm labor. Intraamniotic injection of hypertonic saline is no longer considered appropriate because it has a much higher incidence of serious complications, including death, hyperosmolar crisis, cardiac failure, peritonitis, hemorrhage, and coagulation abnormalities. There are far better medicines available, and saline should no longer be used. Dilation and evacuation (D&E) is a surgical procedure similar in concept to a dilation and curettage (D&C). However, instead of curettage (scraping) to remove the products of conception, various forceps are placed into the uterine cavity to remove the products of conception. D&E is performed for termination of later pregnancies, generally those in the second trimester. Hysterotomy is a surgical procedure in which the uterus is opened transabdominally and the contents evacuated. It is a procedure done for termination of more advanced pregnancies when all other methods of termination are unsuccessful or contraindicated, or, for example, when retained products of conception cannot be expelled with medication or other mechanical means such as D&E.

432. The answer is d. (*Stenchever, pp 185–186.*) Masters and Johnson observed a transudate-like fluid emanating from the vaginal walls during sexual response. This mucoid material, which is sufficient for complete vaginal lubrication, is produced by transudation from the venous plexus surrounding the vagina and appears seconds after the initiation of sexual excitement. No activity by Skene's glands was noted, and production of cervical mucus during sexual stimulation was observed in only a few subjects. Fluid from Bartholin's glands appears long after vaginal lubrication is well established; in addition, it appears to make only a minor contribution to lubrication in the late plateau phase. Uterine and tubal secretions do not contribute to this lubrication.

433. The answer is b. *(Lobo, pp 438–443.)* Sexuality continues despite aging. However, there are physiologic changes that must be recognized. Diminished ovarian function may lower libido, but estrogen replacement therapy (ERT) may help. Sexual dysfunction can be physiologic (e.g., from lowered libido). As with younger patients, however, lowered libido is in most cases treatable. Because aging does not alter the capacity for orgasm or produce vaginismus, a further evaluation should be initiated if these symptoms persist after a postmenopausal woman is placed on ERT.

434. The answer is b. *(Stenchever, pp 188–190.)* This patient presents with vaginismus, defined as involuntary painful spasm of the pelvic muscles and vaginal outlet. It is usually psychogenic. It should be differentiated from frigidity, which implies lack of sexual desire, and dyspareunia, which is defined as pelvic and/or back pain or other discomfort associated with sexual activity. Dyspareunia is frequently associated with pelvic pathology such as endometriosis, pelvic adhesions, or ovarian neoplasms. The pain of vaginismus may be psychogenic in origin, or may be caused by pelvic pathology such as adhesions, endometriosis, or leiomyomas. Treatment of vaginismus is primarily psychotherapeutic, as organic vulvar or pelvic causes (such as atrophy, Bartholin's gland cyst, or abscess) are very rare.

435. The answer is c. *(Stenchever, p 1110.)* Although the estimated incidence of postpill amenorrhea is given as 0.7 to 0.8%, there is no evidence to support the idea that oral contraception causes amenorrhea. Eighty percent of women resume normal periods within 3 months of ceasing use of the pill, and 95 to 98% resume normal ovulation within 1 year. If there were a true relationship between the pill and amenorrhea, an increase would be expected in infertility in the pill-using population. This has not been found. Infertility rates are the same for those who have used the pill and those who have not. Patients who have not resumed normal periods 12 months after stopping use of the pill should be evaluated like any other patients with secondary amenorrhea. Women who have irregular menstrual periods are more likely to develop secondary amenorrhea whether they take the pill or not.

436. The answer is d. (*Stenchever, pp 320–321.*) Absolute contraindications to the use of birth control pills include (1) thromboembolic disorders [deep-venous thrombosis (DVT), cerebrovascular accident (CVA), myocardial infarction (MI), or conditions predisposing to these conditions]; (2) markedly impaired liver function; (3) known or suspected carcinoma of the breast or other estrogen-dependent malignancies; (4) undiagnosed abnormal genital malignancies; (5) undiagnosed abnormal genital bleeding; (6) known or suspected bleeding; (7) known or suspected pregnancy; (8) a history of obstructive jaundice in pregnancy; (9) congenital hyperlipidemia; and (10) obesity in women who are smokers and over age 35. Relative contraindications to the use of the birth control pill require clinical judgment and informed consent. These include (1) migraine headaches; (2) hypertension; (3) uterine leiomyomas; (4) gestational diabetes; (5) elective surgery; and (6) seizure disorders.

437. The answer is a. (*Stenchever, pp 307–311.*) Combination-type oral contraceptives are potent systemic steroids that may cause many detectable alterations in metabolic function, such as increases in binding globulins, bromsulphalein retention, triglycerides and total phospholipids, and a decrease in glucose tolerance. Thus, the benefits of birth control pills must be weighed carefully against the added risks in patients with diabetes, cardiovascular disease, or liver disease. The pill modestly increases HDL cholesterol levels, but should have no direct effect on hemoglobin concentration. In fact, since bleeding volume is generally diminished in birth control pill users, hemoglobin concentration often increases in these patients.

438. The answer is e. (*Stenchever, pp 302–307.*) The two estrogenic compounds used in oral contraceptives are ethinyl estradiol and its 3-methyl ether, mestranol. To become biologically effective, mestranol must be demethylated to ethinyl estradiol, because mestranol does not bind to the estrogenic cytosol receptor. The degree of conversion of mestranol to ethinyl estradiol varies among individuals; however, it is estimated that ethinyl estradiol is about 1.7 times as potent as the same weight of mestranol. The estrogenic component of birth control pills was originally added to control irregular endometrial desquamation resulting in undesirable vaginal bleeding. However, these estrogens imposed possible risks that would not be inherent in the progestational component alone. For example, thrombosis, the most serious side effect of the pill, is directly related to the dose of estrogen. The higher the estrogen dose, the more likely there will be thrombotic complications. The combination pill prevents ovulation by inhibiting gonadotropin secretion and exerting its principal effect on pituitary and hypothalamic centers. Progesterone primarily suppresses LH secretion, while estrogen primarily suppresses FSH secretion. The progestational effect of the pill will always take precedence over the estrogenic effect unless the estrogen dose is dramatically increased. Progestogens are responsible for endometrial changes that result in an environment not conducive to implantation, and production of cervical mucus that retards sperm migration.

439. The answer is b. (*Speroff, p 873.*) The marked effectiveness of the combined oral contraceptive pill, which contains a synthetic estrogen and a progestin, is related to its multiple antifertility actions. The primary effect is to suppress gonadotropins at the time of the midcycle LH surge, thus inhibiting ovulation. The prolonged progestational effect also causes thickening of the cervical mucus and atrophic (not hyperplastic) changes of the endometrium, thus impairing sperm penetrability and ovum implantation, respectively. Progestational agents in oral contraceptives work by a negative feedback mechanism to inhibit the secretion of LH and, as a result, prevent ovulation. They also cause decidualization and atrophy of the endometrium, thereby making implantation impossible. In addition, the cervical mucus, which at ovulation is thin and watery, is changed by the influence of progestational agents to a tenacious compound that severely limits sperm motility. Some evidence indicates that progestational agents may change ovum and sperm migration patterns within the reproductive system. Progestins do not prevent irregular bleeding. Estrogen in birth control pills enhances the negative feedback of the progestins and stabilizes the endometrium to prevent irregular menses. Oral contraceptives have no direct effect on oocyte maturation and do not cause uterotubal obstruction.

440. The answer is a. *(Stenchever, p 344.)* A previous pregnancy with an IUD is not a contraindication to the use of an IUD. The risk of another pregnancy with the IUD in place is not increased. Previous cervical surgery in the face of a normal Pap smear and no cervical stenosis is not a contraindication to IUD use. The Food and Drug Administration (FDA) lists the following contraindications to the use of an IUD: (1) pregnancy; (2) pelvic inflammatory disease—acute, chronic, or recurrent; (3) acute cervicitis; (4) postpartum endometritis or septic abortion; (5) undiagnosed genital bleeding; (6) gynecologic malignancy; (7) congenital anomalies or uterine fibroids that distort the uterine cavity; and (8) copper allergy (for IUDs that contain copper). Other conditions that might preclude IUD insertion include (1) previous ectopic pregnancy; (2) severe cervical stenosis; (3) severe dysmenorrhea; (4) menometrorrhagia; (5) coagulopathies; and (6) congenital or valvular heart disease.

441. The answer is b. *(Stenchever, pp 323–324.)* Oral contraceptives offer many noncontraceptive health benefits. Benign breast disease, both fibroadenomas and fibrocystic changes, are reduced among OCP users. Women who are using combination oral contraceptives are less likely to develop cancer of the endometrium than women who do not use oral contraceptives, probably because the formulations contain a progestogen as well as an estrogen. Since progestogens counteract the stimulatory action of the estrogen on target tissues, women who take oral contraceptives rarely have endometrial hyperplasia and appear to have a lower incidence of nonmalignant cystic disease of the breast. Secondary to the antiestrogenic action of progestin, there is a reduction in the amount of blood loss at the time of endometrial shedding; thus, the development of iron-deficiency anemia is less likely. Users of oral contraceptives are at higher risk for cervical neoplasia, and they definitely require annual screening; however, there is no evidence that the oral contraceptives are the causative factor in this increased risk. A more likely explanation is the presence of confounding factors in contraceptive users that increase the risk, such as multiple sexual partners or regular coitus beginning at an earlier age. Salpingitis, or pelvic inflammatory disease, is also reduced. Functional ovarian cysts are also decreased.

320 Obstetrics and Gynecology

442. The answer is c. (*Speroff, pp 836–849.*) Sterilization has become the most commonly used method of contraception in the United States. In an otherwise uncomplicated pregnancy, a tubal ligation can, if desired, be performed in the immediate postpartum period. Unless the woman has already conceived at the time of the procedure (which is why tubal ligation should generally be performed in the first half of the cycle, the proliferative phase), the contraceptive effect is immediate. Vasectomy in the male, however, should not be considered effective until an examination of the ejaculate is sperm-free on two successive occasions. Tubal ligation can be performed at any time of the ovarian or endometrial cycle, without regard to endometrial development. Most practitioners prefer to perform tubal ligation right after completion of menses (i.e., prior to ovulation) only to obviate the concern that a fertilized oocyte or early embryo could have already passed the ligation area and migrated into the uterus, thus resulting in a pregnancy implanting in the same cycle that the fallopian tubes are ligated.

443. The answer is c. (*Stenchever, p 345.*) Vasectomy is performed by isolating the vas deferens, cutting it, and closing the ends by either fulguration or ligation. Complications that may arise include hematoma in up to 5% of subjects, sperm granulomas (inflammatory responses to sperm leakage), spontaneous reanastomosis, and, rarely, infections. Sexual function following healing is rarely affected.

444–448. The answers are 444-b, 445-a, 446-e, 447-d, 448-c. (*Stenchever, pp 296–346.*) Oral contraceptives are the contraceptive method of choice in the motivated, healthy, monogamous young woman. If the pill is properly used, the failure rate for users is the lowest among women using a reversible method of contraception. However, the use of oral contraceptives is contraindicated in patients with a history of thrombosis. Both condoms and the diaphragm, used in conjunction with spermicides, are effective contraceptives. The diaphragm should carefully fit in the vagina and is therefore not applicable to women with anatomic distortion of the vagina. Latex condoms should not be used in women with a known latex allergy. IUDs are associated with increased risk of salpingitis and therefore should be avoided in patients with a history of pelvic inflammatory disease (PID), multiple sexual partners, or ectopic conception. Although tubal ligation may be considered in the patient with chronic obstructive lung disease, the risk of general anesthesia and surgical intervention in this patient is probably high enough to indicate a more conservative approach, such as the use of an IUD.

449–455. The answers are 449-b, 450-e, 451-c, 452-a, 453-d, 454-d, 455-c. *(Stenchever, pp 296–299.)* There are two methods of describing the effectiveness of contraceptive agents: the theoretical or method effectiveness rate and the actual use effectiveness rate. When comparing different methods, it is important to use comparable figures. The effectiveness of the rhythm method is influenced by the woman's ability to predict the time of ovulation from the regularity of her menses and by her motivation to successfully abstain from intercourse during the 10 days around suspected ovulation. The menstrual and ovulatory irregularities and lapses in the woman's motivation account for a pregnancy rate of 40% with the rhythm method. In contrast to the rhythm method, the IUD requires little or no action on the part of the woman. For this reason the device's actual use effectiveness approaches its maximal theoretical effectiveness, with a pregnancy rate of 3 to 10%. Unrecognized expulsion or misplaced insertion of the IUD are responsible for most failures. The vaginal diaphragm and the condom are barrier contraceptives in that for each act of sexual intercourse they pose a barrier between the sperm ejaculate and the endocervical canal. In theory, both can be very effective. However, both require recurrent motivation for application with each act of intercourse. Lapses in motivation are not uncommon, and there is a pregnancy rate of 15 to 25% for each of these two methods. The condom used with a spermicidal agent is very effective, more so than either used alone. The pregnancy rate with postcoital douching is almost the same as that for unprotected intercourse (80%). This lack of effectiveness is readily explained by the extremely rapid progression of motile sperm into the endocervical canal. Within several minutes of coitus, sperm have ascended the female reproductive tract and can be found within the endocervical mucus, uterus, and fallopian tubes. Coupled with the failure of a vaginal douche to reach the endocervix, this method is essentially useless. Combined oral contraceptive birth control pills are clearly the most effective reversible contraceptive currently available. With correct use, many studies report a contraceptive effectiveness that approaches 100% (pregnancy rate less than 0.1%). This extreme effectiveness is best explained by the pill's multiplicity of actions (i.e., suppression of ovulation, hostility of cervical mucus to sperm penetration, and hostility of atrophic endometrium to the implantation of a conceptus).

Failure to take the pills regularly is responsible for most failures, and in practice pregnancy rates of at least 5% are common.

456–460. The answers are 456-b, 457-b, 458-d, 459-c, 460-b. *(Stenchever, pp 321–323.)* Common side effects of birth control pills include nausea, breakthrough bleeding, bloating, and leg cramps. If these side effects are experienced in the first two or three cycles of pills—when they are most common—the pills may be safely continued, as these effects usually remit spontaneously. On occasion, following correct use of a full cycle of pills, withdrawal bleeding may fail to occur (silent menses). Pregnancy is a very unlikely explanation for this event; therefore, pills should be resumed as usual (after 7 days) just as if bleeding had occurred. However, if a second consecutive period has been missed, pregnancy should be more seriously considered and ruled out by a pregnancy test, medical examination, or both. Women occasionally forget to take pills; however, when only a single pill has been omitted, it can be taken immediately in addition to the usual pill at the usual time. This single-pill omission is associated with little if any loss in effectiveness. If three or more pills are omitted, the pill should be resumed as usual, but an additional contraceptive method (e.g., condoms) should be used through one full cycle. Although most side effects caused by birth control pills can be considered minor, serious side effects do sometimes occur. A painful, swollen calf may signal thrombophlebitis.

Sexual Abuse and Domestic Violence

Questions

DIRECTIONS: Each item below contains a question followed by suggested responses. Select the **one best** response to each question.

461. A 20-year-old woman presents to your office with the complaint of abdominal pain. Through further questioning the woman reveals that she was sexually assaulted at a party 3 weeks ago by a male friend whom she recently started dating. She states that she has not revealed this to anyone else and has not informed the police because she was drinking. Her abdominal and pelvic exams are normal. Which of the following is the best medical treatment to offer this patient?

a. Counsel patient to sue male friend
b. Provide an antidepressant
c. Provide emergency contraception
d. Test for and treat sexually transmitted infections
e. Order CT of the abdomen and pelvis

462. You are a chief resident at a university hospital and are called down to the emergency room at 5:00 A.M. on a Saturday to evaluate an 18-year-old undergraduate who presented to the ER complaining of being a victim of sexual assault while attending a fraternity party the evening before. When you first encounter this patient to take a detailed history, she remains very calm but has trouble remembering the details of the experience. She denies any ingestion of any alcohol or illicit drugs. Which of the following is most likely a component of the acute phase of the rape trauma syndrome?

a. No physical complaints
b. Duration for up to 6 months after the event
c. Always in control of emotions
d. The reaction of the victim may be influenced by victim's relationship to the attacker
e. The victim's coping mechanisms usually remain intact

463. A 36-year-old woman drops by your office unexpectedly and wants to be seen for chronic pelvic pain. She has seen you in the past for well-woman exams and has been treated for chlamydia. She smokes and drinks socially. She has no medical problems or prior surgeries. During questioning her about her chief complaint she reveals that she was sexually assaulted last night at a club after having drinks with some girlfriends. You attempt to take detailed history of the assault; however, the woman's memory seems cloudy and inconsistent. Her physical exam is unremarkable. The victim's inability to think clearly and remember things is best explained by which of the following?

a. Alcohol use
b. Head injury
c. Illicit drug use
d. Rape trauma syndrome

464. You are called to the emergency department to evaluate an 18-year-old woman for a vulvar laceration. She is accompanied by her mother and father. The father explains that the injury was caused by a fall onto the support bar on her bicycle. You interview the woman alone and find out that her father has been sexually assaulting her. Which of the following statements best describes injuries related to sexual assault?

a. Most injuries are considered major and require surgical correction
b. Most injuries require hospitalization
c. More than 50% of victims will have an injury
d. Most injuries occur after the assault has taken place
e. Vaginal and vulvar lacerations are common in virginal victims

465. You are evaluating a rape victim in the emergency department. As a physician, your legal requirement includes which of the following?

a. Identification of the attacker
b. Detailed notation of injuries
c. Delivery of evidence to a law enforcement facility
d. Treating patient even if she refuses
e. Writing the diagnosis of rape in the patient's chart

466. You are an intern working the night shift in the emergency department. During the evaluation of a sexual assault victim, your attending physician asks you to order the appropriate laboratory tests. Which of the following tests should be ordered?

a. HIV, HBsAg, Pap smear, RPR, and urine culture
b. HIV, HBsAg, Pap smear, RPR, and urine pregnancy test
c. Chlamydia and gonorrhea cultures, complete blood count, HIV, HBsAg, Pap smear, and RPR
d. Chlamydia and gonorrhea cultures, HIV, HBsAg, Pap smear, RPR, and urine pregnancy test
e. Chlamydia and gonorrhea cultures, HIV, HBsAg, RPR, urine culture, and urine pregnancy test

467. You are evaluating a 19-year-old woman for a sexual assault. She denies any medical problems or allergies to medications. Her pregnancy test is negative. Which of the following antibiotic prophylaxes do you recommend for sexually transmitted infections?

a. No antibiotic prophylaxis is indicated
b. Flagyl 500 mg PO bid for 7 days
c. Rocephin 250 mg IM
d. Doxycycline 100 mg PO bid for 7 days plus Rocephin 250 mg IM
e. Erythromycin 500 mg PO bid for 7 d

468. During your evaluation of a sexual assault victim in the emergency department, she expresses her fear of becoming pregnant due to the attack. Which of the following is the best method to recommend for emergency contraception?

a. None, because it will cause an abortion and is morally wrong
b. None, because it will be ineffective if taken more than 12 hours after coitus
c. An intrauterine device, because it is 99% effective
d. High-dose oral contraceptive pills
e. Endometrial aspiration

469. After your evaluation and treatment of a rape victim has been completed, you discharge the patient to home. When is the best time to schedule a follow-up appointment for the patient?

a. 24 to 48 h
b. 1 week
c. 6 weeks
d. 12 weeks
e. There is no need for the patient to have any additional follow-up as long as she feels well

470. A rape victim returns to your office 2 months after the attack for a follow-up visit. She informs you that her sleep has improved and she can now be by herself without feeling anxious or panicked. She has also developed new friendships through her church. She states that she is changing jobs and moving to a new town. She feels that with this change she will be in control of her life. The best recommendation you can make for the recovery of this patient is which of the following?

a. Continue counseling
b. Face her attacker to bring closure to this event
c. Get her to accept responsibility for the attack
d. Stop counseling since her recovery is now complete

471. A family medicine physician refers a 19-year-old woman to you for abnormal findings during her well-woman exam. She emigrated to the United States with her family 6 years ago from West Africa. She is not sexually active at this time but has had one partner 2 years ago. She denies any sexually transmitted diseases. She is on nitrofurantoin for recurrent urinary tract infections; otherwise she is healthy. She denies any surgeries, but she remembers undergoing a special ceremony as young child in Africa. Lung, cardiac, breast, and abdominal exam is within normal limits. On pelvic exam you note extensive scarring on the vulva and the labia minora have been removed. The prepuce of the clitous is missing and the clitoris is scarred over. Which of the following is most likely a result of the procedure the patient had in Africa?

a. Amenorrhea
b. Decreased vaginal infections
c. Easier vaginal deliveries
d. Enhanced sexual function
e. Psychosomatic symptoms

472. You are the gynecologist covering the emergency department. The ER physician calls you down to evaluate a 5-year-old girl who was brought in by her mother. The mother is concerned that her daughter may have been sexually molested. She feels this way because her daughter has been acting flirtatious around boys and also because she noted some bloody discharge on her daughter's underwear. The child lives at home with her mother, 1-year-old brother, maternal aunt, and 18-year-old cousin. The child's father is dead and mother is not seeing anyone currently. Which of the following is the most likely abuser?

a. Male stranger
b. Female stranger
c. Male relative
d. Female relative

473. A mother brings in her 16-year-old daughter for an evaluation of chronic abdominal pain. You have seen the girl many times before for various vague complaints over the past year. She has regular cycles that last 4 days with medium to light flow. She denies dysmenorrhea, gastrointestinal symptoms, or feeling depressed. She denies any sexual activity. The mother states that lately she has been doing poorly in school. She denies drug or alcohol use. Her mother thinks it may be related to recent changes at home since the mother's boyfriend moved in. Your exam and lab tests are normal. A previous workup by a gastroenterologist was also negative. Which of the following is the best next step in the management of this patient's symptoms?

a. Initiate biofeedback therapy for chronic pain
b. Order immediate psychiatric evaluation
c. Prescribe antibiotic for chronic gastroenteritis
d. Prescribe antidepressant
e. Question the patient about possible sexual abuse

474. You are called to the pediatric emergency department to evaluate a 7-year-old girl for sexual assault. As a health care provider taking care of this girl, which of the following are you required to do?

a. Administer antibiotics only if testing for infection is positive
b. Demand that the child be placed in foster care pending further investigation
c. Hospitalize the child until the offender has been apprehended
d. Inform the parents that they must notify the police
e. Notify child welfare authorities

475. A 25-year-old G1P0 presents to your office for a routine return OB visit at 30 weeks. On listening to the fetal heart tones, you notice that the patient has a number of bruises on the abdomen. You ask the patient what happened, and she tells you the bruises resulted from a fall she suffered several days earlier, when she slipped on the stairs. The patient returns to your office 3 weeks later for another routine visit, and you note that she has a broken arm in a cast. She states that she fell again. You question her about physical abuse and the patient begins crying and reveals a long-standing history of abuse by her husband. Which of the following is the most likely reason for upper extremity injury in this patient?

a. Injury from being restrained
b. Defensive injury
c. Fall from being pushed
d. Injury related to striking back at her husband

476. You are consulted in the hospital to provide a gynecological exam on a patient who has injuries as the result of an assault by her husband. What percentage of family relationships are violent?

a. 10%
b. 30%
c. 50%
d. 75%
e. 95%

477. You are in the emergency department evaluating a 42-year-old woman who was shot by her husband during an argument. You recognize her because you have treated her numerous times for various complaints. Which of the following is a common characteristic of domestic violence?

a. Victims repeatedly visit clinics and emergency departments for a variety of complaints
b. Victims are reluctant to reveal abuse when their physicians ask them about it
c. The events are isolated and not associated with other abuses
d. The head and neck are rarely areas of injury
e. Signs and symptoms are usually evident, and the correct diagnosis is made most of the time

478. You are evaluating a 36-year-old female in the emergency department for a broken arm. She states that she slipped in the tub. This is the third time you have seen her for a trauma-related injury in the past 6 months. You suspect domestic violence. After treating her broken arm and evaluating her emotional status, which of the following is the next appropriate step in the management of this patient?

a. Confront the patient's partner
b. Discharge her to home
c. Offer counseling and resources
d. Order her to leave her partner
e. Provide an antidepressant

479. You are called to the emergency department to evaluate a 23-year-old G1 who is 6 weeks pregnant and has vaginal bleeding. You have seen her in your office before for her well-woman exam. You had assisted her in receiving counseling and assistance for relationship problems with her verbally abusive boyfriend. She states that they are now married and their relationship has improved. You make the diagnosis of a threatened abortion in the emergency department and schedule the patient for an OB visit at your office in 2 weeks. Which of the following is the normal course of an abusive relationship during pregnancy?

a. Abuse is uncommon during pregnancy
b. An increase is abuse occurs in about 20% of relationships
c. Abuse is usually directed away from the breast and abdomen
d. Pregnant women who are abused usually have fewer complaints
e. Abused women usually receive adequate prenatal care

480. You are seeing a 37-year-old woman in your office for follow-up of an injury related to domestic violence. She states that her husband is over his abusive behavior and is treating her like royalty. He has bought her a new necklace to show how sorry he is about the incident. She has changed her plans to seek counseling and to move out. Which of the following is the most likely outcome in this situation?

a. Abuser accepts responsibility for his behavior
b. Cessation of all abuse
c. Decreased episodes of violence
d. Increasing severity of battering
e. Role reversal with victim taking control of relationship

Sexual Abuse and Domestic Violence

Answers

461. The answer is d. (*Stenchever, pp 205–208.*) The physician's responsibility in the care of a rape victim includes medical, medical-legal, and emotional support. The physician's medical responsibilities include treatment of injuries, testing, and prevention and treatment of both infections and pregnancy. This patient has a normal exam, and a CT is not indicated. The patient should be tested for sexually transmitted diseases and given prophylactic antibiotics to treat such diseases. Also, the patient should be tested for pregnancy and, if she is not pregnant at the time, offered emergency contraception. This patient is not a candidate for an emergency contraceptive, because the sexual assault occurred 3 weeks ago. (Emergency contraception should be given within 72 hours of the event.) Even though there can be long-standing psychological consequences of rape, antidepressants are not indicated at this time in this patient.

462. The answer is d. (*Stenchever, p 206.*) The immediate or acute phase of the rape trauma syndrome can last for hours to days. It is associated with a paralysis of the victim's usual coping mechanisms. The victim's response may be complete emotional breakdown or well-controlled behavior. The actual reaction of the victims will depend on many factors, including use of force, length of attack or how long they were held against their will, and their relationship to the attacker (stranger versus someone close to them). The victim is usually disorganized immediately after the assault and has both physical and emotional complaints.

463. The answer is d. (*Stenchever, p 206.*) As part of the rape trauma syndrome, victims of sexual assault may appear calm, tearful, or agitated, or they may demonstrate a combination of these emotions. In addition, victims of sexual assault may suffer an involuntary loss of cognition wherein they cannot think clearly or remember things.

464. The answer is e. (*Stenchever, p 207.*) Injuries occur in 12 to 40% of sexual assault victims. Most occur when the victim is restrained or physically coerced into the sexual act. Most are minor and require simple repair. Only 1% require major surgical repair and hospitalization. The physician should evaluate for injuries such as abrasions, bruises, scratches, and lacerations on the neck, abdomen, back, buttocks, and extremities, as well as the pelvic area. Lacerations of the vagina and vulva are common in children, virginal victims, and elderly women. If oral penetration was forced, the oropharynx should also be examined.

465. The answer is b. *(Stenchever, pp 208–209.)* Your legal requirement as a physician evaluating a sexual assault victim includes documentation of history, examination and notation of injuries, and collection of clothing and vaginal, rectal, oropharynx, pubic hair samples and fingernail scrapings, as appropriate, for testing. You must submit any specimens to forensic authorities and receive a receipt for the patient's chart. It is important to obtain consent prior to examining and collecting specimens. Since *rape* and *assault* are legally defined terms, they should not be stated as a diagnosis.

466. The answer is e. *(Stenchever, pp 207–208.)* The following are the initial laboratory tests that should be performed at the time of examining a rape victim: gonorrhea and chlamydia cultures from the vagina, anus, and throat; RPR; hepatitis antigens; HIV; U/A; urine C and S; and pregnancy test.

467. The answer is d. *(Stenchever, p 208.)* Antibiotic prophylaxis for gonorrhea and chlamydia should be offered; Rocephin and doxycycline offer good coverage.

468. The answer is d. *(Stenchever, pp 208, 336–337.)* Postcoital contraception (emergency contraception) should be offered to the patient to prevent ovulation/fertilization. This can best be achieved with high-dose combination oral contraceptive and is maximally effective within 3 days of unprotected intercourse.

469. The answer is a. *(Stenchever, pp 207–208.)* The patient should receive follow-up counseling within 24 to 48 hours, and subsequent follow-up appointments can be arranged at 1 and 4 weeks. The patient should not leave without plans for follow-up.

470. The answer is a. *(Stenchever, pp 207–208.)* The reorganization phase of the rape trauma syndrome involves long-term adjustments and may last

332   Obstetrics and Gynecology

for months to years. Flashbacks and nightmares may continue and phobias may develop. Victims may also make many new lifestyle changes (e.g., moving, making new friends, getting a new job). This is an attempt by victims to regain control over their lives. Medical and counseling care should remain nonjudgmental, sensitive, and attuned to the patient's overall well-being. It is important for the patient to continue counseling during this time for full recovery to be achieved.

471. The answer is e. (*Stenchever, p 202.*) Female genital mutilation is a form of sexual abuse recently observed in areas of the world such as Africa, the Middle East, and Southeast Asia. It is often performed by untrained practitioners without anesthesia, usually in early childhood through 14 years of age. Many complications can occur, such as infection, tetanus, shock, hemorrhage, and death. Long-term complications include chronic infection, scar and abscess formation, sterility, obstetrical complications, and incontinence. Psychological problems related to sexual abuse may also be evident, such as anxiety, depression, and sexual dysfunction.

472. The answer is c. (*Stenchever, p 210.*) Approximately 80% of cases of sexual abuse of a child involve a family member. Father-daughter incest accounts for 75% of all cases in which a family member is involved, with the remainder another close relative such as brother, mother, uncle, or cousin.

473. The answer is e. (*Stenchever, p 211.*) Children who have been abused usually exhibit guilt, anger, behavioral problems, unexplained physical symptoms, poor school performance, and sleep disturbances. Physicians who evaluate patients with vague chronic pain syndromes that show no evidence of physical etiology should investigate sexual abuse as a possible contributor. Counseling should be offered as part of the treatment if abuse is encountered.

474. The answer is e. (*Stenchever, p 210.*) In evaluating a child of suspected sexual assault, you should carefully obtain a history and allow the child to say what happened. Techniques of examining a rape victim should be employed (collection of cultures, clothing, hair samples, etc.). The police and child protective services should be notified. Any injuries should be treated, and the child should be hospitalized only if needed based on injuries. Appropriate antibiotic prophylaxis should be given and counseling should be scheduled. The child should be returned to the home only if it is deemed safe.

475. The answer is b. (*Stenchever, p 212.*) The most common sites of injury are the head, neck, chest, abdomen, breast, and upper extremities. An upper extremity may be fractured as the woman attempts to defend herself.

476. The answer is c. (*Stenchever, p 212.*) In the United States it is estimated that at least 50% of family relationships are violent. Most of the offenses are committed by spouses or ex-spouses, and women are the victims in 93% of the cases.

477. The answer is a. (*Stenchever, pp 212–213.*) About 25% of women treated for injuries in emergency departments are victims of domestic violence. Such women usually make repeated visits to clinics and emergency rooms with a variety of somatic complaints. Physicians treating these patients correctly make the diagnosis in only 3% of the cases. Most women report that they would be willing to divulge their domestic abuse to a physician if the physician were to ask. Partner abuse is usually seen in conjunction with other abuses such as elderly abuse and child abuse. Physical injury in cases of domestic violence usually involves the following areas: head and neck, trunk, skin, and extremities.

478. The answer is c. (*Stenchever, pp 214–215.*) As a physician, you should treat the injuries and assess the emotional needs of the patient from a psychiatric standpoint, such as possible depression or anxiety. If such a condition exists, you should refer the patient to a mental health worker. You should investigate the patient's own awareness of her situation and her willingness to take appropriate action. The physician's job is to recognize domestic violence and to ensure counseling for the patient so that she understands her rights and options and can protect herself and her children. A victim of abuse may not leave her situation for economic reasons or fear of retribution.

479. The answer is b. (*Stenchever, p 212.*) Physical abuse is common in pregnancy, occuring in up to 10% of pregnancies. In women who have been previously abused, about 20% will experience an increase in abuse during pregnancy. Abused women usually receive inadequate prenatal care and have more somatic complaints than those who have not been abused. Battering is frequently directed toward the breasts and abdomen.

480. The answer is d. *(Stenchever, p 213.)* Domestic violence attacks usually run in cycles of three phases. Phase 1 consists of a buildup of tension with an escalation of friction between family members. It includes name-calling, intimidation, mild physical abuse. The second phase is the acute battering, which is an uncontrolled discharge of built-up tension. Verbal or physical abuse may occur. Alcohol is usually involved in two-thirds of cases. The third phase occurs after the abuse has taken place. At this time the batterer apologizes, begs forgiveness, and shows remorse. Abusers will offer gifts and make promises to the victim. They are often very charming in this phase. The cycles repeat themselves, with the first phase becoming longer and increasing in intensity; the battering is usually more severe, and the third phase usually decreases in both length and intensity. Batterers are frequently men who refuse to take responsibility for their actions and often blame the victim. As the cycles continue, batterers usually gain more control over their victims.

Ethical and Legal Issues in Obstetrics and Gynecology

Questions

DIRECTIONS: Each item below contains a question followed by suggested responses. Select the **one best** response to each question.

481. Which of the following is not a requirement for hospitals according to the Federal Patient Self-Determination Act?

a. To provide all adults with information about their right to accept or refuse treatment in the event of life-threatening conditions
b. To state the institution's policy on advance directives
c. To prohibit discrimination in care provided to a patient on the basis of the patient's advanced directive
d. To require donation of organs after death
e. To allow patients to decide who has the right to make decisions for them

482. A 31-year-old G3P3 Jehovah's Witness begins to bleed heavily 2 days after a cesarean section. She refuses transfusion and says that she would rather die than receive any blood or blood products. You personally feel that you cannot do nothing and watch her die. Appropriate actions that you can take under these circumstances include which of the following?

a. Telling the patient to find another physician who will care for her
b. Transfusing her forcibly
c. Letting her die, giving only supportive care
d. Getting a court order and transfusing
e. Having the patient's husband sign a release to forcibly transfuse her

483. A physician is being sued for malpractice by the parents of a baby born with cerebral palsy. Which of the following is not a prerequisite for finding the physician guilty of malpractice?

a. A doctor-patient relationship was established
b. The physician owed a duty to the patient
c. The physician breached a duty to the patient
d. The breach of duty caused damage to the plaintiff
e. The physician failed to give expert care to the patient

484. A 27-year-old woman who has previously received no prenatal care presents at term. On ultrasound, she is shown to have a placenta previa, but she refuses to have a cesarean section for any reason. Important points to consider in her management include which of the following?

a. The obstetrician's obligation to the supposedly normal fetus supersedes the obligation to the healthy mother
b. The inclusion of several people in this complex situation raises the legal risk to the physician
c. Child abuse statutes require the physician to get a court order to force a cesarean section
d. Court-ordered cesarean sections have almost always been determined to achieve the best management
e. A hospital ethics committee should be convened to evaluate the situation

485. Your 36-year-old patient is admitted to the hospital for induction of labor at 42 weeks gestation. She provides the hospital with her living will at the time of her admission. She signed the will 5 years ago, but she says to her nurse that she still wants to abide by the will. She has also signed an organ donor card allowing the harvesting of her organs in the event of her death. Why is her living will not valid for this hospitalization?

a. In the event that she becomes delerious during labor, she will be unable to change her mind
b. She is pregnant
c. It has been too many years since the signing of the will
d. Signing an organ donor card automatically invalidates a living will
e. Her husband may decide later on that he disagrees with her living will

Questions 486–490

Your patient is a 44-year-old G4P4 with symptomatic uterine fibroids that are unresponsive to medical therapy. The patient has severe menorrhagia to the point that when she menstruates, she cannot leave the house. You recommend to her that she undergo a total abdominal hysterectomy. You counsel her that she may need a blood transfusion if she has a large blood loss during the surgical procedure. Her current hematocrit is 25.0. The patient is a Jehovah's Witness who adamantly refuses to have a blood transfusion, even if it results in her death.

486. Which of the following is not an ethical concern that needs to be considered when working through this case?

a. Legal issues
b. Patient preferences
c. Quality-of-life issues
d. Medical indications

487. The patient's insurance company refuses to pay for the surgical procedure. Which of the following ethical areas is involved?

a. Autonomy
b. Justice
c. Contextual issue
d. Patient preference
e. Quality of life

488. Respect for the patient's autonomy or own wishes requires that which of the following be assessed?

a. The needs of society
b. The duty not to inflict harm
c. The impact that the treatment will have on the patient's quality of life
d. Consideration of what is the best treatment
e. The patient's personal values

489. Prior to performing the abdominal hysterectomy, you must obtain the patient's informed consent. Which of the following is not a key element of informed consent?

a. The patient must have the ability to comprehend medical information
b. Alternatives to the procedure must be presented
c. If the patient is incapable of providing consent, the procedure cannot be performed
d. The risks of the procedure must be presented
e. The benefits of the procedure must be presented

490. The patient requests that you do not talk at all to her husband about her medical care. This request falls under which of the following ethical concepts?

a. Informed consent
b. Confidentiality
c. Nonmaleficence
d. Advanced directive

DIRECTIONS: Each group of questions below consists of lettered options followed by a set of numbered items. For each numbered item, select the **one** lettered option with which it is **most** closely associated. Each lettered option may be used once, more than once, or not at all.

Questions 491–500

Match the ethical concern or principal with the appropriate definition.

a. Patient preferences
b. Beneficence
c. Quality of life
d. Nonmaleficence
e. Autonomy
f. Medical indication
g. Contextual issues
h. Justice

491. The duty not to inflict harm or injury

492. The duty to promote the good of the patient

493. Giving the patient his or her due

494. Respect of the patient's right to self-determination

495. What does the patient want?

496. What is the best treatment?

497. What impact will the proposed treatment have on the patient's life?

498. What are the needs of society?

499. What are the treatment alternatives?

500. What impact will lack of the proposed treatment have on the patient's life?

Ethical and Legal Issues in Obstetrics and Gynecology

Answers

481. The answer is d. *(Scott, pp 939–954.)* Hospitals must now inform patients about their rights to accept or refuse terminal care. Such information has to be documented in the patient's chart. The patient has the option to make a clear assignment of who can make decisions if the patient cannot. Patients are not required to allow organ donation.

482. The answer is c. *(ACOG, Committee Opinion 55.)* Determination of ethical conduct in doctor-patient relationships can sometimes be very difficult for the physician who is confronted with a patient's autonomy in making a decision that the physician finds incomprehensible. However, the autonomy of the patient who is oriented and alert must be respected even if it means in effect that the patient is committing suicide. The obtaining of a court order to transfuse an adult against his or her will is almost never an acceptable option and leads to a tremendously slippery slope of the doctor's control of the patient's behavior. A patient's spouse also does not have legal authority to make decisions for the patient if the patient is competent, awake, and alert. The situation is different when a child is involved, and then societal interests can occasionally override parental autonomy. It would be inappropriate for a physician to abandon a patient without obtaining suitable coverage from another qualified physician. Transfusing forcibly is assault and battery; thus, in this case, the physician must adhere to the patient's wishes and, if need be, let her die.

483. The answer is e. *(Ransom, 2000, pp 786–792.)* Negligence law governs conduct and embraces acts of both commission and omission (i.e., what a person did or failed to do). In general, the law expects all persons to conduct themselves in a fashion that does not expose others to an unreasonable risk of harm. In a fiduciary relationship such as the physician-patient relationship, the physician is held to a higher standard of behavior because of the imbalance of knowledge. In general, the real gist of negligence is not carelessness or ineptitude, but rather, how unreasonable was the risk of harm to the patient caused by the physician's action? Thus physicians are held accountable to a standard of care that asks the question, "What would the reasonable physician do under this specific set of circumstances?" The physician is not held accountable to the level of the leading experts in any given field, but rather to the prevailing standards among average practitioners. When a doctor-patient relationship is established, the defendant owes a duty to the patient. If the defendant breaches that duty—that is, acts in a way that is inconsistent with the standard of care and that can be shown to have caused damage directly to the patient (*proximate damage*)—then the physician may be held liable for compensation.

484. The answer is e. *(Gleicher, pp 206–210.)* When confronted by a complex situation in which there are conflicting values and rights, getting the most people involved is the best approach to reduce risk and to come up with the best, most defensible answer under the current circumstances. The obstetrician should employ whatever departmental or hospital resources are available. A standing ethics committee or an ad hoc committee to deal with such complex situations is often available and will minimize the ultimate medicolegal problems that can ensue when bad outcomes seem likely. The obstetrician must further recognize that he or she has two patients, but that it is not clear, nor is it legislated, whose interests take priority. However, general ethical opinion is that the mother generally should come first. Most court-ordered cesarean sections have been performed on patients who were estranged from the medical system, and this sets a very bad precedent for further state intervention in doctor-patient relationships and maternal rights. Child abuse statutes do not at this point require a court order to force a cesarean section even for a healthy fetus, and a court order would almost never be appropriate.

485. The answer is b. *(Scott, pp 939–954.)* Living wills represent the chance for patients to declare their wishes in advance of situations in which they become no longer competent to do so. They are revocable by the patient at any time and are automatically invalid if the patient is pregnant, as another being is involved. Living wills can be set aside if a long period has elapsed since their drafting and the wishes are not known to be current. Also, there is the potential for conflict if the patient has signed a donor card and prolongation of life would be needed to carry out those wishes. Generally, such action would not be honored unless relatively expeditious arrangements were possible.

486–490.   The answers are 486-a, 487-b, 488-e, 489-c, 490-b. (*Beckmann, pp 33–37. ACOG, Committee Opinion 237.*) Patient preferences, quality-of-life issues, and medical indications are all examples of ethical concerns that must be taken into account when working through ethical dilemmas. Consideration of legal issues is not a factor in ethical decision making. If the patient's insurance company refuses to pay for the indicated procedure (in this case, hysterectomy), the ethical principle of justice (the patient should be given her due) is being challenged. Autonomy is the ethical principle whereby the patient has the right to self-determination. Therefore, the needs of society (a contextual issue) are not considered as a factor of autonomy. Informed consent requires that the patient be able to understand the risks, benefits, and alternatives of a particular medical procedure. If the patient is unable to understand the medical information, a legal guardian can be assigned to make those decisions for him or her. A patient's desire not to have his or her medical history discussed with anyone else involves the ethical concept of confidentiality.

491–500.   The answers are 491-d, 492-b, 493-h, 494-e, 495-a, 496-f, 497-c, 498-g, 499-f, 500-c. (*Beckmann, p 34.*)

Bibliography

Adashi EY, Rock JA, Rosenwaks Z (eds): *Reproductive Endocrinology, Surgery, and Technology,* vols 1 and 2. Philadelphia, Lippincott-Raven, 1996.

American College of Obstetricians and Gynecologists: *Patient Choice: Maternal-Fetal Conflict.* Committee Opinion 55, October 1987.

American College of Obstetricians and Gynecologists: *Informed Refusal.* Committee Opinion 237, June 2000.

American College of Obstetricians and Gynecologists: *Circumcision.* Committee Opinion 260, October 2001.

American College of Obstetricians and Gynecologists: *Primary and Preventive Care: Periodic Assessments.* Committee Opinion 292, November 2003.

American College of Obstetricians and Gynecologists: *Premature Rupture of Membranes.* Practice Bulletin 1, June 1998.

American College of Obstetricians and Gynecologists: *Prevention of Rh and Alloimmunization.* Practice Bulletin 4, May 1999.

American College of Obstetricians and Gynecologists: *Vaginal Birth After Previous Cesarean Delivery.* Practice Bulletin 5, July 1999.

American College of Obstetricians and Gynecologists: *Thrombocytopenia in Pregnancy.* Practice Bulletin 6, September 1999.

American College of Obstetricians and Gynecologists: *Management of Herpes in Pregnancy.* Practice Bulletin 8, October 1999.

American College of Obstetricians and Gynecologists: *Antepartum Fetal Surveillance.* Practice Bulletin 9, October 1999.

American College of Obstetricians and Gynecologists: *Induction of Labor.* Practice Bulletin 10, November 1999.

American College of Obstetricians and Gynecologists: *Operative Vaginal Delivery.* Practice Bulletin 17, June 2000.

American College of Obstetricians and Gynecologists: *Gestational Diabetes.* Practice Bulletin 30, September 2001.

American College of Obstetricians and Gynecologists: *Polycystic Ovary Syndrome.* Practice Bulletin 41, December 2002.

American College of Obstetricians and Gynecologists: *Fetal Heart Rate Patterns: Monitoring, Interpretation, and Management.* Technical Bulletin 207, July 1995.

American College of Obstetricians and Gynecologists: *Health Maintenance for Perimenopausal Women.* Technical Bulletin 210, August 1995.

American College of Obstetricians and Gynecologists: *Diagnosis and Management of Preeclampsia and Eclampsia.* Practice Bulletin No.33, January 2002.

American College of Obstetricians and Gynecologists: *Cervical Insufficiency.* Practice Bulletin No. 48 November 2003.

Beckmann CRB, et al (eds): *Obstetrics and Gynecology,* 4/e. Philadelphia, Lippincott, Williams & Wilkins, 2002.

Benacerraf BR (ed): *Ultrasound of Fetal Syndromes.* Philadelphia, Churchill Livingstone, 1998.

Cunningham FG, et al (eds): *Williams Obstetrics,* 22/e. New York, McGraw-Hill, 2005.

DeCherney AH, Nathan L. (eds): *Current Obstetric and Gynecologic Diagnosis and Treatment,* 9/e. New York, Large Medical Books/McGraw-Hill, 2003.

Dewan DM, Hood DD (eds): *Practical Obstetric Anesthesia.* Philadelphia, Saunders, 1997.

DiSaia PJ, Creasman WT (eds): *Clinical Gynecologic Oncology,* 5/e. St. Louis, Mosby, 1997.

Droegemueller, et al (eds): *Comprehensive Gynecology,* 3/e. St. Louis, Mosby, 1997.

Fleisher AC, et al (eds): *Principles and Practice of Ultrasonography in Obstetrics and Gynecology,* 5/e. Stamford, CT, Appleton & Lange, 1996.

Gabbe SG, et al (eds): *Obstetrics: Normal and Problem Pregnancies,* 2/e. New York, Churchill Livingstone, 1991.

Gleicher N, et al (eds): *Principles and Practice of Medical Therapy in Pregnancy,* 3/e. Stamford, CT, Appleton & Lange, 1998.

Griffiths CT, Silverstone A, Tobias J, Benjamin E (eds): *Gynecologic Oncology.* London, Mosby-Wolfe, 1997.

Hankins GDV, et al (eds): *Operative Obstetrics.* Norwalk, CT, Appleton & Lange, 1995.

Hoskins WJ, Perez CA, Young RC (eds): *Principles and Practice of Gynecologic Oncology,* 2/e. Philadelphia, Lippincott, 1997.

Jaffe R, Bui TH (eds): *Textbook of Fetal Ultrasonography.* London, Parthenon, 1999.

James DK, et al (eds): *High Risk Pregnancy: Management Options,* 2/e. London, Saunders, 1999.

Jones KL (ed): Smith's *Recognizable Patterns of Human Malformations,* 5/e. Philadelphia, Saunders, 1997.

Keye WR, et al (eds): *Infertility: Evaluation and Treatment.* Philadelphia, Saunders, 1995.

Korf BR (ed): *Human Genetics: A Problem-Based Approach.* Cambridge, MA, Blackwell Science, 1996.

Lobo RA (ed): *Treatment of the Postmenopausal Woman,* 2/e. Philadelphia, Lippincott, Williams & Wilkins, 1999.

Postgraduate Obstetrics and Gynecology, 22:25, December 2002.

Queenan JT (ed): *Management of High Risk Pregnancy,* 4/e. Malden, MA, Blackwell Science, 1999.

Ransom SB, Dombrowski MP, McNeeley SG, Moghissi K, Munkarah AR (eds): *Practical Strategies in Obstetrics and Gynecology.* Philadelphia, Saunders, 2000.

Ransom SB, McNeeley SG (eds): *Gynecology for the Primary Care Provider.* Philadelphia, Saunders, 1997.

Reece EA, et al (eds): *Medicine of the Fetus and Mother,* 2/e, Philadelphia, Lippincott, 1999.

Rock JA, Thompson JD (eds): *TeLinde's Operative Gynecology,* 8/e. Philadelphia, Lippincott-Raven, 1997.

Rodeck CH, Whittle MJ (eds): *Fetal Medicine: Basic Science and Clinical Practice.* London, Churchill Livingstone, 1999.

Scott JR, et al (eds): *Danforth's Obstetrics and Gynecology,* 8/e. Philadelphia, Lippincott-Raven, 1999.

Speroff L, Glass RH, Kase NG (eds): *Clinical Gynecologic Endocrinology and Infertility,* 7/e. Baltimore, Lippincott, Williams & Wilkins, 2005.

Stenchever MA, Droegemueller W, Herbst AL, Mishell DR (eds): *Comprehensive Gynecology,* 4/e. St. Louis, Mosby, 2002.

Thompson JD, Rock JA. (eds): *TeLinde's Operative Gynecology,* 7/e. Philadelphia, Lippincott, 1992.

Timor-Tritsch JE, Monteagudo A, Cohen HL (eds): *Ultrasonography of the Prenatal and Neonatal Brain.* Stamford, CT, Appleton & Lange, 1996.

Zatuchni GI, Slupik RI: *Obstetrics and Gynecology Drug Handbook.* St. Louis, Mosby, 1996.

Index

Notes

Notes